The Complete Book of
Men's
Health

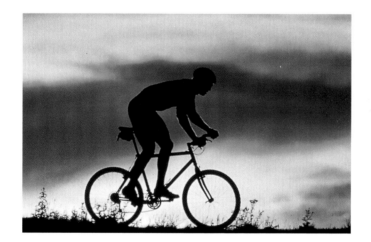

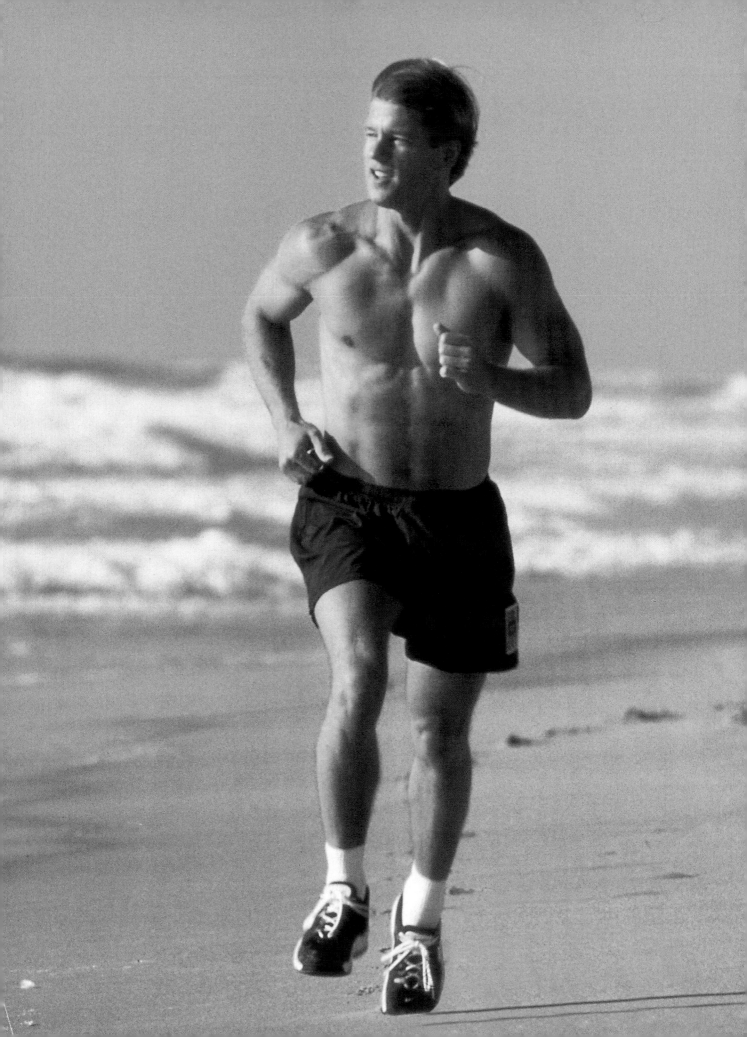

The Complete Book of
Men's Health

The Definitive, Illustrated Guide to Healthy Living, Exercise, and Sex

By the Editors of **Men'sHealth.** Books

Reviewed by Kenneth A. Goldberg, M.D., medical director of the
Male Health Institute at Baylor Health Center, Irving-Coppell, Texas

RODALE

SEX AND VALUES AT RODALE

We believe that an active and healthy sex life, based on mutual consent and respect between partners, is an important component of physical and mental well-being. We also respect that sex is a private matter and that each person has a different opinion of what sexual practices or levels of discourse are appropriate. Rodale is committed to offering responsible, practical advice about sexual matters, supported by accredited professionals and legitimate scientific research. Our goal—for sex and all other topics—is to publish information that empowers people's lives.

First published in Great Britain in 1999 by Mitchell Beazley, an imprint of Octopus Publishing Group Ltd, Michelin House, 81 Fulham Road, London SW3 6RB

Library of Congress Cataloging-in-Publication Data
The complete book of men's health : the definitive, illustrated guide
to healthy living, exercise, and sex / by the editors of Men's
Health Books
p. cm.
Includes index.
ISBN 0–87596–528–8 hardcover
ISBN 1–57954–298–0 paperback
1. Men—Health and hygiene. 2. Physical fitness for men.
3. Exercise. 4. Hygiene, Sexual. I. Men's Health Books.
RA777.8.C66   1998
613'.04234—DC21   98–8658

Distributed to the book trade by St. Martin's Press
8 10 9 7   hardcover
4 6 8 10 9 7 5 3   paperback

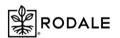

RODALE

WE **INSPIRE** AND **ENABLE** PEOPLE TO IMPROVE
THEIR LIVES AND THE WORLD AROUND THEM

CONTRIBUTING WRITERS
Jack Forem, Kelly Garrett, Christopher Hall, Doug Hill, Diane Kozak,
Richard Laliberte, Susan Paterno

RODALE HEALTH AND FITNESS BOOKS
Men's Health Magazine Editor In Chief: **Michael Lafavore**
Men's Health Books Managing Editor: **Jack Croft**
Vice President and Editorial Director: **Debora T. Yost**
Executive Editor: **Neil Wertheimer**
Design and Production Director: **Michael Ward**
Research Manager: **Ann Gossy Yermish**
Copy Manager: **Lisa D. Andruscavage**
Book Manufacturing Director: **Helen Clogston**
Design Coordinator: **Tanja Lipinski-Cole**
Associate Art Director: **Charles Beasley**
Manufacturing Manager: **Mark Krahforst**
Manufacturing Coordinator: **Melinda B. Rizzo**

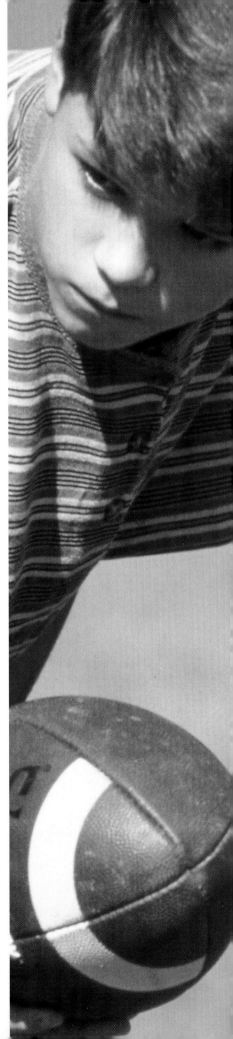

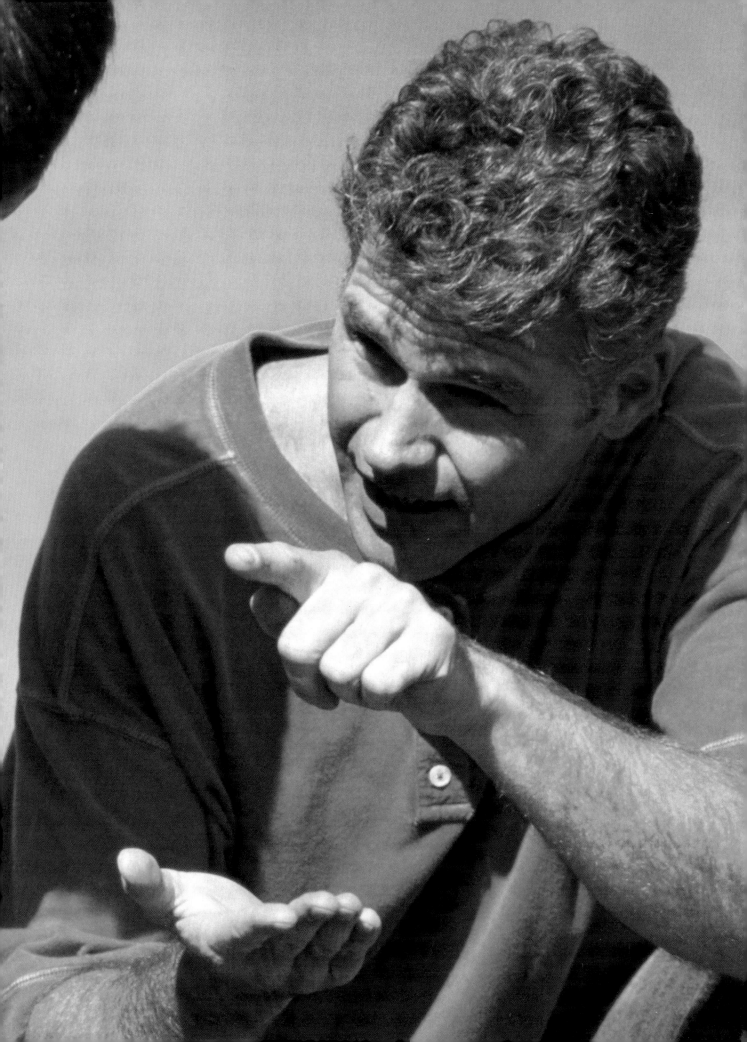

Contents

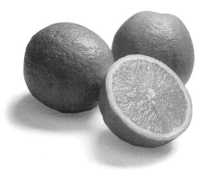

Healthy Living Guide

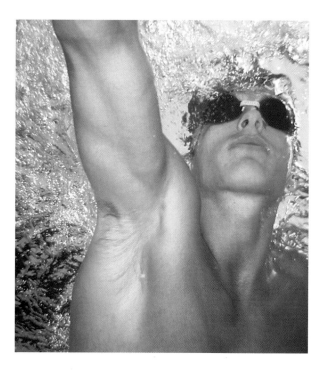

Male Health Concerns

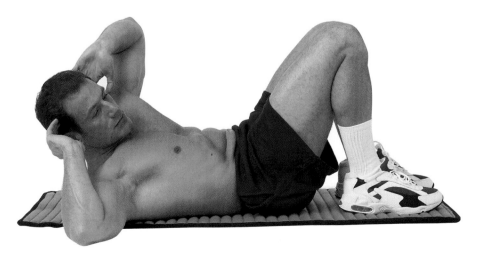

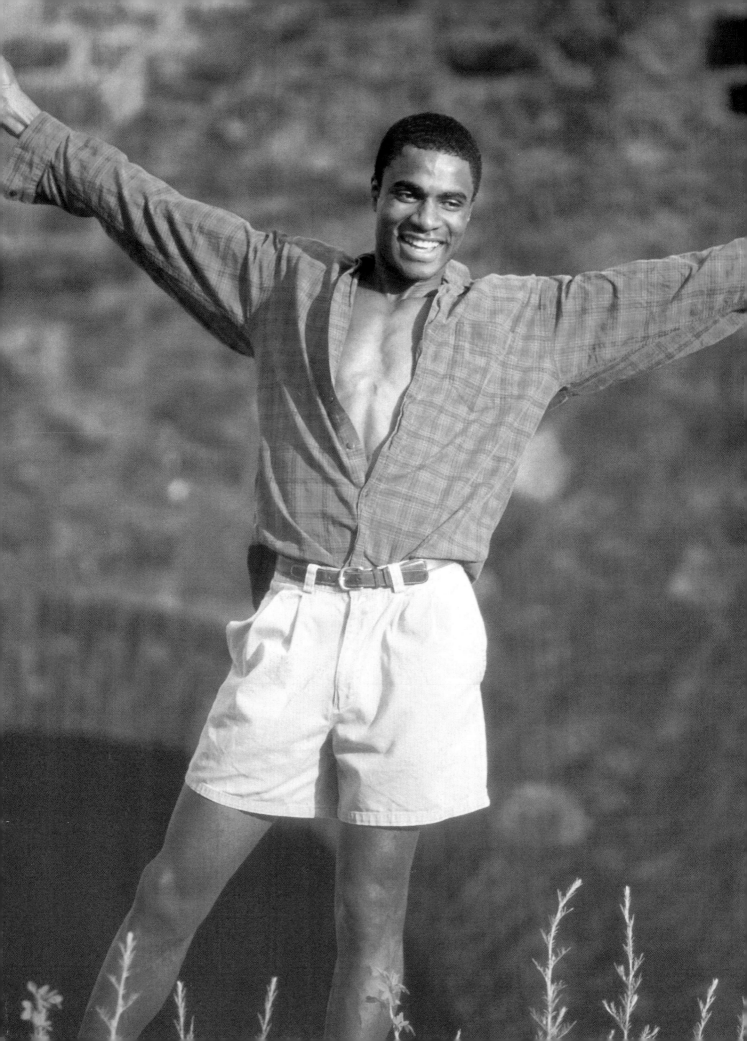

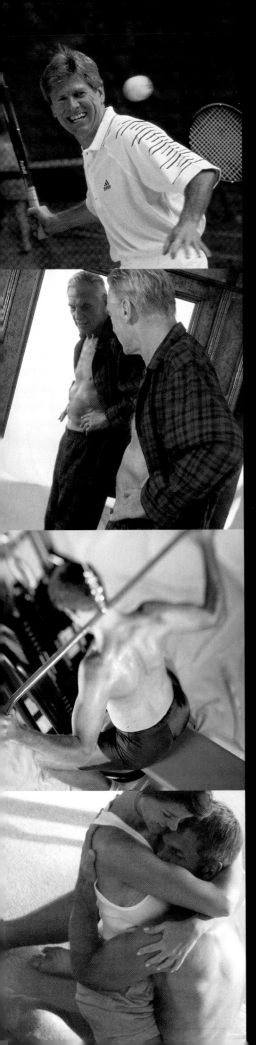

Healthy Living Guide

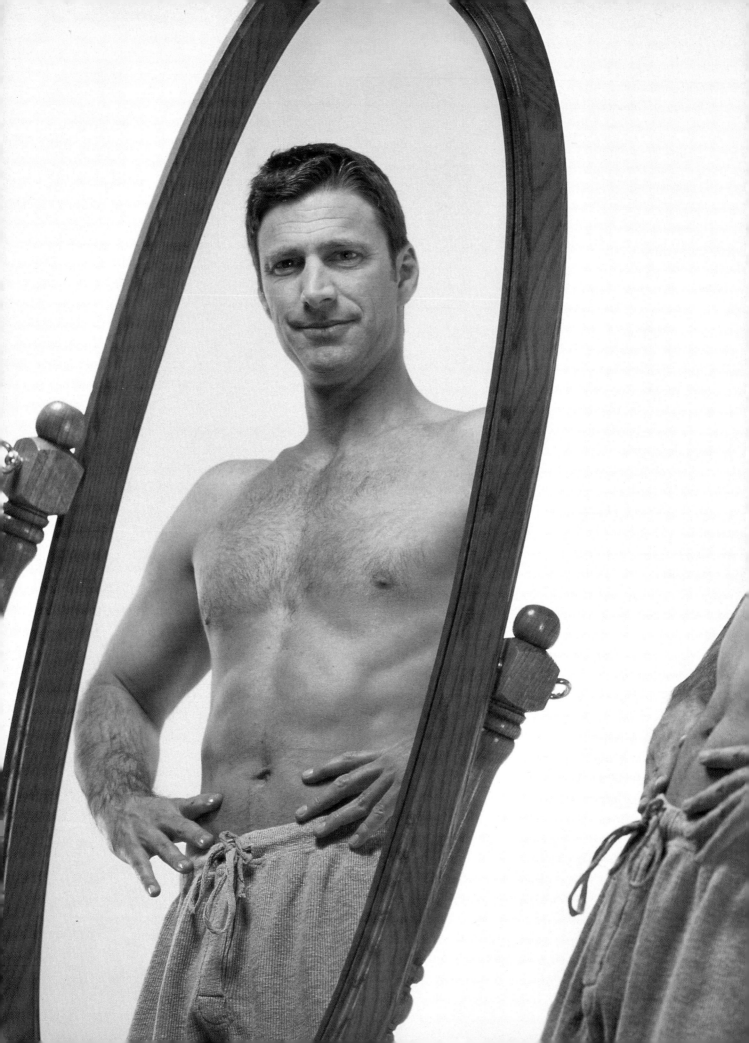

Ways to a Better Lifestyle

A Man's Life

Marriage, children, career, mortgage, bills: Remember when your biggest concern in life was how to score a hot date? With the added responsibilities that age inevitably brings, comes the potential for a much deeper sense of fulfillment, but only if you're willing to work for it.

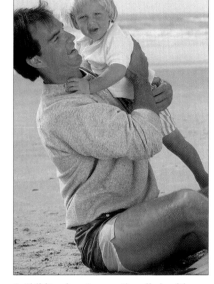

▲ *Child's play: An emotionally healthy man balances family and work needs.*

Take Control of Your Life

Being in control of your life means first understanding why you feel out of control at times.

Is your schedule so tight that a request to pick up the dry-cleaning or a quart of milk makes you lash out like a steroid-laden linebacker? If you complain about the small ways you're asked to help family or friends in need, stop and ask yourself why. If taking out the trash or fixing dinner is such a burden on your time, imagine what will happen if a real crisis occurs, like a serious illness, a layoff, or a crumbling relationship? A crisis will challenge your values system; and the only way to take control of your life is to understand and act on those values.

Time to Take Stock

The first step to understanding your values is to assess them. Hand on heart, many men will put family, God, and community at the top of the list of what they cherish most. But actions speak louder than words. How you spend your time and money tells you where your values are.

Examine your checkbook and day planner. To an increasing degree, work has replaced God and family as the thing that we worship and love most. If work is your god, you may never be satisfied.

It may seem paradoxical, but on the job is not a place where most men feel in control, even though that's where they spend much of their time. At work, many (perhaps most) men learn to keep their emotions in check, to strive for power, promotion, kudos, and money, to worry less about what's right and more about how to make themselves look good in the eyes of others. Often, too, men will sacrifice developing other, more humane values in order to work on increasing the mental muscles that lead to more money and status.

But a life out of balance can lead to a whole host of problems, including preventing you from developing the very people skills you'll likely need to achieve the career stature you crave. Besides, there's a life out there to be lived. Says Edwin M. Greenberg,

---

Are You a Workaholic?

Hard work, commitment, and dedication, which were once the keys to prosperity, have become an unhealthy obsession for more and more men. Self-confessed workaholics speak of using work as a way of coping with life, just as alcoholics use alcohol. You could be a workaholic if:

• You work late nights, weekends, and always bring work home.

• You take work to bed with you.

• You feel guilty when not working.

• You refuse to take vacations.

• Your list of priorities fails to include family, friends, and relaxation.

• You've started to forget family birthdays and anniversaries.

• You have few friends or hobbies, and not much social life, outside of work.

• You live mainly on junk food.

• Your job gives you headaches, backaches, or stomach aches.

• You're chained to beepers, cell phones, and laptop computers.

• It bothers you to ask for help with work, no matter how big the task.

• You think a task won't be done right unless you do it yourself.

• You work to escape problems at home or in your personal life.

• Your own expectations are your greatest source of pressure.

• You accept more work even when you're overcommitted.

• Work is your drug of choice; challenge gives you a high you can't achieve in relationships or other activities.

Ph.D., a clinical psychologist in Los Angeles, "You want to enjoy yourself between here and the journey's end—which is death."

BE ACCEPTING

Take a good look at your primary relationships, especially with your family. Men tend to apply the rule of their own law at home, says Dr. Greenberg, and their authoritarian approach can often leave their loved ones feeling like foot soldiers in a war of words.

Work on trying to be "accepting, able to tolerate uncertainty and ambiguity. Allow the kids and your wife to find their own path without you dictating the outcome," says Dr. Greenberg. Becoming a kinder, gentler guy may require practicing different skills than you've honed in the workplace.

Give Yourself a Break

Take better care of yourself, too. Learn to appreciate the benefits of relaxation and leisure time, if for no other reason than to maximize your performance on the job. Get away for regular vacations to recharge your batteries. Pursue a hobby you can lose yourself in, if only for a few hours every week.

Studies show that work performance diminishes for those who refuse to take regular, daily breaks. Try to change your environment for 15 minutes or a half-hour if possible every day. Go for a walk out of doors. If that's not possible, find a place where you're comfortable and imagine yourself somewhere you enjoy, like a Hawaiian beach or a tropical rainforest. You want a short but complete break from your work. If you pause only to spend your 15-minute

Did You Know?

Marriage is good for your health. A study of 16 Western countries demonstrated that the overall mortality rate among unmarried men was around twice as high as that among married men. As well, married men were found to have fewer mental and physical illnesses and were generally happier than unmarried men.

break thinking about how to solve a work-related problem, you're not getting the rest you need.

Your reward will be a more fulfilling and longer life. In only the past few years, life expectancy for men has risen from 70 to 72, according to the Bureau of Health Statistics, thanks in part to more and more men taking better care of themselves mentally, physically, and spiritually.

Why Women Live Longer than Men

We've come a long way since 1919 when American men lived to be just 54 and women 56. Improvements in medical science, together with better sanitation and housing, have increased average life expectancy to 72 for men, 79 for women. Of course, many developing countries still have a long way to go— in parts of Africa, for example, men and women are lucky to make it into their forties (see table, right).

Worldwide, with very few exceptions, women outlive men. Why? Well, in Western countries at least, it seems that men are their own worst enemies. We tend to smoke and drink more than women, and have generally unhealthier lifestyles. Women seek medical help more readily than men. Stress, too, is a contributor to the biggest killer of men, cardiovascular disease. Many men seek relaxation in booze, which has its own gloomy health consequences. And the fearlessness we celebrate in daredevils like Evel Knievel and Chuck Yeager can lead to risk-taking behavior that may end in disaster, such as driving too fast.

▲ In rich and poor countries alike, life expectancy is generally higher for women than for men. Myanmar is the exception here, possibly because of high rates of death in childbirth.

Men   Women

A Healthy Lifestyle

Having a healthy lifestyle means living a balanced life, and finding joy in your physical, intellectual, and spiritual well-being, without neglecting one for the other. That prescription, we admit, is a lot easier to give than it is to follow, but it's well worth taking up the challenge and dumping those bad habits.

Breaking Bad Habits

Many of us have developed a host of unhealthy habits that are useful for coping with the stresses of everyday life. Even if we want to change, we often revert to these familiar ways during times of crisis.

Part of living a healthy life means breaking free from bad habits. And that takes time. Give the new habits you're trying to acquire at least two or three weeks before expecting to see some improvement. Better yet, try to practice your new, healthy habits for 90 days. If you do, you'll be living a much healthier and more satisfying life.

DON'T LET SMOKE GET IN YOUR EYES
First and most important: If you're a smoker, quit now. It's the fastest and easiest way to improve your health. By now, you're familiar with all the antismoking arguments, so we won't insult your intelligence by trotting them out again here. But consider this: Would the billion-dollar, politically powerful tobacco companies allow death warnings on cigarette packages if there was even the remotest possibility that smoking doesn't kill you? Not a chance. The sooner you quit, the longer you'll live, studies show.

EAT WELL TO STAY WELL
Poor nutrition, especially a diet high in saturated fat— dairy products, red meat, junk food—leads to cardiovascular disease, the number-one killer of men. Eating foods rich in saturated fat results in increased blood levels of cholesterol, a fatty liquid, which begins to build up on the walls of arteries, eventually clogging them like a drain full of grease.

Too much fat will have you looking like the Pillsbury doughboy, eventually sapping your energy and causing more health problems. Have a good look at your current diet.
• Are there too many fatty foods?
• Do you tend to eat large quantities of junk food?
• Are fruit and vegetables low down on the list of foods you eat?

A nutritious diet is based on generous amounts of filling, energy-rich foods such as pasta, bread, and rice, and plenty of fresh fruit and vegetables. For protein, choose lean meat, fish, legumes (such as pinto and navy beans), and low-fat dairy products. Avoid butter, and stick to moderate amounts of low-fat versions of milk, ice cream, yogurt, and cheese. Limit your oil intake, always choosing monounsaturated oils (such as olive or canola) and low-fat, oil-based products like margarine.

Don't forget plain old water—we're two-thirds water after all. We lose water constantly through sweating, urinating, and breathing, requiring us to replenish the supply or risk

What's on the Menu?

Ready for lunch? How about stir-fried locusts? Or would you prefer a bowl of salted clay, or grasshopper stew?

Around the world, each culture has its favored food items (as on the menu above), as well as its taboos. Some choices appear wise and survival-based, rejecting items that are poisonous, indigestible, or taste downright evil.

Other choices are unfortunate. The taste for clay in some countries of the Middle East promotes anemia and retarded development in children; a taboo against fish in parts of Africa and Mexico leaves the local people lacking in protein.

But there's no need to feel superior. In the West, we can choose among an enormous variety of foods, the envy of the rest of the world. The problem is that we often choose the wrong things: too much red meat, salt, sugar, not enough fiber.

The lesson is that the mindset of our culture isn't always right. Try not to unthinkingly swallow what the culture dishes up. Take the initiative and decide on the menu that's right for your good health.

dehydration. Make sure you always drink when you're thirsty, since thirst monitors the body's need for more fluids. Doctors also recommend drinking at least six to eight eight-ounce glasses of water daily. Keep a big glass or sports water bottle nearby during the day and sip from it. You'll be surprised at how much you drink.

EXERCISE FOR LONGER LIFE

Exercise helps you live longer, relieves stress, staves off diseases like colds and flu—it can even put a spark in your sex life. All you have to do is find 30 minutes three times a week to do some form of aerobic exercise like walking, jogging, swimming, or biking.

Before starting a fitness program—especially if it has been years since you saw the inside of a gym—make sure you consult with a doctor.

Top 10 Tips for Total Health

Kenneth A. Goldberg, M.D., medical director of the Male Health Institute at Baylor Health Center, Irving-Coppell, Texas, advises the following:

1 Don't smoke. It's not good for your lungs (or heart) or anybody else's.

2 Cut calories, limit fat, sugar, and salt in your diet, add fiber, and eat more complex carbohydrates.

3 Practice moderation in all things, especially alcohol consumption.

4 Exercise regularly—and stick with it.

5 Maintain a healthy weight: being overweight aggravates high blood pressure and heart disease.

6 Exercise your mind: Read, have a good conversation with a friend, learn something new, connect with some power greater than yourself.

7 Have a positive attitude. Learn to laugh at petty annoyances.

8 Monitor your health: See your doctor for regular checkups and do self-exams monthly.

9 Ditto your dentist. Brush your teeth, tongue, and the roof of your mouth, and be sure to floss regularly.

10 Get some sleep. Experts say men need more than 7 but fewer than 10 hours, depending on their genetic predisposition.

PROTECT YOURSELF FROM THE SUN

Skin cancer is most easily avoided with sunscreen and common sense. If possible, stay out of the sun from 10:00 A.M. to 3:00 P.M. when cancer-causing ultraviolet (UV) rays are strongest. If you have to be outdoors, be sure to wear sunscreen and a hat. Never use a tanning parlor—the UV light might give you a tan to die for.

Don't Let the Sun Catch You Frying

One of life's great pleasures is sunbathing on a pristine beach, feeling the warmth of the rays on your upturned face. Sunbathing can be addictive, but like other addictions, it's best to break the habit.

Sunlight contains ultraviolet (UV) radiation, which can cause damage to eyes and skin, including cataracts, skin cancer, and premature aging. Anyone with fair skin ought to avoid the sun when it's at its fiercest: between 10:00 A.M. and 4:00 P.M. For others, and for fair-skinned risk-takers, a hat, sunglasses with UV protection, and a sunscreen will protect you from overexposure.

Sunscreens or sunblocks come in lotions, creams, and gels. They contain chemicals that partially block UV rays, allowing you to stay in the sun longer without burning. Use one with a sun protection factor (SPF) of at least 30. The higher the SPF, the longer you can stay in the sun before burning. Apply sunscreen liberally to all exposed skin—including the top of your head if you're losing your hair—30 minutes before going out, and reapply every two hours.

UVA Rays

Weaker than UVB, these rays are not blocked by the ozone layer. They're more likely to tan you than burn, but play it safe and use protection.

UVB Rays

These powerful rays are only partly filtered by the ozone layer. They'll burn you if you're not careful, and sunburn increases your risk of developing skin cancer.

UVC Rays

This very intense type of UV light is—thankfully—completely blocked by Earth's ozone layer.

O Z O N E   L A Y E R

Sunlight Is Strongest:
• From 10:00 A.M. to 4:00 P.M.
• In mid-summer
• At high altitudes
• Near the equator

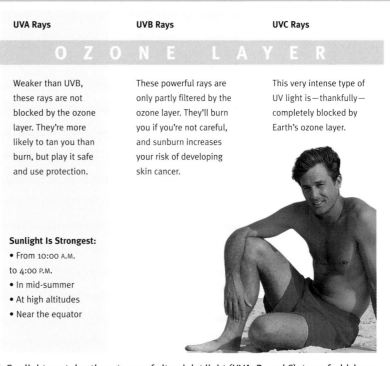

▲ *Sunlight contains three types of ultraviolet light (UVA, B, and C), two of which are at least partially blocked by the ozone layer. What gets through, however, can cause sunburn, wrinkles, and skin cancer. You owe it to yourself to take precautions.*

DRINK IN MODERATION

A little bit of booze can be a good thing. Moderate drinking protects against heart disease. But imbibing more than about two glasses of beer or wine a day will have the opposite effect on your health. Heavy drinking over a long period of time can do a great deal of harm to your physical, mental, professional, domestic, and social well-being. Keep your drinking within safe limits and stick to them.

GRILL THE DOC

Heart disease and cancer are the top two killers of men, and the chances of you contracting either can be greatly reduced with good, preventive medical care. Yet for many guys, going to the doctor is about as appealing as having a tooth pulled without anesthetic. Who among us hasn't trembled at the prospect of a rectal exam or upon hearing those five feared words: "Turn your head and cough," while having a cold hand cupped around our testicles?

You need to feel comfortable with your doctor, so choosing the best one for your needs is important. Ask friends for recommendations.

Boost Your Body's Defenses

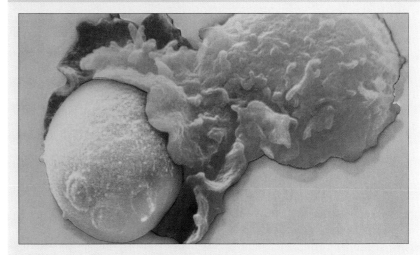

▲ *Like an alien being, a white blood cell (shown here in blue) starts to engulf an invader, in this case a yeast spore. The spore will soon be completely digested.*

Treat your body's immune system well and it will squelch any attempt at invasion from foreign organisms and cancerous changes.

The immune system is made up of special cells (including white blood cells) and proteins (called antibodies) that help fight off invading bodies like bacteria, fungi, and viruses, and also certain poisons. The system also plays a role in the control of cancer by recognizing and destroying cells that grow out of control.

A good, low-fat diet is one of the key ways to ensure a strong immune system. This means eating lots of grains, fruit, and vegetables. You should also consider some dietary insurance in the form of supplements containing the B-complex vitamins, plus vitamins A, C, and E, and iron and zinc.

A healthy way of life is the other factor in keeping the immune system happy. That includes defusing stress by learning to relax, exercising regularly, and catching the sleep you need.

Women Doctors: Good for Your Health?

Women see male doctors all the time, and for the most intimate examinations, such as Pap tests, breast examinations, gynecological exams, you name it. By contrast, some men won't go to a woman doctor for a flu shot. Squeamishness or prejudice, whatever the cause, these men are definitely missing out.

Studies indicate that women doctors outrank their male counterparts when it comes to communication skills. They typically spend more time with their patients and are more likely to address not just strictly medical concerns, but also the social and environmental issues that affect health, such as work, family, and relationships. They even smile and nod more often.

And it seems that men who go to female physicians tend to communicate more freely. For example, one study conducted by researchers at the Health Institute of the New England Medical Center found that men who went to female doctors provided over twice as much information as those seeing male physicians.

Female doctors also appear to be more prevention-oriented than male doctors. In a study of almost 2,000 patients led by researchers at the St. Louis University School of Public Health, those who went to women physicians were 56 percent more likely to have their blood cholesterol checked than patients who went to male physicians.

A good physician will take time to explain the cause of your illness in a way that helps you understand the reason for the treatment. If he or she is hurrying off to the next appointment before doing so, try another doctor. Keep looking until you find one you like.

KNOW YOUR BODY

Many of us give our bodies about as much thought as what we ate for lunch last week. Which is to say, little or none. This attitude creates a tendency to ignore the distress signals the body sends out. Hence, we seek medical help only when the pain makes a hot poker in the eye seem like a blessed relief, or when the wound or ailment has become so ghastly that women faint and children run away at the sight of it.

If you feel pain for prolonged periods of time or develop unfamiliar lumps, sores, or aches that don't disappear in a few days, call the doctor. Even when you're feeling fine, take a moment or two to examine yourself every month. Check your testicles for lumps. Look over your moles, too, for changes in size and color. Anything unusual warrants a call to the doctor to determine whether an office visit is necessary.

Also make sure that you know your family's history of diseases and disorders. That knowledge will help you and your doctor determine what symptoms you need to monitor even more carefully.

GET YOUR ZZZS

Don't scrimp on sleep. Studies show nearly half of all men sleep fewer than the eight hours a night most need. If you fall asleep easily during the day—you put your head down and you're in the Z-zone—you need more sleep. If for some reason you

can't get more sleep at night, then try taking short naps during the day. Even as little as 30 minutes helps refresh and reverse a deficit.

ROLL WITH LIFE'S PUNCHES

Finally, don't neglect your mental health. Learn to relax. Find a few minutes every day for yourself in a quiet place to read or reflect on the day's events. Take up hobbies you can enjoy alone or with others.

Take yourself less seriously and learn to laugh at life's absurdities, suggests Los Angeles psychologist Edwin M. Greenberg, Ph.D. Humor is a great antidote to the pressures and seriousness of much of our lives, Dr. Greenberg says. And don't be afraid to be yourself, he adds. Studies show that people who are more unconventional and less traditional—"rebels who march to the beat of their own drum"—tend to be healthier.

It's Official: Sex, Drugs, and Alcohol Are Good for You

Sex, drugs, and alcohol are good for you? Absolutely, when you choose your drugs and drink as carefully as you choose your lovers.

Sex can relieve stress, relax your body, help you sleep, stimulate your nervous system, boost your immune system, and keep you on an emotional even keel. Be careful, though, when choosing your partners. In this era of genital herpes and AIDS, one night of passion can haunt you forever. Always use a condom.

Medical researchers have shown that 325 milligrams of aspirin—the typical

tablet size—every other day, can reduce the risk of a heart attack by preventing blood clots. It also reduces the risk of colon cancer and some of the harmful effects of smoking. Before starting an aspirin regimen, however, discuss the pros and cons with your doctor. With any medications, always follow the directions carefully.

Numerous studies show that alcohol can protect you against heart disease. The key is moderate drinking. You should have no more than 1 ounce of alcohol a day. That's two 12-ounce beers, one to two glasses of wine, or one shot of hard liquor.

Your Good Friend Caffeine

A lot of us wouldn't be able to start the day without caffeine. There's nothing like that heart-pumping cup of coffee in the morning, is there? Caffeine, the magic ingredient in coffee, is a mild stimulant that's also found in tea, chocolate, soft drinks, pain relievers, and diet pills. Research has shown that it can improve mental alertness, reaction time, concentration, reasoning, and memory. It can also alleviate some types of headache by constricting blood vessels in the head.

There is a downside, however. Caffeine may cause you to experience anxiety, sleep disturbance, irritability, muscle tremors, heartburn, lack of concentration, and diarrhea. More insidious is caffeine dependence. Chronic users have experienced

withdrawal symptoms, including headaches, nausea, vomiting, and lack of energy when they stop drinking coffee. Finally, caffeine adversely affects some people when mixed with certain medications.

Should you cut back? It's hard to put a limit on daily caffeine consumption because reactions to it are so very individual. For some people, one cup of coffee may be too much, while others can drink half a dozen cups and have no problems. The best advice is to cut back if the coffee seems to be making you nervous or irritable, or if you're having trouble sleeping.

▶ *The old heart-starter is probably doing you no harm—if you can keep consumption within reasonable limits.*

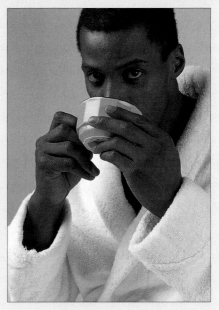

Changing Your Lifestyle

Most of us can benefit from a change in lifestyle, even a fairly minor one like cutting down on fatty foods. Sometimes, though, drastic changes are called for, changes that amount to a lifestyle makeover. Such a break with past habits may be difficult at first, but the long-term rewards are incalculable.

> **"Life is about more than just maintaining oneself, it is about extending oneself. Otherwise living is only not dying."**
> Simone de Beauvoir, French writer

Is a Change in the Wind?

If you choose to give up smoking, to eat a nutritious diet, to exercise, and to get regular medical checkups, you'll reap the benefits of greater productivity and a longer life, says Southern California psychologist Dennis A. Chernekoff, Ph.D., who specializes in counseling men. "Care for yourself well and learn to function well in the world and that will lead you to a sense of contentment, and allow you to function at your very best," he says.

Some men, however, need more than just these sorts of changes.

Henry David Thoreau once observed that "most men lead lives of quiet desperation." If that sounds like you, there's no reason to continue feeling that way. Men become desperate largely because their values are out of sync with their actions, says Dr. Chernekoff. Ranking your values and attempting to live according to what's most important to you is the first step toward a healthy lifestyle.

On the other hand, if you choose to work 12 hours a day, go home, flop yourself down in front of the television, and guzzle a six-pack while scarfing down a half-frozen pizza,

desperation may be unavoidable. The important thing to remember is this: You run your life, and you can choose to live differently.

You and Your Emotions

Choosing to live a better, healthier life is likely to require a different mental approach than the one that you've used to get to this point.

First of all, it requires paying more attention to your emotions. "Most men are disconnected from their emotional side," says Dr. Chernekoff, who sees the consequences in his patients who suffer from withering

Do You Need to Change Your Lifestyle?

The way you spend your time defines your values. Examine your answers to the following questions. If you answer yes to five or more of them, you may want to consider making some lifestyle changes.

• Are you often bored?

• Do you think others find you boring?

• Have you turned down invitations to socialize so often that you're no longer included?

• Do you spend more than 10 hours a day sleeping?

• Do you watch more than an hour of television daily?

• Have you forgotten the title of the last book you read for fun?

• Do you define vacation as a time to spend catching up on work?

• Do you eat mostly things you can hold in your hand while writing, talking on the phone, or driving?

• Does your calendar or electronic timekeeper dictate where you go and what you do every moment of your waking hours?

• Do you forget the names and ages of your children? Do your children call you Mr. Daddy? Do you forget your mother's birthday? Your anniversary?

• Do you have trouble remembering when you last saw your neighborhood in daylight?

• Are you oversnacking, oversmoking, overeating, overdrinking, overdoing, or overconsuming anything?

• Do you volunteer to do extra tasks at work rather than go home and face what you'll find there?

• Are you taking aspirin, antacids, and painkillers or nonprescription medication on a regular basis?

• Do you have an office with a view that's totally wasted on you?

• Can you discriminate between hunger and anxiety?

• Do you have anxiety attacks if work is delegated to anyone but you?

• Are you ignoring aches and pains that probably ought to be treated? Are you avoiding regular physical examinations in places that could lead to real trouble later on ?

• Do you often feel as though something is missing in your life?

• Have you forgotten the last time you went to a movie, the theater, or a sporting event?

relationships and diminished satisfaction in their jobs and careers. The reason is simple: Men largely define themselves by their work.

LIFE IN THE CORPORATE JUNGLE
Especially in today's corporate environment of hostile takeovers, downsizing, and outsourcing, men learn quickly that survival—not to mention promotion and higher pay—has little to do with exhibiting traits valued by family and friends.

Dr. Chernekoff says that men in such situations tend to shut down their emotional side. They become harder, tougher. That's a course of action that has a terrible impact on relationships. "Eventually," he explains, "we become robotic in our interactions. If production is the only value that matters to you, then you've achieved it. But what if you also value experiencing joy and being with others, if you want to look at a sunset, or hold hands and feel good? If that's also important to

you, then you have to consciously cultivate your emotional side."

If you value spending time with your family and your friends, then you can choose to turn down jobs or promotions that will take you away from them for 12 hours a day. Although many men chase higher and higher salaries looking for greater security, "money will not guarantee internal peace or a sense of well-being," Dr. Chernekoff warns.

EMOTIONAL RESCUE
Men often believe their families care most for the paycheck they bring home, when in fact, wives and children usually want more time from the men they love, not more money, Dr. Chernekoff has found. He says that many men choose punishing careers and climb corporate ladders because it fulfills an emotionally immature notion about toughness. The strongest men are those who consciously create their own value system and act on it, he adds.

Hobbies can help fulfill the need all humans have to create. Since so much of your day is devoted to production, leave time at the end to discover something new or to improve yourself. Maybe it's woodworking or rebuilding a car engine, or flying model airplanes—anything that can take your mind off work. But you've got to be honest with yourself. If you're going to the garage to escape your family or hide out, then it's destructive, Dr. Chernekoff says.

Slowing Down the Aging Process

Feeling a little time-worn? Don't we all. Like rust, time never sleeps. The clock's always running whether we like it or not, and let's face it, we *don't* like it! You can't stop the march of time, but it is possible to slow its inevitable effects on your body and mind.

How We Age

The first gray hair, the first wrinkle, the start of an expanding waistline: Most of us disregard the initial signs of aging until at a certain point—maybe in our late thirties or early forties—they simply can no longer be so easily shrugged off.

Your hair (if you've got any) is now salt-and-pepper, you can't take the stairs two at a time any more, and young women in the office look past you to the Brad Pitt lookalike. That's when the aging process hits home. So, what happens when we age?

Many facets of aging are still not completely understood, but basically your body starts to wear out. Cells either no longer renew themselves as well as they used to, or don't renew themselves at all.

Take skin, for example: As a youth, when your skin got old, it was quickly replaced with a new hide. But about the time you turned 30, the old skin began to hang on longer and longer. Genetics and your inclination to sunbathe determine how deeply crevices will sink into your face and body.

> "I think it is the food. I eat corn, rice, and vegetables—not much meat. I get up early and go to sleep before nine. I don't drink or smoke, but some other old people do."
>
> Huang Bohan, of Bama, China, on how he lived to be 105

Hair begins to lose its color by the time men hit middle age, when the body's supply of pigment begins to decrease. Couple that with a genetic predisposition to gray, and pretty soon those few wisps of white have become a head full of powder.

Beginning in your late twenties, your metabolic rate slows down, and with it the rate at which you burn calories. You can maintain the same diet and exercise regimen at age 30

The Elusive Fountain of Youth

In the sixteenth century, Ponce de Leon sailed for North America in search of the island of Bimini where he hoped to find the rejuvenating Fountain of Youth. He found Florida instead. Ever since, hucksters and snake oil salesmen from around the world have marketed an array of useless products with an equally useless guarantee of youthfulness and immortality.

The remedies for aging have ranged from Kickapoo Indian medicine to honey, castor oil, vinegar, yogurt, molasses, garlic, wheat germ, royal jelly, milk, and brewer's yeast. Lethal dosages of vitamins, a macrobiotic diet, teas made from sarsaparilla, and ginseng—over the years all have been touted as suppliers of endless youthful energy. More recently, purveyors of a wide variety of high-tech preservation systems have promised immortality to the truly affluent.

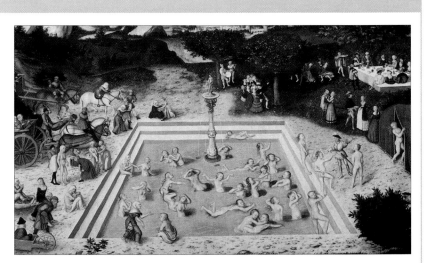

Advocates of cryonics, for instance, will put your body on ice and revive you when science finds a cure for the ailment that killed you. Let the buyer beware, however. Apart from living a healthy life, the truth is that little else will help you escape the ravages of time.

▲ *For centuries explorers sought the legendary Fountain of Youth. This is a fanciful sixteenth-century view of how the fountain's waters rejuvenated the elderly.*

Aging's Outer Limits

There's a common belief that medical science has increased the human lifespan. Unfortunately, that's not true. The reality is that the human body is only built to last about 120 years. Few of us reach that age because of diseases and accidents.

What medical science *has* done—combined with improved sanitation and housing—is to increase the average life expectancy. We've now got an excellent chance of living longer than our grandparents. There's still a cap on our lifespan, but medical science has allowed us to live more of it. Increasing the lifespan itself is still the stuff of science fiction.

▶ *More and more of us are living to a happy old age, but despite science's best efforts, the lifespan has a limit.*

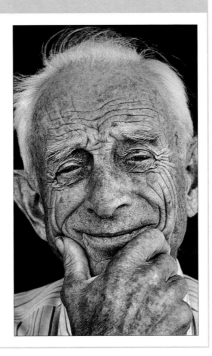

that you did at age 20 and still gain extra pounds. Before you know it, you've got a middle-age pot belly.

Less visibly, many of your vital organs are in decline. Cells in the kidney, brain, heart muscle, and lens of the eye don't renew themselves, so once they wear out, the body can't replace them.

Men also age due to hormonal changes. These begin toward the end of your forties, when there's a very noticeable decline in testosterone, a decline that continues throughout the rest of your life. Testosterone acts like fertilizer: It goes to the skeleton, the muscles, and the brain to stimulate growth. As the supply diminishes, the skeletal system and the muscles gradually weaken.

Stress is another big reason why men age. We weren't built to cope with the constant stress of modern life, just short bursts of it that allow for recovery time. Many men are under day-to-day stress, both at work and at home. That damages heart and muscle tissue, adding to the normal physiological declines of aging.

Look and Feel Young

There's no way to bring the aging process to a complete halt. You can, however, slow it down, so that you'll look and feel your best at every stage of your life. The recipe for staying young is simple: Eat a moderate, low-fat diet, exercise regularly, protect yourself from the sun, reduce stress levels, stay mentally active, and sit back and enjoy the passing of time.

GO LOW-FAT

A slower metabolism from your late twenties onward means you'll have an expanding waistline if you don't cut your calorie intake. Switch to a diet that's low in fat. That doesn't mean you can never eat Mexican food, hamburgers, or steak again. A moderate amount of these foods is okay. What you should be doing is switching the emphasis of your diet away from fat and protein toward grains, fruit, and vegetables.

EXERCISE

It takes surprisingly little to maintain age-inhibiting fitness—exercise five times a week to increase your heart rate 20 percent for at least 30 minutes. It's not so hard to find the time, either. Bring sneakers to work and walk for 45 minutes at lunch instead of going out for a high-fat meal. Exercise will leave you feeling more relaxed and cheerful, and it also helps you sleep better.

How Wrinkle-Resistant Are You?

Genetics and your lifestyle choices are perhaps the most important indicators of how soon wrinkles will appear and whether the crevices on your face and body resemble the Grand Canyon.

Do you spend a lot of time in the sun? Smoke? Drink alcohol? Live in a city or town with heavy air pollution? Are you fair-skinned? Are you related to Keith Richards? For every yes answer, your chances of delaying the onset of wrinkles diminishes significantly.

The sun is your skin's worst enemy, regardless of the weather or the season. You can slow down the wrinkling process if you use a sunscreen with a sun protection factor (SPF) of 30 or more every day, year-round, on all exposed skin.

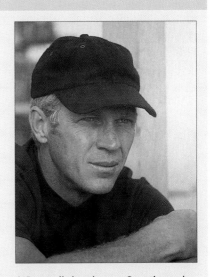

▲ *Ruggedly handsome: Genetics and sunbathing are the two big factors that determine how wrinkled you'll become.*

SUNBATHING EQUALS WRINKLES

Exposure to the sun's ultraviolet rays worsens the effects of aging skin. The best and most effective way to prevent wrinkles is to always go outside covered, either with clothes and hat or a sunscreen with a sun protection factor (SPF) of 30 or higher.

HEAD OFF STRESS

To reduce stress you might need something as simple as an occasional 15-minute break away from the office during the workday. Go for a stroll outside. Bigger problems, however, need more complex solutions. Maybe you're chasing money and power too much, and need to reassess your values. Do you really need such an expensive car? The big-screen television? The luxury home or condo? The five-star restaurants? Take a walk on the beach instead. You may live longer to enjoy what's truly meaningful.

KEEP MENTALLY YOUNG

We've all met people who seem as if they're old before their time. It's not physical so much as mental: Their attitudes, outlook on life, interests, general knowledge (or lack of)—all seem more appropriate to somebody many years older.

Avoid this fate by exercising your mind. Read as much as you can, stay well-informed about current events, argue politics and religion, take up challenging hobbies and pastimes—mental workouts like these will maintain and increase your mental agility and capacity for learning.

If You Want to Cover Up

Not every man can take the irreversible signs of aging with equanimity. It's easy to say that you should accept those gray hairs and wrinkles as badges of honor, that they make you look distinguished. There are times, however, when you just want some camouflage. Here are some suggestions.

IRONING OUT WRINKLES

Some cosmetics manufacturers say their skin-care products can reverse or prevent wrinkles. They'll prevent

---

Down with Free Radicals!

Think of free radicals, a molecular by-product of breathing, as guerrilla warriors infiltrating your body on orders from the Grim Reaper. Free radicals are unstable and highly reactive, in need of electrons to survive. So they take electrons from body tissue, leaving damaged cells behind. Those damaged cells lead to the diseases of aging: clogged arteries, cataracts, cancer, and so on.

The Good News about Antioxidants
You can fight back with counterterrorist vitamins called antioxidants, natural enzymes that eliminate free radicals. Some researchers have found preliminary evidence to suggest antioxidants may combat the tissue oxidation (or "rusting") that free radicals cause.

The principal antioxidants are vitamins C and E; beta-carotene, which the body turns into vitamin A; and the mineral selenium, which works in tandem with vitamin E. Other antioxidants include vitamin B_6, thiamin, lecithin, and zinc. When taken in doses slightly higher than the government's recommended daily allowance, these nutrients may "slow down the aging process," according to gerontologist John Walsh, Ph.D. "And slow down the damage aging causes to your body. Even I take them," he says.

Where to Find Antioxidants
Antioxidants are found mainly in fruit, vegetables, and whole-grain cereals, although certain animal-derived foods also contain useful amounts. Natural sources include red, orange, yellow, and deep-green vegetables; oats, wheat, rice, and corn; garlic and onions; liver, kidney, fish, shellfish, red meat, and poultry; and citrus fruit and berries.

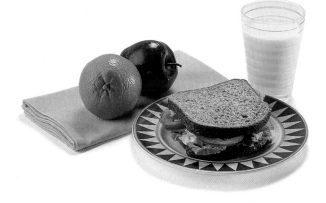

◄ *Antioxidants are everywhere, found in a wide range of foods. Take a bite out of this tasty free-radical-fighting lunch: Chicken (vitamin B_6), lettuce (beta-carotene), and tomatoes (beta-carotene and vitamin C) on whole-grain bread (vitamins B_6 and E), with fresh fruit (vitamin C). Wash it all down with a selenium-rich glass of cold milk.*

Flatten That Stomach

If the bulge around your middle has taken on a life of its own, you're probably willing to do what it takes to make permanent changes in your physique. To combat unwanted girth, try the following:

• Switch to a low-fat diet that includes plenty of carbohydrates, fruit, and vegetables.

• Stand up straight and suck in your gut. Toned abdominal muscles can improve posture, and vice versa.

• Do fat-burning aerobic exercise: Try tennis, running, swimming, a rowing machine.

• Start doing abdominal exercises, but don't think a few crunches by themselves are going to give you washboard abs. For full details, see "The Total Abdominal Workout" on page 110.

Keep Your Mental Powers Sharp

By the time you reach 45, your brain is losing 50,000 cells a day from the cerebral cortex, the part where "smart" lives. Your hippocampus, a ridge of tissue in the brain where memories are processed, has begun to decline. You may find yourself forgetting dates and appointments, wondering how to get to a place you visited only a month earlier. Not to worry though; your memory will still serve you, it's just moving more slowly. And besides, as the cells diminish, your head full of knowledge and experience—called wisdom— continues to grow.

Remember, too, that keeping the mind stimulated can help preserve intellectual function. Play word games, work on puzzles, read the newspaper, learn woodworking or a foreign language. Keep offering your mind new experiences: Travel; join a church, club, or civic organization; learn to adapt to change; interact with people who are smarter than you.

Because stress, anxiety, and depression are debilitating to the mind, try to readjust your attitude when you feel the onset of the blues. Take time out to relax. Make leisure part of your life. See a happy movie, think of something funny, sing an upbeat song— whatever helps to lift you out of the funk.

A well-balanced diet and a consistent program of exercise also helps keep brain cells functioning at optimal levels. Remember, too, don't panic. Your memory may be slowing down, but you have increasingly more information to recall as time goes by.

▶ *Keep in touch: Reading the paper counts as part of a mental exercise program.*

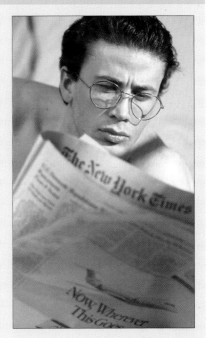

wrinkles only if they contain sunscreen, but mostly they'll just plump up the skin to give the appearance of fewer wrinkles, with impermanent results. There is one product that *does* work, however: The prescription topical skin cream Retin-A will help eliminate and reduce fine wrinkles if applied daily. There's a drawback, though: Retin-A makes your skin extremely sensitive to the sun's ultraviolet rays, and you will be more susceptible to skin cancer.

DISGUISING GRAY HAIR

Coloring your hair will get rid of the gray. A professional hair-care specialist will probably do a better job than you. But if you opt to do it yourself, don't make the mistake that many guys do by going too dark. Choose a shade a little bit lighter than what you want your hair to be, and if you still think it is too light, work your way up to darker hues.

WHAT TO DO ABOUT BALDNESS

Baldness makes men look older. If it really bothers you, don't comb one side of your remaining hair over your naked pate; it always looks fake. Instead, get an appropriate, stylish haircut—usually a short one—to look your best. If you want to cover up those shiny spaces, you have two options: hair transplants (they're expensive) or taking either the drug minoxidil (it's not always effective) or the oral drug Propecia.

Stopping Gray Hairs

As far as researchers know, the only way to stop hair from graying is to stop time. Though some studies have shown smoking may contribute to an increase in gray hair, there is no conclusive evidence. Researchers do know that melanin, which gives hair its color, diminishes with age. When the melanin stops, hair loses color, turns white, and becomes coarser and duller.

Those who want to turn back the clock might consider first giving up smoking, then trying a few nontraditional choices, like hair dyes and color. Be aware, though, that applying chemical color—be it temporary or permanent— may mean you have to color or keep closely shaved your facial hair. As a last resort, daring men might want to try shaving their heads. Apart from these solutions, though, perhaps the best way to deal with gray hair is to keep it well-groomed.

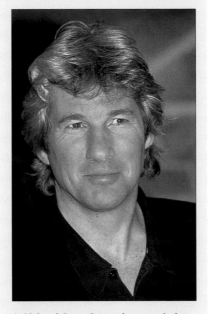

▲ *Richard Gere shows that gray hair can be sexy. A good cut on healthy hair can make you look vibrant.*

Sleep Easy

We spend about a third of our lives asleep, yet scientists still aren't sure why we need it. What we do know is that if you go without it, your creativity, memory, critical thinking, and physical performance deteriorate. Compelling reasons, if ever they were needed, for getting some quality shut-eye.

Symptoms of Problem Sleep	
• Nervousness	• Fatigue
• Memory lapses	• Snoring
• Mood swings	• Hallucinations
• Grogginess	• Lethargy

Why You Need to Sleep

"I'll have plenty of time to sleep when I'm dead," you rationalize, your bloodshot eyes glancing from the report you're writing toward the clock that you *think* reads 1:00 A.M. You're not sure what it says, really, since your vision is so blurred and you're having a hard time focusing and thinking clearly.

These are symptoms of sleep deprivation. So is being dependent on an alarm clock. If you need an alarm to rouse you in the morning, you're not getting enough shut-eye.

And why is sleep so important? Without adequate sleep, human performance diminishes significantly, researchers say. Scientists have yet to figure why sleep is so important physiologically, but they do know what happens when you fail to get enough of it. First, you feel sleepy. Then, you begin a rapid decline in mood, performance, creativity, and critical thinking abilities. In the extreme, no amount of willpower can keep humans awake.

As far as we know, no one has ever died from staying awake, although plenty of lab animals have succumbed to researcher-induced sleep deprivation, according to James B. Maas, Ph.D., professor of psychiatry at Cornell University and author of *The Sleep Advantage*.

How Much Sleep?

The optimal amount of sleep for an average adult man is "at least an hour more than what you're used to getting," says Dr. Maas. The average man sleeps about seven hours a night. By contrast, most men need between eight and nine hours of sleep to stay fully alert—a little more or less depending on your genetic predisposition. When you try to get by with less, you miss out on the most important sleep cycle, the one that occurs between the seventh and eighth hours of sleep.

During that time, you enter the final stage of sleep, when the brain's neural network is stimulated, the equivalent of recharging the brain's batteries, Dr. Maas says. The recharge allows you to retain and gain new ideas and insights, strengthen memory, acquire new mental material of different kinds. If you fail to stimulate the neural network, says Dr. Maas, the brain begins to deteriorate.

To give your brain the rest you need for peak performance during working hours, you need about four or five 90-minute sleep cycles a night, a combination of deep and REM, or rapid eye movement, sleep.

Dr. Maas is among a group of researchers who believe REM sleep stimulates the metabolism to release chemicals into the brain that make learning easier. Men who believe they can scrimp on sleep are depriving themselves of peak performance,

10 Ways to Better Sleep

1 Go to bed and get up at the same time every day, regardless of whether you have to go to work.

2 Abstain from alcohol and cigarettes for at least two hours before bedtime. Don't drink coffee later than five hours before turning in.

3 Make your bedroom cozy and restful. Don't eat, work, or watch TV in it.

4 If you're having trouble falling asleep, don't just toss and turn. Get out of bed, go into another room, and read or do relaxation exercises until you feel sleepy.

5 Try to avoid sleep-inducing drugs if you can. Using drugs allows you to maintain bad habits you should be trying to break.

6 Try not to eat a heavy meal before you go to bed.

7 Regular exercise will help tire you out, promoting good sleep. Be sure you finish exercising at least three hours before bed.

8 Play some relaxing music, let some fresh air into the room, turn off the phone, and allow your body and mind to wind down at least 30 minutes before you want to fall asleep.

9 Take a 15- to 30-minute nap during the day if you feel you're sleep deprived.

10 Don't rob yourself of adequate rest day after day by working late. When you've reached the limit of your productivity, say good-night.

What Your Brain Is Doing While You Sleep

The electrical activity in your brain alters while you sleep (shown in black on the clocks), depending on the stage of sleep you're in. When measured with a monitor, this activity looks like waves. Hence, the two types of sleep we experience are called slow-wave (deep) sleep, and REM (rapid eye movement) sleep, associated with dreaming.

When you first go to bed, you experience slow-wave (also called non-REM) sleep, which is usually divided into four progressively deeper stages as the brainwave frequency becomes slower. At the same time, your body temperature, metabolism, blood pressure, pulse rate, and respiration all drop.

Every 90 minutes or so after the fourth stage of slow-wave sleep, you experience a period of REM sleep, lasting from 5 to 30 minutes. REM sleep is less restful than slow-wave sleep—the brainwave activity is similar to when you're awake. Your pulse, blood pressure, and breathing become irregular and your eyes dart rapidly back and forth beneath your closed eyelids.

As the night progresses, most of us will pass through four or five sleep cycles, although illnesses and sleep disorders can disturb the pattern and prevent you reaching the deepest, most restful sleep stages.

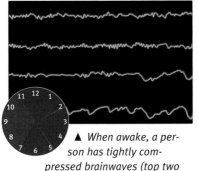

▲ When awake, a person has tightly compressed brainwaves (top two lines, above). Most of us wake up for short periods (see red areas on clock).

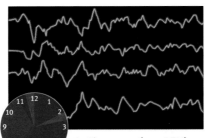

▲ Slow-wave (non-REM) sleep has brainwaves that are high and broad. There is little eye motion (bottom two lines). This is stage four, the deepest stage of sleep (in red).

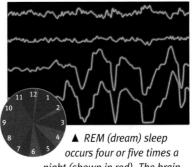

▲ REM (dream) sleep occurs four or five times a night (shown in red). The brainwaves are similar to those generated while awake. Eye movement is dramatic.

because they're missing the neural stimulation needed for memory and problem-solving, Dr. Maas says.

Solve Your Sleep Problems

If you answer yes to one or more of the following questions, you probably need more sleep:
• Do you suffer more than a minor dip in alertness in the afternoon? Do you feel drowsy, start to nod off, have a hard time focusing on a task?
• Do you fall asleep within five minutes of going to bed? Well-rested people take about 10 to 20 minutes to fall asleep.
• Do you turn off the alarm on the weekends and find yourself sleeping for several hours more than during the week?

Dr. Maas offers a few suggestions to find your way back to life among the rested. First, make sure you go to bed and wake up at the same time every day, weekends included. Next, set your bedtime 20 minutes earlier every night until you have a day with no feeling of midday sleepiness. That's how to figure your daily optimal sleep level. At the same time you're weaning yourself from the alarm clock, if you're getting sufficient sleep your body will awaken naturally every morning. If you want to rise early, subtract your optimal sleep level from the hour you want to awaken and go to bed at that time.

Sleep through Your Life

Around age six, the pineal gland at the base of the brain is secreting the highest levels of sleep-inducing melatonin into the bloodstream, allowing for the kind of deep sleep we covet but experience too rarely.

Levels of melatonin secretions remain fairly constant throughout childhood, but begin a steady decline in the teenage years. At about age 30, sleep becomes lighter. Deep, restful slow-wave sleep diminishes. It is during slow-wave sleep that the human growth hormone, which is believed to rejuvenate the body and repair the previous day's wear and tear, circulates at its highest level, experts say.

Though many men 65 and older report that they need less sleep, some experts disagree. They say the elderly have the same sleep requirements as middle-age men, but illness, medications, and the ailments of old age, particularly hardening of the arteries, decrease their ability to sustain long periods of deep sleep. By age 65, many men get as little as 30 minutes of slow-wave sleep a night.

If you live a healthy lifestyle now, centered around a low-fat diet and moderate exercise, you'll be better able to maintain the levels of sleep your body requires to rejuvenate yourself as you age.

How to Reduce Stress and Save Time

Live fast, die young, leave a handsome corpse: It's the mantra of the stress maniac. And it's also very true. Every minute that you think you save by hurrying can lead to one more minute taken off the end of your life. Every minute you relax might be one more to savor in the sunset years.

What Is Stress?

Stress is the result of an experience that causes upset, anger, frustration, or repulsion. It is anything that creates tension and uncertainty, like worrying about what else you need to do right now, or what your work colleagues will think if you don't get the promotion, or everything that you didn't do today that you need to do tomorrow.

Everyone has pressure in their life that makes them feel stressed out, ranging from screaming bosses and howling babies to overtaxed bank accounts, and clueless coworkers. If your enjoyment of life is hampered by stress, your body may be sending you warning signals that you're under too much duress.

WARNING SYMPTOMS
Here are some early warning signs of harmful stress. Heed them—ignoring them can make them get worse.
• Difficulty falling asleep
• Inability to concentrate
• Lapses of concentration

• Reduced interest in sex
• Eating when not hungry
• Smoking more
• Drinking more alcohol
• Recurrent headaches
• Increasing irritability, impatience, and loss of temper
• Constantly feeling lethargic

When You're All Revved Up with Nowhere to Go

The fight-or-flight response places your body on red alert: Your pulse quickens, blood pressure jumps, and muscles become tense. You're primed for action. But this instinctive reaction to threat is inappropriate for most situations these days, when the cause of the "threat" isn't physical. The stress from worrying about a business presentation, for example, has no ready physical release. The stress stays with you, potentially putting your health at risk.

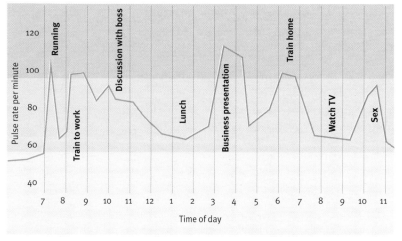

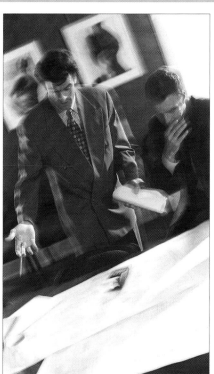

▲ *The chart shows how the pulse rate—a measure of the fight-or-flight response— reacts to both physical and emotional causes over the course of a typical working day.*

Fight or Flight?

Programmed into every one of us is the fight-or-flight response. When the brain thinks a crisis is approaching, it sends out alarm signals in the form of chemical messengers known as neurotransmitters. These trigger the production of hormones whose purpose is to put the whole body on red alert. Here's what happens.

• Your heart rate increases and your blood vessels dilate.

• Your blood pressure rises.

• Your muscles become tense.

• Your digestive system shuts down.

• You start to sweat more.

• Your breathing becomes faster.

The brain is preparing the body to either fight the perceived threat or flee from it.

This served prehistoric humans well. When confronted by a saber-toothed tiger or some cranky cavemen from the neighboring tribe, for instance, the fight-or-flight response gave our flat-headed ancestors a good chance of survival.

These days, it's still essential for surviving life-threatening situations. Say, for instance, you're in rush-hour traffic and somebody swerves in front of you. Stress will heighten your reactions and swiftly kick your self-protective instincts into gear, making your response sharper and quicker than it would be normally. The fight-or-flight response comes in handy when dealing with work challenges such as crucial business meetings or imminent deadlines.

Our body's natural reaction to stress, however, is far less appropriate for dealing with the day-to-day stresses and strains of contemporary urban life. For example, there's no physical outlet for the stress and tension that builds up when your train is 20 minutes late or you're stuck in a traffic jam. The physical pressure builds up and finds no release, leading in some cases to illness.

Take the Stress Test

Your life is a product of the choices you make. Are you choosing stress and anxiety? Or are you opting to feel relaxed and in control? Do the stress test below to see. If you answer yes to most of the questions under "Healthy Choices," congratulations! You're managing stress well. If, however, you find yourself answering yes to more than five of the "Unhealthy Choices," then it's time to think about making some important changes in your life.

Unhealthy Choices

• Do you often get nervous, angry, or upset over small disappointments or problems?

• Do you live with a sense of apprehension that your life is about to take a turn for the worst? Do you suffer from fear, anxiety, or panic?

• Do you suffer from recurring headaches? Do your back and neck muscles ache constantly?

• Do you chain smoke your way through the day?

• Are you overworked, lonely, isolated?

• Do you try to boost your energy with caffeine and sugar?

• Do you find yourself regularly suffering from loss of sleep, shallow breathing, stomach, or intestinal problems, and/or high blood pressure?

• Are you constantly criticizing and finding fault with other people? Do people dread working with you? Are you difficult to get along with?

• Do you raise your voice a lot, talking over other people?

• Is your anger often out of proportion to circumstances?

• Do you often find it almost impossible to admit mistakes and/or to apologize to others?

• Do you see your job as a burden rather than a challenge?

• Do you hold grudges? Do you often find yourself obsessing over wrongs you feel others have done you? Do you feel victimized?

Healthy Choices

• Are you confident that you're giving your best efforts, and that your best is good enough?

• Do you remember to walk away from your desk for reasons other than nature's call, getting more work, or visiting the snack machines?

• Do you regularly pray, meditate, or participate in any form of religious or spiritual activity?

• Do you have reasonable goals and objectives for your life?

• Do you ask for help readily?

• Do you kiss your wife, hug your kids, or pat your pet when you get home?

• Do you have hobbies? Read books, listen to music? Do you ever share a joke or a laugh with others? Do you find pleasure in the little things in life?

• Are you a good driver? Do you avoid reckless driving, antagonizing other motorists, and excessive speed on the roadways?

• Do you leave your job at the door when you get home in the evenings?

• Do you know your limitations? Do you accept them?

• Does your list of priorities include family, friends, and fun? Are *you* anywhere on the list?

• Do you take time out during the day for exercise, meals, and relaxation?

• Do you look forward to going to work? Do you volunteer to help others? Do you offer subordinates praise and encouragement?

How Stress Feeds Your Waistline

Go out on any city sidewalk during rush hour and you'll see the results of our stressed-out culture on the bodies of the men whose bellies precede them. High-fat diets and lack of exercise combined with stress can equal one bulging spare tire. Why?

When the brain perceives a threat, it immediately calls on the adrenal glands to send out the defenses. The adrenals, which are located on top of the kidneys, pump a hormone called cortisol into the bloodstream. The action of cortisol is to deposit fat into the body, which is meant to produce the energy needed to flee or fight the danger.

The challenges and pressures of modern life—traffic jams, rotten relationships, bellowing bosses—can trigger the adrenals, which call for more fat deposits. If the fat goes unused, it accumulates, usually around the abdomen. Guys with big bellies (apple shapes) are at a greater risk of cardiovascular disease than those who have large buttocks or thighs (pears).

Medical researchers have found, for example, that high levels of stress experienced over long periods of time slow down the immune system, making you vulnerable to a host of minor infections, and possibly to some forms of cancer.

Chronic stress can also aggravate or directly cause a wide range of diseases and ailments, including high blood pressure, diabetes, acne, digestive disorders, infertility, headaches, impotence, ulcers, poor sleep, back pain, and asthma. Excessive stress can also plunge you into emotional turmoil, affecting both your relationships and your mental health. In extreme cases, it may even lead to anxiety disorders and depression.

Your Attitude to Stress

Stress is also a matter of interpretation, many experts say. If you manage your life poorly, allowing yourself to become obsessed about work or money or status, life's challenges will weigh on you a lot more heavily than the next man. That's why the demands of a job might overwhelm one guy, yet the same workload might stimulate another.

A hectic workload can also help you to become better organized as you figure out a way to manage the overload sensibly. Stress from a boring, dead-end job might motivate you to spread your wings. Fear of poverty or failure can prompt you to to enrol in a course to increase your employment skills, or else to work harder when you feel like quitting.

In the same way, anxiety over the prospect of a serious illness might force you to see a doctor or a dentist on a regular basis.

Stress and your reactions to it, then, are just another way that life is like poker: You may be dealt a bad hand, but how you play it is entirely up to you.

How to Reduce Stress

Three factors—regular exercise, a nutritious diet, and good sleeping patterns—form the basic building blocks of healthy living that will ensure that your mind and body are able to fight off stress and worry more easily. Get that trio into shape and you can embark on a stress-prevention program that involves

Is Stress Making You Sick?

The unhealthy effects of stress show up all over the body, anywhere from the skin to your internal organs. Unrelenting stress can also depress your immune system, making you more susceptible to minor infections such as colds and flu.

Heart Disease
Anxiety can cause your blood vessels to constrict and your heart rate to increase, eventually leading to high blood pressure and heart disease.

Digestive Disorders
Stress is known to contribute to—and maybe even cause—gastrointestinal disorders like irritable bowel syndrome, along with its symptoms of diarrhea, cramps, gas, and heartburn.

Body Odor
Stress increases sweat production, which often leads to bacterial growth under your arms and on your feet, causing odor.

Dental Problems
Stress causes some people to grind and clench their teeth, which can eventually lead to cracks, painful infection, and expensive dental work.

Aches and Pains
Stress can aggravate back pain, and prolonged tension in the neck and shoulders can lead to headaches.

Mental Problems
In its more advanced stages, stress can cause lack of concentration or memory loss.

Sexual Difficulties
Stress can reduce interest in sex and aggravate erection problems.

Skin Disorders
In some people, stress causes the skin to break out in a rash.

Laugh to Relax

Laughter is the medicine that helps heal the stressed-out soul. Medical scientists take laughter so seriously that they've conducted extensive research on it. They say that adults laugh only 15 times a day on average, while children laugh 400 times daily.

What do kids know instinctively that grown-ups have long forgotten? How to play, that's what. When adults forgo play and focus exclusively on work, the resulting stress often leads to a variety of symptoms, including

muscular pain. When you play and laugh, the laughter releases chemicals in the brain called endorphins, which help to relax muscles and relieve pain.

Because you can't always control what happens in life, try to shift your focus to controlling your response to challenges and problems. Use humor to defuse difficult situations, and try not to take small annoyances seriously.

► *Stress-busting endorphins are released by the brain whenever you laugh.*

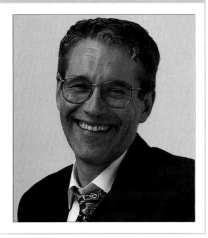

identifying the problem, talking the situation over, and finding a long-lasting solution.

EXERCISE, SLEEP, AND DIET
Regular exercise not only keeps you fit, it rids the body of stress-related hormones. Engage in an activity for 30 minutes or more three times a week and choose something that you'll like doing and stick with— cycling, swimming, golf, tennis, running, brisk walking, gardening.

Sleep is a terrific stress antidote. Although many men discount its importance, studies show that insufficient sleep leaves you less productive and feeling frazzled. If you're unable to get as much shut-eye as your body needs, consider napping. Even 30 minutes will refresh you and make you more alert.

Eating a balanced diet ensures that you're getting all the nutrients you need. A little alcohol can be a good stress-reliever: It can help relax muscles and alter perceptions to help you see the crisis in a more positive light. "We tend to see the negative more positively after a drink,"

says Larry Feldman, Ph.D., psychologist and author of *Feeling Good Again.* But he also warns alcohol can be used as a crutch, especially if you don't fix the problem that caused the tension in the first place.

IDENTIFYING THE PROBLEM
It may be easy to see what's causing the problem. Maybe your job is too fast-paced, and too much is expected of you. On the other hand, it isn't always those who travel in life's fast lane who become stressed. People in mundane, low-grade jobs have little

Eat Well to Stay Stress-Free

You can minimize the effects of stress by eating foods that restore depleted nutrients. Complex carbohydrates and proteins are believed to enhance mental performance in stressful situations. Some people choose to avoid foods with caffeine and lots of sugar, since although those ingredients may provide bursts of energy, they'll leave you feeling worn out and restless a few hours later. Alcohol, too, can mask the symptoms of stress, but leave you feeling even worse when its soothing effect wears off.

Foods to Eat
Complex carbohydrates (starches), such as rice, pasta, potatoes, bread, and popcorn, trigger the production of

serotonin in the brain, which helps to relieve stress and give the body a steady source of energy.

Proteins like meat, fish, and poultry are believed to enhance mental performance and provide amino acids to help repair damage to the body's cells.

Fruit, such as citrus fruit, bananas, cantaloupe, strawberries, kiwi fruit, peaches, apricots, and tomatoes are rich in vitamins and beta-carotene. They provide vital nutrients and help repair damage to the body caused by stress.

Vegetables, such as bell peppers, beets, lima beans, squash, broccoli, carrots, spinach, parsley, and other green leafy vegetables, provide vitamins and

nutrients. Milk (preferably low in fat), whole bran, nuts, and wheat germ are sources of potassium, a mineral that helps muscles relax.

Foods to Avoid
Products containing caffeine, such as chocolate, coffee, tea, and soft drinks. Caffeine can destroy B and C vitamins.

Sugary foods like candy boost energy, but can leave you feeling lethargic and irritable. The empty calories can lead to excessive weight gain, diabetes, and other health-threatening conditions.

Alcohol can impair judgment and slow reflexes. It creates a chemical imbalance that can lead to increased tension and anxiety.

control over their work, which can be repetitive and unsatisfying.

Sometimes it may be hard to identify exactly what's causing the stress. To pinpoint the problem, the next time you feel anxious, make a note of the circumstances, and see if a pattern emerges.

DEALING WITH THE PROBLEM

Women generally cope with stress better than men. That's because they're more likely to open up to others about their problems. In contrast, men tend to conceal their troubles as tightly as a winning poker hand, increasing their anxiety in the process. So, once you've worked out who or what is at the heart of your stress problem, talk the issue over with your partner or a friend, or with the person who's causing the problem.

Be positive and you probably can work out a constructive solution. Let's say your opinions aren't sought at work and you are bored with your current job. You'll get nowhere if you simply confront the boss with "I'm bored" or "I want more interesting work." Instead, offer a concrete, workable proposal.

How to Manage Your Time More Effectively

Complementing stress-prevention techniques is time management, a way of taking control of your life. If you have no idea where the day goes, you're a good candidate to keep track on a piece of paper of how you spend your time, accounting for all 24 hours. Try to identify the time-wasters. Here are some of the most important ones.

- Interruptions, especially phone calls
- Indecision
- Not having a plan for the day
- Not having an organized desk
- Not being able to say no to unreasonable demands
- Not being able to ask for or to accept help when it's offered
- Moving from task to task without finishing anything
- Shooting the bull too much
- Poor communications
- Meetings that take too long

Find your top time-wasters and start doing something about them. To guide you, follow these principles.

- Don't procrastinate. Prioritize the tasks you want to accomplish, setting realistic goals. Write them down so you've got a plan for the day. Then go through the list, finishing one job before moving to the next.

- Any unfinished tasks should be transferred to the following day's plan. Make a note of anything that interfered with your work, together with a way to rectify it. You may need more secretarial help, for example.

- Divide large projects into more manageable chunks and delegate work to others when you can.

- Take regular breaks during the working day. You'll come back to the task feeling refreshed, and may even be able to find a new angle to solve a problem that had previously frustrated you. Get a change of scenery, by going for a walk, for example.

GET YOUR VALUES RIGHT

If a high-flying job has you wound tighter than a baseball, maybe it's time to downshift into a less fast-paced position. This is a big step that will require some reflection on what you value most in life. Ask yourself these questions.

- What do you want out of life?
- What really matters to you? Expensive cars? Costly vacation homes?
- Do you value the time you spend with your partner, your kids, or by yourself pursuing creative or athletic ventures?

Write down your priorities, then make a list of how you spend your time. Compare the two lists. Does the way you spend your time reflect your priorities? If the lists are far apart, you need some serious attitude adjustment which may involve a career change.

CARVE OUT TIME FOR YOURSELF

An important part of time management is allowing time for yourself. Try to limit your television-watching to about five or six hours a week and

---

Tips for a Stress-Free Life

- Give yourself a break. Take time out for family, fun, and relaxation. Remember, all work and no play makes Jack a coronary risk.

- Eat healthy foods, exercise, get plenty of sleep, reduce caffeine and alcohol consumption, quit smoking.

- Not every fight is worth winning. Stand your ground when you're right, but learn to yield.

- Talk things out. If you're worried or under pressure, share it with a close friend, family member, professional counselor, or clergyman.

- Learn new skills. Keep your mind stimulated and active.

- Make a daily list of things to do. Be reasonable about what you can really accomplish in a given time. Make sure to allot enough time to each task, then add a little extra time for the unexpected.

- Set realistic goals for your life, and prioritize how you will spend your resources. Live within your means.

- If you need to, cry. Find a private place and let the tears flow. It helps vent emotional pressure.

- Do something for someone else; it will help get your mind off your own troubles. Volunteer around the house or in the community.

---

replace it with creative, enriching, or fun activities, avoiding anything that becomes stressful and too competitive. "Form the habit of doing something that nourishes yourself," advises Dr. Feldman.

This principle extends to vacations as well. Many men in high-powered jobs have high-powered vacations, forcing themselves awake by sunrise, filling every moment with appointments, activities, or competitions, often topping off the day with calls to the office and a few faxes before going to bed.

Vacations are for resting and recharging batteries. Stop trying so hard. Sit in the breeze and read a book. Tell the office to call only in an emergency. Better yet, don't tell them where you are—give your vacation number to a trusted friend or relative and have him screen your office calls to separate emergency from nuisance.

RELAXATION EXERCISES

The best defense against stress is a strong offense. Dr. Feldman offers some fast and simple tension-control exercises he says will reduce the negative effects of stress if you practice them diligently.

Stop working and begin counting backwards to yourself from 40. Do this five times a day. After you say each number, repeat the word relax. Like this: 40 relax, 39 relax, 38 relax, and so on. When you finally get to zero, repeat the process four times. It takes about four minutes and it allows you to break completely from your work without ever getting up from your chair.

Dr. Feldman also suggests doing brief breathing exercises. Take a deep breath and exhale four or five times. Repeat every two hours.

Though it might seem difficult to find a place to be alone during the day, consider going to the men's

10 Ways to Relax

1 Breathe deeply, inhaling through your nose. Hold your breath for 10 seconds, then exhale. You should feel your stomach expand with each breath. Sometimes closing your eyes or focusing on a pleasant place or a view helps.

2 Laugh. We don't mean a little snicker or a smirk, but a laugh that originates in the belly and forces itself out almost against your will. To help make you laugh, see a comedian, read a humorous story, watch a film or television comedy.

3 Let go of negative thoughts. When you leave your office, tell yourself: "I'm through for the day." Don't bring work-related problems home with you. If the problems continue to dog your thoughts, say "stop" or "delete" or "cancel" and make that the word that reminds you to banish work-related aggravations from your thoughts.

4 Pray or meditate. Involve yourself in some form of spiritual activity. Set aside 20 to 30 minutes a day to commune with God or nature or something that will put you in realistic perspective with the universe.

5 Relax each part of your body, starting with your feet. Do this by focusing all your thoughts and attention on relaxing your toes. When your toes feel relaxed, move to your ankles, your legs, and so forth, until you reach your head.

6 Get up and stretch to help break physical tension. Stand up, walk around your desk or the room. Gently roll your head from side to side a few times. Roll your shoulders forward, then backward.

7 Place your fingers and thumbs on your scalp, apply as much pressure as is comfortable, and massage gently.

8 Pick on a pillow. Pound one to release physical tension, or scream into one to relieve pent-up pressure. In extreme cases, you may want to throw it or drop-kick it across the room.

9 Indulge yourself by soaking in a warm tub for 15 minutes or so.

10 Find an activity that you like. Jogging, trekking, writing, or *anything* works as long as you've chosen it because it interests you. Avoid choosing something related to work or anything else that might be stressful.

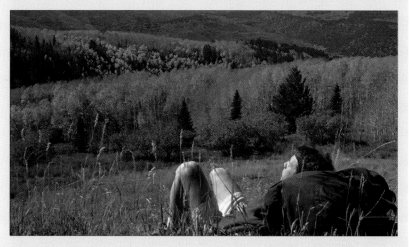

▲ *Fight stress with a relaxing activity. A day on the trail not only gives you fresh air and exercise but also helps put worries in perspective.*

room and sitting on the toilet, he says, or practicing meditation in your car a few minutes before or after work or in between appointments. Other forms of longer medi-

tation are helpful to your overall well-being, including yoga, tai chi, and transcendental meditation. See also "10 Ways to Relax" for some more relaxation suggestions.

Good-Looking Skin

It's your biggest organ, and it regularly gets bruised, scratched, battered, and fried. It's also one of your main erogenous zones. Yet chances are, you probably give barely a thought to your skin. Maybe it's time for a change of attitude. After all, how good you look depends on how well you care for it.

You've Got a Hide

The skin accounts for 16 percent of your total weight. A square inch has about 600 sweat glands, 100 oil-secreting glands, 60 or so hairs, 20 blood vessels, and countless nerve endings. It's waterproof; it stretches every which way; and it automatically renews itself. As a conduit for the sense of touch, it's a major link to the outside world. And it's almost maintenance-free.

Caring for skin is one of those things that divides the sexes: Women spend many hours and thousands of dollars on skin products while men hardly think about theirs at all. But guys only need to have an understanding of what skin is and follow a few minimal steps to keep it healthy.

The Right Stuff for Your Skin

It used to be that cosmetic companies marketed only to women. Then they realized they were neglecting an enormous, untapped demographic: men. And so the onslaught began with a media blitz hawking hundreds of skin-care products geared toward guys. Despite the claims of these companies, over-the-counter products do nothing at all to reverse damaged skin or a wrinkled brow. "It's all bull," says dermatologist Jerome Z. Litt, M.D. "Men really don't have to do much to care for their skin."

That said, moisturizers will temporarily make skin look less dry and wrinkled.

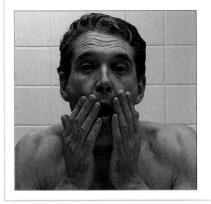

But by far the best skin-care regimen is a well-balanced diet. Beyond that, Dr. Litt's recommendations include using a mild soap. Men with body-odor problems should use an antibacterial soap like Safeguard, Dial, or Coast on the genital area and underarms. Here are some other tips.

• If your skin is dry or flaky, use a mild cleansing soap like Neutrogena and follow that up by applying a non-emollient-based moisturizer such as Moisturel.

• For mild forms of eczema, a type of dermatitis, use Moisturel or a product like it. The main ingredients are water and glycerin.

• If you have sensitive skin, try a mild cleanser like Cetaphil. Avoid using fatted soaps or anything containing emollients (a heavy-duty moisturizer) or cold cream, especially if your skin leans toward the oily end of the spectrum. Emollients tend to clog up the pores and cause small whiteheads to appear, Dr. Litt says.

◄ *Male skin care: Splash on some water and wash with a mild soap cleanser.*

Tips for Good-Looking Skin

• Keep your skin clean. Wash your face thoroughly with a mild soap and water. Avoid rubbing or pulling on it, which is why using your hands to wash is preferable to using wash cloths, sponges, brushes, or loofahs. Wash your neck and ears, too.

• The rules of general good health apply to preserving your skin: Don't smoke (it causes wrinkles), drink alcohol in moderation, do some form of aerobic exercise, and eat a healthy diet that includes plenty of fruit, vegetables, and grains. Drink six to eight glasses of water a day.

• Reduce your stress levels by practicing relaxation exercises or meditation for 15 minutes a day.

• Exposure to the sun causes damage and wrinkles. Limit skin damage by staying out of the sun whenever possible. Wear a sunscreen (SPF 30 and above) when you go outside, fair weather or not. Protect all of your exposed skin—lips, eyes (use wraparound sunglasses that block UV rays), ears, hands. There is no such thing as a healthy tan.

• Examine your face periodically for moles or other indications of skin cancer. If you have a growth or discoloration that changes size or color, see a physician.

Introducing Your Skin

The skin consists of several layers. The epidermis, or outer layer, sits on top of the dermis. The dermis contains the blood vessels that nourish the skin, hair follicles, and sebaceous (oil) and sweat glands.

The top layer of skin is composed of dead cells bound together to make the surface tough and waterproof. It sheds itself constantly—an estimated 400 pounds worth over a lifetime—replenished by the living cells below. Any product you put on your skin,

Your skin comes in three layers. The thin outer layer, the epidermis, is what you see. It absorbs punishment, from the sun and the elements, and from bruising sports and careless behavior. The top of the epidermis is made up of dead cells that form a durable and waterproof surface. The body constantly sheds the dead cells, replacing old cells with new. The next layer, the dermis, is the thickest part of the skin. The dermis contains a fibrous substance called collagen, which keeps the skin supple. It also has hair roots or follicles, sweat, sebaceous, and apocrine glands, nerves, blood vessels, and fat. (Sebaceous glands contain the oily substance sebum, which lubricates skin and hair, while apocrine glands secrete sweat.) The smallest layer of skin, found below the dermis, is the subcutaneous fatty layer.

▶ *The skin you see (the epidermis) is the outermost of three layers.*

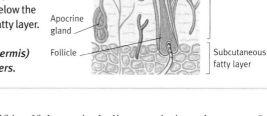

such as a moisturizer, will do nothing to alter the chemistry of the layer of living cells in the dermis, though it may plump up the outer layer of dead cells temporarily, giving you a boyish, Dick Clark appeal.

Look Your Best

Looking after your skin is not that difficult, nor does it involve using expensive lotions and potions.

Tobacco smoke and the sun's ultraviolet light are the two biggest dangers to your skin's health, not to mention your general health. So, do your skin—and yourself—a favor: If you smoke, give up; and limit your exposure to the sun. For full advice on keeping your hide healthy, see "Tips for Good-Looking Skin."

FIRST-AID FOR SKIN PROBLEMS

Treat small cuts, scrapes, and burns with an over-the-counter antibacterial cream such as Polysporin or Bacetracin. For a mild case of sunburn, avoid spray-on products or creams. Instead, sit in a lukewarm tub and soak. Severe sunburn should be treated by a doctor.

Skin Ailments

You might think your days of agonizing over pimples would be a memory as distant as the senior prom. But oily skin can cause acne eruptions on a guy's face and chest well into his thirties, forties, and fifties. If the acne persists, see a dermatologist. Other skin problems, like rosacea and dermatitis, should be diagnosed and treated by a physician.

Rosacea causes blood vessels to surface on the nose. Though no one knows why, this condition occurs almost exclusively in men. Rosacea is easily treated with topical creams and oral antibiotics.

Dermatitis is the generic name for any skin inflammation. There are hundreds of such inflammations, including psoriasis and eczema. See a doctor if you have a recurring rash that doesn't respond to over-the-counter remedies.

SCARS

The majority of cuts, especially small ones, heal without scarring. If large wounds are treated improperly, they tend to leave scars—fibrous flesh and discolored skin. You can help stop scarring by never picking scabs and by seeing a doctor if the wound is deep or jagged.

Acne: Not Just a Teenager's Problem

Those ugly zits probably played havoc with your self-confidence when you were in your teens. But for some men, acne doesn't end there: About 1 in 100 men in his forties has outbreaks on the back, chest, and face. As well, whiteheads and other small pimples may continue to appear throughout life, depending on factors like illness, stress, and oily skin.

Acne appears when sebum (an oily goop made by sebaceous glands in the skin) plugs up pores around hair follicles. Bacteria start to grow and the pores become inflamed and infected. The increase in sebum is probably linked to a surge in the production of male hormones, which is why boys get it worse than girls.

What about the perception that eating certain foods—chocolate, french fries and sweets, for example—will cause an attack of acne? Studies have shown there's no connection between eating these foods and an eruption of pimples, says Joseph P. Bark, M.D., dermatologist and author of *Your Skin: An Owner's Guide*. Given the slow speed at which food is broken down by the body, it is virtually impossible that the chocolate bar you enjoyed yesterday afternoon is responsible for that pimple on your chin this morning.

For severe acne attacks, see a dermatologist, who may prescribe medications such as antibiotics, which attack the infection, and isotretinoin (Accutane), which works by shrinking sebaceous glands and reducing sebum production. To help prevent pimples, try an over-the-counter gel that contains benzoyl peroxide, especially if you have oily skin. Resist the temptation to squeeze pimples—you could worsen the infection and cause scarring.

Keep Your Hair Healthy

"I'm not really balding," you say. "I've just got a high forehead." Nice try. Hair loss is inevitable for many of us, but there are ways to make the best of the bad hand you've been dealt. Switch your focus from worrying about shedding hair to taking steps to revitalize what you've got.

The Folly of Follicles

Hair is formed from a protein called keratin and grows from follicles in the skin. The root, the only live part of the hair, grows and pushes the dead hair shaft out of the skin, and a new strand is born. Men lose anywhere from 30 to 100 head hairs a day in a natural sloughing process.

Hair loss on that scale isn't noticed because you've got somewhere around 100,000 hairs on your scalp. Loss becomes noticeable only when you lose in excess of 200 hairs a day for several months.

A number of factors can lead to hair loss, including stress, illness, scalp infections, and drugs. But by far the most common cause is male-pattern baldness, which is genetically determined. If your father is

bald, you've got a pretty good chance of going the same way.

Testosterone, the very hormone that makes you male, is at the root of the problem. In men who are genetically programmed for baldness, chemical receptors in the hair follicles convert testosterone to dihydro-testosterone. This chemical causes the follicles to produce thin and downy hair, which is not thick or long enough to hide the scalp. Hence, the naked noggin.

WHAT YOU CAN DO ABOUT BALDNESS

The majority of men come to a grudging acceptance of their wide open spaces. The rest of you have three options: You can disguise it, you can have micrograft transplantation, or you can use drugs.

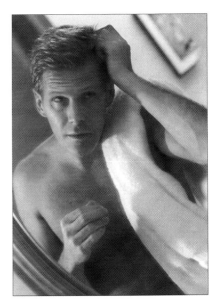

▲ Well-kept, glossy hair—even with hair loss—announces you as a healthy, well-groomed individual.

A little bit of crafty styling goes a long way when it comes to camouflaging hair loss. Men with thinning hair have found that soft body waves and weaves add volume and texture, giving the appearance of having more hair than they really do. Those with extensive loss might consider purchasing a custom-made hairpiece.

Dealing with Hair Loss

Before you tear out your remaining hair, there are options. A good hair stylist will recommend a style that best covers the bald patches, or give your hair a body wave to make it look thicker. He or she can also suggest hair-care products that make the most of the hair that's left. And if there isn't much, there's always the Kojak style.

Alternatively, there's hair replacement which, says Steven Victor, M.D., dermatologist and hair replacement specialist, can work on anyone but requires a skilled physician. It's expensive and time-consuming, but the result is that you get more hair up there.

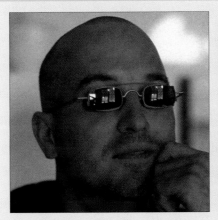

▲ Shave it off—shave it all off. This look has sex appeal and is up-to-date.

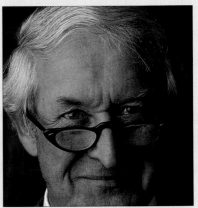

▲ This style gives the illusion of a good head of hair, but avoid if the hair is sparse.

Note "custom-made." Don't bother with cheap, mass-produced types. You'll only make people laugh.

Hair replacement treatments have become more popular as a way to permanently regrow hair. Before technology refined the technique, treated men left the doctor's office looking like they'd just undergone brain surgery. Today, men are able to shampoo the next day. Be warned, a realistic head of hair is expensive.

Minoxidil, marketed as Rogaine, is a drug that's been shown to encourage regrowth in about one-third of the men who try it. Of the other two-thirds, some have fuzz return and others have no change. It seems to work best on men just starting to lose hair or those with fine hair, and has no effect on completely bald spots. The oral drug Propecia stops loss and can produce regrowth. Both drugs must be used permanently.

How to Care for Your Hair

"There's a lot more to hair than just keeping it," says Francisco Gavili, a hair stylist with the Vidal Sassoon salon in New York. Your hair makes a statement: When hair is stylish and healthy-looking—even if there's little left on top—it says to the world that you're well-groomed, confident, and healthy. Yet, as Gavili notes, to the extent that men think about hair at all, most believe their hair to be healthy only when they've got a head full of it. You can keep what you've got on top in tip-top shape by following these precepts: Get a good

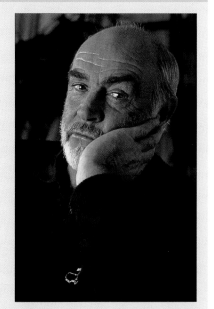
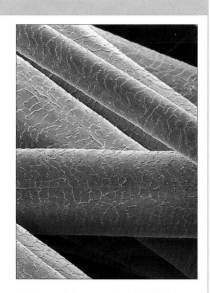

Find the Right Haircut

Remember haircuts when you were a kid? You went on a Saturday without an appointment, waited a few minutes until the chair was free, hopped up, and watched while the barber buzzed the top, sides, and back of your head. Five minutes later you and Dad were out the door and heading for the hardware store. Most men want that kind of convenience as adults, but they'd like a better end result up on top. That's why many men eschew barbers for stylists. The most important factor that makes a specific style suitable is your facial structure. Here's a range of face shapes and the styles that suit them.

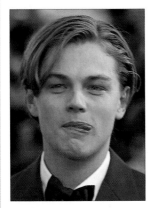

▲ *Leonardo DiCaprio's tousled fringe and off-center part balance his strongly heart-shaped face.*

Square
A good style is wide on top, flat at the sides, perhaps with longer hair at the back.

Triangle
A triangular face is widest at the jawline, narrowest at the forehead. A good style is full at the top and narrower through the sides.

Heart
The cut should draw the eye away from the narrow chin, maybe by being left fuller in the back or by bangs. Part off-center.

Diamond
Go for a cut that's fuller in the back to offset the narrow chin. Part off-center to disguise a narrow forehead.

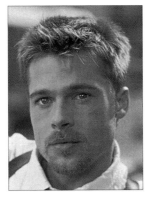

▲ *Brad Pitt's squarish face is complemented by a rounded cut that's full and wide on top, flatter at the sides.*

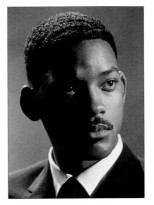

▲ *The closely cropped look sported by Will Smith in* Men in Black *ably complements his round face.*

Round
Two contrasting styles work well: the first, long and narrow through the sides, adds height; the other is cut close all over.

Oblong
Suitable hairstyles use a layered cut with full sides and a flat top.

Pear
The cut should give fullness to the top and breadth to the forehead. Bangs can create the illusion of width.

Sharp rectangle
Try asymmetrical styles that widen the face and add interest. Bangs work well. Leave the sides full, and keep it short at the back.

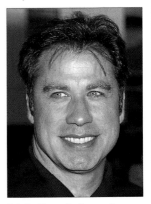

▲ *John Travolta has a sharp rectangular face. The hair is kept short, while bangs create an illusion of width.*

---

cut, wash, and condition regularly, treat your hair gently, and use an appropriate styling product to keep your hair looking good all day.

GET THE STYLE RIGHT

You'll need a professional stylist to create the right cut for you, so shop around. The right cut is one that best matches your hair—its texture, color, part, wave, and so on—with your features. A good style should also be easy to care for. You should get your hair cut frequently—every four to six weeks—to keep the style in shape and stop the hair's ends from drying out. Your stylist will also be able to advise you about hair-care products as well as giving you the cut you deserve.

KEEP IT CLEAN

Women say there are few bigger turn-offs in a man than lank, greasy hair. So shampoo every day, unless your scalp is extremely dry. Not only will your hair look fuller, but a daily wash keeps dandruff at bay.

Select a mild shampoo—look for words like "low pH" on the label. Many products are too harsh, warns Los Angeles stylist Renee Durslag, and will leave hair dry and brittle. With so many shampoos, condition-ers, hairsprays, mousses, thickeners, and gels on the market, it's hard to know what to buy. Ask friends and your stylist for recommendations, and try different products until you find the ones that work for you.

WHY YOU NEED A CONDITIONER

Another must, even for short hair, is a weekly conditioner. Men who spend a lot of time in the sun, at the beach, or in the pool need a daily, deep conditioner to combat dryness. Since overuse of conditioners tends to make hair limp, flat, and harder to style, men with fine or oily hair need only a light application weekly.

How much you use and how often you use it depends, again, on your hair and scalp. If your hair seems too limp, cut back on the conditioner; if it seems coarse and dry, use more.

BE GENTLE

Try to avoid excessive tugging and brushing, since it pulls, twists, and damages hair, leaving the ends split. The same goes for drying your hair. If you usually just towel-dry it, use the towel gently and don't scrape it across the scalp. Blow dryers should be used on a high to medium heat setting, but turn the airflow down to low and keep the nozzle six inches from your head.

KEEP IT IN PLACE

Gels and mousse give you the convenience of styling your hair with a blow dryer, spritzing it with a little spray, and forgetting about combing for the rest of the day. How much and what product you'll use depends on your hair texture, type of scalp, and preferred look. Mousse is better for wavy, longer hair. Gels are good for styling short hair.

Be careful, though, when using styling products. Gels, mousses, and hairspray can build up in your hair, leaving it dull and limp. Use a clarifying shampoo once a week to strip away the buildup. If you use a lot of styling products, stylists recommend a clarifying shampoo twice a week, since the buildup can also lead to dandruff. Don't, however, use a clarifying shampoo instead of a regular mild one, since overuse dries out the hair, leaving it unmanageable.

A Permanent Solution

The very idea of a man dying his hair or having a permanent would have been unthinkable at one time. These days, guys are more receptive, and an increasing number are finding out what these procedures can do

for them. As with anything that relates to hair, look for a good stylist who can advise you on what's available and the possible drawbacks.

Body waves make straight hair wavy or curly. You don't have to end up with corkscrew curls, though. A soft body wave is a subtle way to add body and texture to fine, straight hair, or thinning hair.

Dyes can also be used discreetly in a process called weaving. The stylist weaves the dye through your hair to give the illusion of natural color and highlights. You'll also find lots of do-it-yourself products in stores—always follow the directions on the package.

Bleaching is the harshest of the hair-altering procedures. It sucks the color out of the hair. Several problems arise if you try to bleach your own hair. The bleach, much like what you'd use for laundry, is caustic and can damage skin, scalp, and eyes. If done carelessly, hair might emerge bright orange or yellow.

How to Choose a Stylist

• Ask friends for referrals.

• Try out a likely barbershop or salon, and ask questions. How long have they been in business? If you're interested, find out how much experience they have with coloring and waving hair.

• Go for a stylist who listens to you about how you care for your hair, and what you like and don't like about it. Listen to the way he or she suggests something different to your usual cut. Is it a dialogue, or do you feel like you're being forced into it?

• Choose someone you feel relaxed with. "The stylist should make the client feel comfortable," says Los Angles hair stylist Renee Durslag. "If you feel otherwise, go somewhere else."

• Stick with the stylist who keeps you coming back for more. If you like what he or she does with your hair—month after month—then you've found the right person.

Beating Body Hair

A lot of men complain about excessive back or chest hair, especially body builders who need a smooth surface to compete well. Other men, too, dislike carrying a hairy rug on their backs.

More common is the tendency for men to sprout hair from the nose, ears, and eyebrows as they age. The easiest and safest way to remove such hair is to clip it back with a pair of small, sharp scissors. Furry eyebrows are a little more difficult since clipping leaves telltale stubble.

For those harder-to-clip places, you have a few options—shaving, bleaching, depilatories, tweezing, waxing, or electrolysis. Only electrolysis removes hair permanently. Choosing one over another is a matter of personal preference. Here are some things to consider.

• Shaving can cause ingrown hairs and stubbly, coarse regrowth of fine hairs and a five o'clock shadow.

• Clipping with a pair of round-ended clippers deals with the odd rogue hair, or with nasal hairs. Hairs tend to regrow coarser.

• Bleaching is not recommended for summer. Tanned skin against white hair looks unnatural.

• Depilatories are chemical concoctions that dissolve fine hairs but leave behind coarse ones. They can cause burns if done improperly.

• Tweezing plucks hairs individually. Regrowth is coarse and thick.

• Waxing is like tweezing on a massive scale. A skin-care specialist covers a small area in warm wax, allows it to harden and cool, then rips it off, tearing out unwanted hair with it. Ouch!

• Electrolysis permanently removes hair by sending a small jolt of electricity to kill individual follicles. It is relatively painless, but requires repeated treatments and can become expensive.

How to Smell Clean and Fresh

Scientists who study such things estimate that it takes 6 to 12 seconds to make a first impression. Unless, of course, the guy making the impression has body odor. Then, it takes just one whiff. Here's how to make sure every impression you make—whether it's the first or the fiftieth—is pleasant.

A Fresh Start

Guys who smell bad often have no idea a foul cloud is shadowing them. The reason: They're habituated to the stench. It's the rest of us who suffer. Like bad breath, body odor is the last thing people will tell you about. They'll tell everybody else in the office that you're as ripe as a rotting fish, but nobody will know quite how to break the bad news to you.

If you have even the slightest suspicion that your body reeks, do something about it. The solution may be as easy as showering every day and washing your clothes.

You have to understand where to concentrate your scrubbing efforts. Secretions from your sweat glands are actually odorless. What makes you smell is the bacteria that multiplies in the sweat. The strongest odor comes from the armpits and the genitals, where apocrine glands are located. Unlike the rest of the body's sweat glands, which exude a sort of salt water inhospitable to the growth of bacteria, the apocrine glands secrete a milky fluid filled with the kinds of proteins and fats bacteria thrive on.

The longer you allow the sweat to sit and stew, the more pungent you become. That's why the number-one rule of smelling fresh is to take a shower or bath every day. If your lifestyle or the climate makes you sweat a lot, shower more often.

Daily bathing with a deodorant soap is adequate for the typical guy. Avoid using a deodorant soap on your face, however, warns Jerome Z. Litt, M.D., assistant clinical professor of dermatology at Case Western Reserve University School of Medicine in Cleveland, Ohio. "It can leave a residue and dry out skin." Try not to scrub too hard, either, since skin irritation also encourages bacterial growth. If you're overweight, make sure you wash inside folds of fat where bacteria can thrive.

Obesity and eating the wrong foods can aggravate sweating and body odor. Certain foods cause proteins and oils to sweat out of your pores and onto your skin, feeding the bacteria what they need to grow big and strong. Foods to watch out for include anything spicy or fishy, including onions and garlic.

QUIZ

Q. At what time of day is your sense of smell sharpest?

A. The afternoon. That's something that you should take into consideration when shopping for cologne or perfume.

Q. How many distinctive odors can your nose detect?

A. About 4,000.

Meanwhile, in Club Ped...

The feet have more sweat glands than the underarms. Combine the moisture they exude with the dark warmth of your shoes and you've created a Club Ped playground for trillions of bacteria that break down into compounds that—well—stink. Co-conspirators with these bacterial culprits are your shoes, which give the little evildoers sanctuary to breed. Here's how to put your best foot forward.

• If you've got a chronic foot odor problem, wash your feet daily with an antibacterial soap such as Dial or Safeguard to help kill the bacteria.

• Dry your feet thoroughly, especially between your toes. Then put on socks and shoes.

• Consider using foot powder and antiperspirant sprays and deodorants to mask the odor.

• Wear cotton or other natural fiber socks and deodorant shoe inserts.

• Let your shoes air out after each time you wear them, preferably for 24 hours or more.

▶ *The moist warmth of socks and shoes makes feet prime targets for bacteria.*

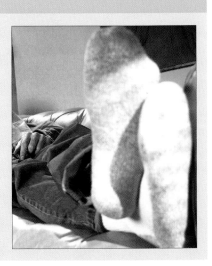

A Man's Guide to Aftershaves and Colognes

As animals, our scent defines us. The cosmetic industry knows this well, and has zeroed in on the crucial link between smell and sex by launching hundreds of aftershaves and colognes. In prehistoric times, cavemen relied on their unique aromatic musk, a combination of sweat, dead animal skins, and decaying food that somehow attracted mates. Today, that same combination of odors would ensure the death of your gene pool. So how to choose the right scent for you?

Look for one that fits your lifestyle and environment. Musk, for instance, conveys sensual and sexy, perhaps an inappropriate memorandum to send to co-workers. For the office, try something light, like a citrus smell, and save the heavier message for dates and parties. Other good scent types include woodsy, spicy, and fruity.

Your body's natural scent will mix with the cologne or aftershave to give you your own unique smell. That's why it's important to try a few scents before choosing one. Trying a scent is as easy as finding your way to the nearest department store's cosmetic section and asking a clerk for assistance. The clerk will spritz your arm; give it a few seconds to dry, then smell. Make sure you try a few brands before deciding.

The best-known men's lines include Hugo Boss, Armani, Georgio, Polo, Guess, Eternity, and CK, which can cost a considerable chunk of change.

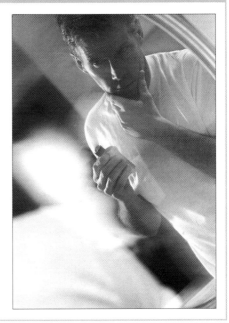

▶ *A good aftershave has a scent that suits your lifestyle and surroundings.*

Masking Body Odors

Been sweating over the question of how a deodorant differs from an antiperspirant? Deodorants mask odor with a mild perfume and contain chemicals that slow the growth of bacteria. They don't reduce the amount of sweat.

Antiperspirants reduce sweat secretions by up to 40 percent. Their active ingredient is usually aluminum chloride, which reacts with proteins in your sweat to form a gel that partially blocks sweat pores.

Since deodorants and antiperspirants might cause your skin to break out, make sure you stop using them at the first sign of redness. Change brands until you find one compatible with your skin. Remember never to apply either deodorant or antiperspirant to broken skin.

If all deodorants and antiperspirants tend to irritate your skin, try using one of the over-the-counter antibacterial creams, such as Neosporin, to kill the bacteria. For a more natural approach, there is sodium bicarbonate, or baking soda. Not only does baking soda kill the odor-causing bacteria, it absorbs sweat as well. Apply it directly to your armpits or mix it first with talcum powder. As a last resort, you might try shaving your armpits, since the hair gives the bacteria a better breeding ground.

Is It Your Clothes?

If you take a shower every day and you still smell bad, you may have a clothes-washing or changing problem. Bacteria reside in clothes, too, Dr. Litt points out. Those bacteria then invade the glands and the cycle of growth and decay begins again, only this time your clothes are rancid, too. That's the reason your mother told you to change your underwear and socks every day. Change your shirt and pants while you're at it.

And don't neglect proper washing. Follow loading instructions on your washing machine. The more clothes you try to shove in the washer, the less likely they'll come out fresh-smelling, clean, and bacteria-free.

Pheromones: Sex Smells

Did you ever meet someone and feel a certain chemistry between the two of you? Pheromones may be the reason. In nature, these chemical attractants are routinely used by animals to meet and mate.

Does the same thing apply to us? Science does not yet fully understand human sexual chemistry, but there is evidence to suggest that pheromones play some part in sexual attraction. Researchers have found that these odors are important enough to have a sense organ—the vomeronasal in the nose—dedicated to detecting them.

Pheromones are secreted by the apocrine glands, located under the armpits and in the genital area. Their effect may be greatly diminished by bathing daily to eliminate body odor—also caused in part by the apocrine glands. But think carefully before you enhance your natural odor by not washing for a while – there's a thin line between smelling ruggedly sexy and smelling downright bad.

How to Have Fresh Breath

You just had to have your favorite garlicky meal last night and now you're paying for it. Whenever you get close to anyone, they wince and the conversation ebbs. Halitosis is socially awkward at the best of times, an unmitigated disaster at others. Here's how to eliminate rhino breath from your life.

How Not to Be Sniffed At

Bad breath can usually be traced to food eaten recently. Anything fishy, spicy (including onions, pastrami, hot peppers, salami, pepperoni, and our old friend, garlic) or fatty, especially milk products and meats, sets off a chemical reaction in the stomach that causes the lungs to secrete an odor.

Typically, the odor lasts anywhere from 24 to 48 hours, says William M. Dorfman, D.D.S., a Los Angeles cosmetic dentist who specializes in treating bad breath. Brushing teeth and using mouthwash might mask the odor temporarily, but it won't take it away.

Gum diseases such as gingivitis and periodontitis can also cause bad breath. If you haven't already done so, develop good brushing and flossing habits. Brush your tongue in addition to your teeth and gums. Swish water around your mouth. Use only a mouthwash that is alcohol-free. And if you smoke, bad breath is another reason to give up.

Chronic Halitosis

What if you're among the millions of men who suffer from chronic bad breath? How would you know? It's a good question, Dr. Dorfman says. People on the receiving end of bad breath are generally loathe to mention it—even your spouse and best friend would rather have you discover it for yourself. So try a little experiment. Get a cotton ball and rub it around your tongue, gums, and mouth. Now smell it. Do you feel like keeling over? Perhaps you've found the reason for those unexplained canceled dates and shortened conversations.

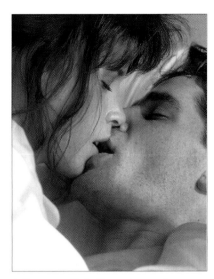

▲ *Your mouth is the gateway for many sensual pleasures. Keep it fresh.*

About 90 percent of the time, chronic bad breath is caused by a buildup of smelly bacteria at the back of the tongue, where most people forget to brush, says Dr. Dorfman. What you smell is volatile sulfur compounds, the same stuff that makes rotten eggs smell bad. The bacteria love to hide and multiply in dark, hard-to-reach places, which is why flossing is so important. Flossing removes the plaque and bacteria that grow in between the teeth, places where brushes miss.

Make sure, too, that you visit your dentist twice a year to get your teeth cleaned. Apart from anything else, this will prevent gum disease, which is another common reason for bad breath. Leftover food particles become plaque and tartar in your mouth—bacteria that decay and cause bad breath.

In a healthy mouth, the dead cells normally sloughed off in the course of a day are shed into the saliva, swallowed, and digested without causing bad breath. In an unhealthy mouth, an overabundance of plaque

---

Five Tips for Better Breath

1 Rinse your mouth with 8 ounces of water mixed with a half-teaspoon of salt. Use as an emergency measure to fix a breath problem at work.

2 A teaspoon of baking soda mixed with a glass of water makes a good homemade breath-freshener. You can also use baking soda mixed with water to brush your teeth.

3 Using a fluoride toothpaste, brush your teeth thoroughly (aim for three times a day), and include the back of your tongue and the roof of your mouth.

Don't forget to floss. Get regular dental checkups and professional cleanings.

4 Equal parts of 3 percent hydrogen peroxide and water swished around in your mouth for about 30 seconds can help neutralize the acidic bacteria that contribute to bad breath. (Limit the use of hydrogen peroxide to two times a week, dentists suggest.)

5 In a pinch, mouthwash; sugar-free mints, candies, or gum; and breath-fresheners will mask odor—but only for a few minutes.

How to Floss Your Teeth

Flossing is an important part of dental hygiene: It removes the plaque that a toothbrush can't reach. There are literally dozens of types of floss on the market. All do a good job, so pick one you find easiest to use. Wide floss, which is also called dental tape, is good if you have wide spaces between your teeth or a lot of bridgework. Waxed floss is easier to slide between tight teeth than unwaxed floss. "Spongy" types of floss fray less than most other flosses.

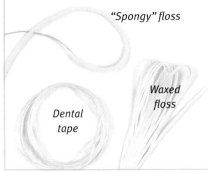

"Spongy" floss

Waxed floss

Dental tape

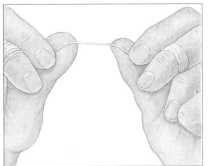

1 Take an 18-inch piece of floss and wind 6 to 8 inches of it lightly around your middle finger, taking care not to cut off your circulation. Wind the rest of the floss around the same finger of your opposite hand. Hold the floss with your index fingers and your thumbs. Gently move about an inch of the floss between your two front teeth. then make a C shape by bending the floss around one tooth.

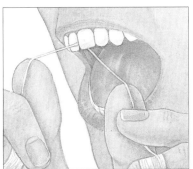

2 Slide the floss between your teeth toward your gums, and go slightly under the gumline. Slide the floss up and down between your tooth and gumline, but don't use a sawing motion. Remove the floss from between your front teeth and unwind another clean piece from one of your fingers. Place the floss between one of your front teeth and its neighbor, then repeat the procedure as above. Continue with the rest of your teeth.

decreases saliva, leaving you with dry mouth and morning breath.

Dentists recommend this four-step breath-freshening routine for sufferers of bad breath.

- Get a good cleaning.
- Floss daily.
- Brush your teeth three times a day.
- Use a tongue scraper.

BREATH-FRESHENERS
Dr. Dorfman warns against using breath-fresheners, breath-freshening sweets, or commercial mouthwashes for anything other than temporarily masking the odor. The products that fight rather than mask odor are only available through dentists, he says, including BreathRx, a new product that kills bacteria while neutralizing volatile sulfur compounds.

Other Causes of Bad Breath

Sometimes bad breath is a genetic condition, Dr. Dorfman warns. This might require special mouth rinses and a more rigorous dental program

available only through your dentist. Be aware, too, that smoking, certain illnesses, such as diabetes and liver failure, and medical treatments can cause chronic bad breath.

Your dentist is the best person to determine if yours is a medical or a

genetic problem. Technological advances have equipped many dentists with a special instrument designed to measure the amount of volatile sulfur compounds in your mouth. It's used to pinpoint your problem and monitor improvements.

Is This What's behind Your Bad Breath?

Unless there's an illness or a genetic predisposition, the causes of bad breath are found mainly in the mouth. Here's an oral survey.

Gum Disease
Gums become red, soft, and swollen, and often bleed. Caused by a large buildup of plaque and tartar at the gumline or by rough brushing or flossing.

Tooth Decay
Bacteria eat away at a tooth. The decay is caused by plaque.

Bacteria on the Tongue
The back of the tongue is where most people forget to brush, which is why it's the prime spot for a buildup of smelly bacteria.

Food Fragments
Small pieces of food stuck between teeth are ripe for attack by odor-producing bacteria.

Plaque
A combination of food particles, bacteria, and saliva. It forms a microscopic film over teeth.

Tartar
A hard substance that sticks between gums and teeth. It's what plaque turns into when you don't brush or floss adequately.

Exhaled Breath
The breath from your lungs may be scented by cigarette smoke or by a recent fishy, onion-rich, fatty, or garlicky meal.

Keep Your Teeth in Good Shape

Most men have heard a dental horror story, and a fair number have actually experienced one. Whether it's these stories, lack of time, or downright laziness, the fact is that many guys go for years without seeing a dentist. They are selling themselves short: A healthy smile is your best calling card.

Teeting Troubles

It's a dim and painful memory: A small child in a big seat trying to tell the dentist through cotton, tubes, and pointy chrome instruments: "It hurthhhzzz, it hurthzzz!" only to be drowned out by whooshing sounds and ignored by the guy in the white coat. A bad day at the dentist's can prevent you from returning for regular checkups, which is the worst thing you can do for your teeth.

Keeping your choppers in good shape should be a matter of routine, just like shaving. Too many guys ignore their teeth, however, until they see or feel a problem. If you feel pain, have bleeding gums, or notice any chips and cracks in your teeth, "you should have seen a dentist a year ago," says Philadelphia dentist Jonathan Scharf, D.M.D., past president of the American Academy of Cosmetic Dentistry.

The first rule of good dental health: See a dentist at least once a year for a thorough cleaning. Because most people score below average on dental hygiene, many dentists will recommend twice yearly cleanings, a preventive measure covered by lots of insurance companies. The reason: Years of poor brushing and flossing will quickly lead to bleeding gums, decay, and infections that, if ignored, can cause irreversible bone damage and tooth loss requiring expensive and extensive repair.

THE PLAQUE PROBLEM

Plaque causes the two biggest problems—tooth decay and gum disease.

Anatomy of a Tooth

The external part of the tooth is divided into two parts, the crown and the root. The visible portion of the tooth is covered with enamel, which covers several interior layers. Directly underneath the enamel is the dentin, a slightly elastic tissue. It makes up the largest part of the tooth. In the center of the tooth is the pulp, the soft tissue inside the dentin. It contains nerves and blood vessels which enter the root of the tooth by a small canal, the root canal. When an untreated cavity, fracture, or other injury exposes the pulp, bacteria often will seep in and grow, causing infection. This can damage and kill the pulp, causing pain and pressure when you chew or drink hot or cold beverages.

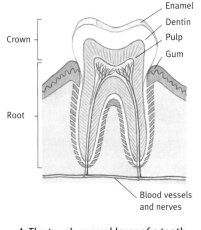

Crown
Root

Enamel
Dentin
Pulp
Gum

Blood vessels and nerves

▲ *The tough enamel layer of a tooth protects other, more sensitive layers.*

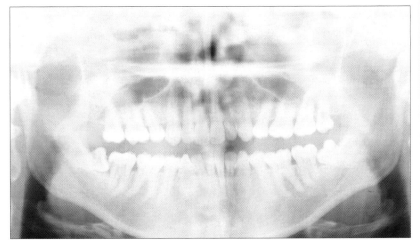

▲ *Dentists use x-rays to diagnose problems. In this one, fillings show up as bright spots.*

How to Brush Your Teeth

Dentists say that too many men have too many preventable dental problems. So, we're going to risk insulting your intelligence by going back to basics.

To remove plaque and food debris from the inner, outer, and biting surfaces of your teeth you should brush at least twice (but preferably three times) a day for two to three minutes each time. And here's a tip for keeping from brushing too hard: Hold your toothbrush between your thumb and index finger, just like you hold a pen. Now here's how dental hygienists say you should brush.

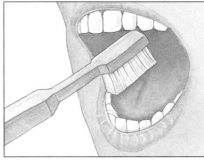

1 Place the head of the brush at a 45-degree angle against your gumline. Clean the front teeth by moving the brush in small circles.

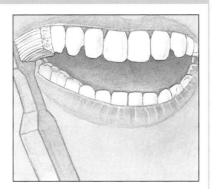

2 Brush the outer surface of the upper and lower back teeth, making sure that the brush is kept angled against the gumline.

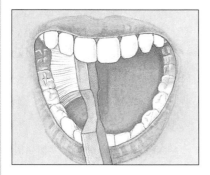

3 Clean the inside surfaces of the lower teeth, using small circular movements. Remember to maintain the 45-degree angle with the gumline.

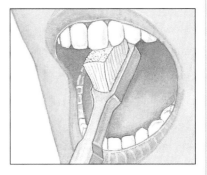

4 Brush the biting surfaces of the upper teeth, using to-and-fro strokes. Repeat to clean the biting surfaces of the lower teeth.

5 Use an up-and-down stroke to clean the inner surfaces of the front teeth, tilting the brush vertically to make access easier.

Plaque is a microscopic film formed by bacteria that expand and multiply by feeding on all the leftover food in your warm, moist mouth. Picture maggots in a trash can. Brushing and flossing removes the food that feeds the bacteria. If left to thrive, plaque turns into a sticky residue on the teeth and gums that hardens into tartar and eventually destroys healthy tissue and the enamel outer covering of your teeth.

Often, the enamel doesn't have the strength to hold off the bacterial barbarians, who invade the tooth's next layer, the dentin. Without a counterattack by the lab-coated cavalry (your dentist and hygienist), the bacteria attack the tooth's inner layer—the pulp—causing pain and infection, and possibly leaving you with an urgent need for expensive root-canal surgery.

TOOTH WHITENING
Staining, a far less serious problem than tooth decay or gum disease, is caused mainly by coffee and tea drinking, and smoking. It's possible to whiten teeth with no ill effects or changes to the tooth structure. Going to a dentist is best. He or she will use a mixture of strong chemicals that extract the stain or undesired color from the teeth, restoring those coveted pearly whites. Over-the-counter teeth whiteners will give only temporary results.

Oral Hygiene: A Primer
Everybody knows you should brush at least twice a day, especially after meals. You should also floss every night. We know you were taught to brush as a kid, but maybe it's time for a little refresher course (see also "How to Brush Your Teeth").

Choose a brush that has a relatively small head (roughly 1 inch by ½ inch) and soft nylon bristles. Brush in an elliptical or circular pattern with the bristles at a 45-degree angle to the gumline. Most people brush for less than a minute, but to destroy cavity-causing bacteria, dentists and hygienists suggest spending a little longer, between two and three minutes.

Choosing a Brush

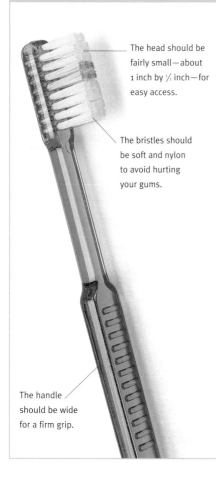

The head should be fairly small—about 1 inch by ½ inch—for easy access.

The bristles should be soft and nylon to avoid hurting your gums.

The handle should be wide for a firm grip.

The array of toothbrushes available on the market can be a little daunting. This is what the American Academy for General Dentistry says to look for in a good toothbrush and how to get the most out of it.

• Choose one with a small head to make it easy to move the brush around inside your mouth.

• Change your toothbrush every three to four months, before the bristles become frayed or splayed. Old toothbrushes are ineffective and can harbor the bacteria that cause gum disease.

• Change your toothbrush after an illness. The bacteria could be lurking in the brush.

• If you have manual dexterity problems, nascent gum disease, or limited tolerance for dental hygienists chastising you about your poor brushing habits, consider purchasing an electric toothbrush. Two of the better models are Sonic and Braun, dentists say. Some models have an alarm that's meant to let you know that you should be moving on to the next part of your mouth.

Many dentists recommend electric toothbrushes for patients. Though they don't do a better job than a manual toothbrush used correctly, it's the "used correctly" part most people have trouble with. Misusing an electric toothbrush is pretty hard to do, since it's the dental equivalent of a point-and-shoot camera. Just place the brush on the teeth, push the button and wait for the beep that tells you to move the brush to the next part of the mouth. Some even shut off automatically.

But no matter how diligently you brushed, food remains wedged between your teeth. That's why you need to floss. It's important to do so before bed every night, so that the sugar bugs don't have a chance to destroy the gum tissue and make you, quite literally, long in the tooth. Flossing is a fairly simple procedure, and it's detailed on page 33.

If your gums bleed from brushing or flossing, you should see a dentist or hygienist for a thorough checkup and cleaning.

Are Amalgam Fillings Safe?

First, the good news. There appears to be little conclusive evidence that amalgam fillings are dangerous. Now, the bad news: No one can guarantee their safety, either.

Amalgam, or silver fillings, consist of about 35 percent silver, 13 percent tin, 2 percent copper, and 50 percent mercury. They are popular among dentists and patients because they are less expensive than other materials and are extremely durable, able to stand up to the chewing–grinding motions of molars and bicuspids.

It's the mercury in amalgam fillings that causes concern. Mercury, the silvery metallic liquid in thermometers, is poisonous. When you chew, small amounts of mercury vapor may be released from the fillings. Studies have shown some people with

amalgam fillings have had more mercury in their blood and urine than those without fillings. Though no studies have shown fillings to cause serious illness, high levels of mercury in the blood can cause kidney or lung damage, memory loss, vision impairment, and high blood pressure.

Research is still being done into the potential health risks of amalgam fillings. At the same time, dental scientists are discovering stronger mercury-free composite fillings (a white-colored combination of plastic, porcelain, and acrylic), used now by some dentists to replace amalgams.

The way to avoid problems with amalgam fillings is to avoid needing them. Careful brushing and flossing, as well as regular visits to the dentist, will likely make the controversy moot—at least for you.

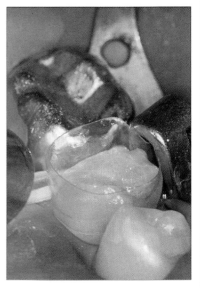

▲ Composite fillings are becoming more and more popular. Here, a new filling is hardened using "blue" light.

Don't Forget the Mouth Guard

Guys play rough, which you know if you've played football, boxing, hockey, lacrosse—even basketball. "You'd be absolutely foolish to play any contact sport without a mouth guard," says cosmetic dentist Jonathan Scharf, D.M.D., who has seen his share of toothless warriors. It can happen at any time: A competitor crashes into your jaw, causing the upper and lower teeth to smash together. The next thing you know you're spitting out bloody biters.

Why risk it? Go to any sporting goods store and pick up a mouth guard. All you have to do is plop it in boiling water to soften it, let it cool down, then put it in your mouth to mold it to your bite. Not only do mouth guards have a rating system to help you determine which strength is best for your level of activity, many also carry insurance liability policies that will pay for dental work if the guard fails to do the job.

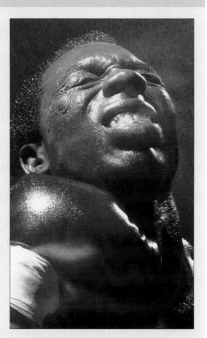
▲ Mouth guards are required in boxing—for obvious reasons.

Gum Disease

About 70 percent of all adult tooth loss is due to gum disease, also called periodontal disease. It's a condition that afflicts three out of four people to some degree or another.

Gum disease is chronic inflammation and infection of the gums and surrounding tissue, caused by poor brushing and flossing habits and a genetic predisposition. Early warning signs include red, swollen, or tender gums, bleeding while brushing or flossing, gums that pull away from the teeth, pus between the gum and tooth, and persistent bad breath. Gum disease is a silent attacker: There may be no discomfort or pain until the disease has spread so far that the tooth is unsalvageable. That's why dentists advise frequent dental exams.

ROOT-CANAL SURGERY

You need to have root-canal surgery whenever the pulp becomes severely infected, causing damage or killing the tissue. Since teeth don't heal without treatment, the infection will spread, the bone around the tooth will begin to degenerate, and the tooth may fall out. Before the tooth goes, however, most people experience such extreme pain that they find themselves begging the dentist to yank it. Most dentists counsel patients to try to keep as many natural teeth as possible, so the usual step before extraction is root-canal surgery.

This is what you should expect during root-canal surgery, according to the American Academy of General Dentistry.

First, the dentist gives you a local anesthetic through a needle into the gum, then places a rubber sheet—a dental dam—around the tooth to isolate it. A hole is drilled all the way from the crown to the pulp chamber.

The diseased and dead pulp is cleaned out—along with infected root-canal tissue—and an antibiotic paste and a temporary filling are packed into it. Some days later, you go back to the dentist to have the filling removed and the canals checked for sterility.

When no infection can be detected, the dentist goes ahead and fills the cavity with a sealing paste or a rubberlike substance. The roots of the tooth are then sealed with cement.

Do You Grind Your Teeth?

Most men learn that they grind their teeth after a nudge to the ribs in the middle of the night and a stern warning from a sleepless mate: "You're making too much noise!" Teeth grinding (the medical name is bruxism) occurs in one out of four people and often leads to eroded teeth and a dull ache in the jaw.

Stress and nervous tension are usually why we grind. Some other warning signs might signal a problem: Do you bite your fingernails? Pencils? Chew the inside of your mouth? If you do, then you may unknowingly grind your teeth, too.

Often, teeth grinders aren't diagnosed until the damage is done. Here are some telltale signs of bruxism.

• The tips of your teeth look flat.

• The enamel is so worn that the dentin is exposed and your tooth is sensitive to hot and cold liquids.

• Your jaw pops and clicks.

If you are diagnosed with teeth grinding, you'll probably be advised to keep your mouth as relaxed as possible. Relax your tongue, allowing it to rest comfortably on or near the roof of your mouth. Keep your teeth apart, lips shut.

If that doesn't work, the dentist can make you a night guard to minimize damage to your teeth and jaw. The best way to fight grinding, though, is to embark on an overall stress-reduction program.

How to Keep Your Nails Well-Groomed

Nails—the things on the ends of your fingers, remember? Maybe you don't care about the look of your fingernails—and toenails —but your honey probably does. The sight of stained and tattered fingernails or overgrown, fungus-encrusted toenails is not what most women would consider a turn-on.

Nailing Nasty Nails

Taking care of your nails is a strictly low-maintenance job. It takes little time or effort, but can pay off big, especially with the lady (or ladies) in you life. First, keep your nails short by using nail scissors or clippers. It's easiest to cut your nails after a bath or shower when they are slightly softer. Remember to cut them in a curve, following the natural shape of your finger tips.

You may suffer from hangnails from time to time. Hangnails, in

fact, have nothing to do with nails. They're caused when a sliver of dry skin splits from the cuticle or skin surrounding the nail, dies, and gets snagged on anything from paper to sweaters and hair. Don't bite, pull, tug, or remove hangnails. Instead, trim them with nail scissors or clippers. Avoid ripping out living skin. It can bleed and become infected.

Apply moisturizer to your nails twice daily to keep hangnails from appearing. Moisturizer is key to keeping your nails and hands well tended, manicurists say. Any brand will do. If your cuticles are white and cracking, your hands are excessively dry and you'll need to use a heavy, sticky moisturizer until they soften up. If you have soft skin and supple cuticles, a lighter formula should do the trick.

Ever notice how more women than men wear rubber gloves when washing the dishes? They do it for an understandable reason. In some people, water softens nails and causes them to break off. Gloves also protect against the effects of liquid detergent. Unless you're planning to grow your nails long, water is nothing to worry about.

The Right Way to Trim Your Nails

It's best to trim your nails after bathing or showering when the nail is at its softest. A well-trimmed fingernail has a small edge of white peeking up over a rosy nail bed. When trimming, use nail clippers or scissors and follow the natural shape of the nail. Cut the nail either straight across (if your fingertips are squarish) or with a slight oval curve (if they're curved).

You'll likely notice sharp edges after clipping. To smooth out the points, use an emery board and file from the corner to the center. Though it may seem more natural to move from the center to the corner, it risks causing the nails to flake and become brittle, often leaving tiny slivers of nails you'll need to keep trimmed short with clippers.

Before you trim your toenails, look at them. Most have a groove where nail and skin meet snugly. To avoid ingrown toenails, never trim below that groove. Cut straight across and just above it.

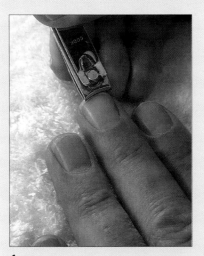

1 Cut the nail either straight across if your fingertips are squarish, or with a slight curve if they're more rounded.

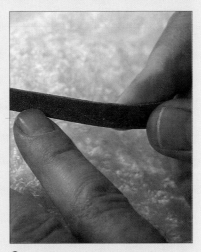

2 Finish off the job by smoothing the nail with an emery board. Start from the corner and move to the center.

10 Tips for Neat Nails

1 Don't groom nails with your teeth.

2 Keep nails short. Use the right tools: scissors or clippers.

3 Using a nail file, file the tip smooth. Round off the edges so they blend into the top.

4 Massage hand lotion or nail cream into cuticles every day.

5 Gently push cuticles back with a moist towel. Never cut cuticles or push them back too hard.

6 Soak yellow nails for 10 to 15 minutes in a solution of equal parts warm water and hydrogen peroxide, then scrub gently with a soft nail brush.

7 Dehydration causes nails to chip, crack, and peel. Massage petroleum jelly into nails to help prevent dryness, preferably before bed so it can be absorbed undisturbed while you sleep.

8 Keep a nail file handy as a quick-fix for problems like nicks and breaks, and to keep edges smooth. A fine-textured one is easiest to use.

9 Eat a healthy, balanced diet.

10 Nicotine from cigarettes stains nails. You know what to do.

HOW TO HAVE CLEAN NAILS

Guys sometimes clean their fingernails with an amazing assortment of knives and other sharp objects. We understand the temptation. But for safety reasons, don't do it. Instead, put a few drops of regular laundry bleach in a bowl of water and dish soap, then scrub with a brush. For less stubborn stains, sprinkle laundry detergent onto your nails and scrub. Be sure to follow up the routine with moisturizer to avoid dry, cracking skin and brittle nails.

Another reason to avoid knives, ice picks, and Philips-head screwdrivers as nail cleaners is that these objects may puncture the nail, leaving it susceptible to bacterial growth and fungal infections.

STOP BITING!

A lot of us gnaw at our nails like a dog with a favorite bone. Southern California manicurist Patti Garcia says many of her male clients do so because of stress. Usually it's because they gave up a bad habit such as smoking. Find some other oral gratification like chewing gum, Garcia suggests. As unpalatable as it may seem, Garcia recommends chewing on a plastic coffee stir stick as a nail substitute. It feels almost the same as a fingernail in your mouth, and leaves your nails intact.

FUNGAL PROBLEMS

Fingernails sometimes turn fungal. Using an antibacterial soap will help prevent infections; if your fingernails start to turn green, or a yellow or white spot appears to grow larger with time, try an over-the-counter antifungal cream. If that doesn't work, see a dermatologist to get a proper diagnosis. With some fungal infections, only a prescription drug will clear up the problem.

Nearly all nail-related fungal problems occur in the toenails. People affected usually have a genetic tendency to fight off the fungus poorly—about 10 percent of the population. To help reduce fungus, try following a few commonsense measures to keep your feet dry.

• Always step out of the shower onto a clean, absorbent cotton mat.

• Try drying your feet with a blow-dryer, and dusting your toes with antifungal powder.

• If the weather and your workplace permit it, wear sandals without socks. Otherwise, wear shoes that are made from either leather or canvas—materials that allow air to circulate around your feet.

• Do whatever possible to keep your feet dry and clean.

BLACKENED NAILS

Nails blacken when blood vessels break under the nail plate. Blackened fingernails occur when a malfunctioning hammer misses its target. Blackened toenails often come after continual play of stop-and-start sports such as tennis. Leave the nail alone and let it fall off on its own. If you're in a lot of pain, see a doctor.

Ingrown Toenails

Tight shoes cause ingrown toenails, a condition so called because the nail "grows into" the toe, cutting the skin and causing pain and infection.

The solution? Wear better-fitting shoes. Make sure there's a half-inch space between your big toe and the end of the shoe: There should be enough room for you to wiggle your toes. Also, try to avoid choosing pointed shoes, which tend to squeeze toes together. Go for round- or square-toed styles instead.

Trimming toenails to below the groove where the skin of the toe and the nail meet can exacerbate the problem, encouraging the sharp end of the nail to grow into, instead of over, the groove. Some people may have a genetic predisposition for ingrown toenails, and they appear to be most prevalent among those with wide feet.

Ingrown toenail

Inflamed skin

▲ *An ingrown toenail curves under the skin at the sides of the toe, causing a painful inflammation.*

Shaving and Beard Care

Perhaps the most visible sign of the passage from boy to man is the appearance of facial hair. Shaving, of course, is the ritual that marks the passage. Nicks and yelps of pain have probably been around since prehistoric man. Today, thankfully, we have a wide array of products to assure the perfect shave.

The Ultimate Shave

Are you electric or wet? Some people like the convenience of an electric razor, while others prefer the closeness of a shave that wet razors give. A wet blade undoubtedly provides the closest shave, which is why men with sensitive skin often prefer an electric razor.

Electric razors are best for men with chronic ingrown hairs or any other skin malady of the face, such as acne. Unlike wet razors, electric ones don't remove the top layer of skin. That has its pluses and its minuses. Men who use wet razors take off the dead skin daily, making their faces feel smooth. But the blade's nicks and scratches can also cause rashes. Electric razors reduce irritants and thus aggravation.

Make sure your face is dry when you use an electric shaver, as shaving while wet irritates the skin and gives a substandard shave. And don't be surprised if the razor leaves behind more stubble than you'd like. You can always keep the shaver in your briefcase and duck into the men's room for a quick touch-up.

A constant problem for most men who prefer wet razors is nicks, cuts, and skin irritation. Here are a few tips recommended by barbers that will reduce the possibility of irritating your skin.

• If your face tends to become red after shaving, soak it before and after in cool water instead of warm. (You can either splash your face continually or wrap it for a few minutes in a towel or washcloth.)

• The best time to shave is right after taking a bath or a shower when your skin is moist.

• Most important is to cut with the grain of the hair, even in hard-to-reach places. Shaving against the way the hair grows often results in reddish bumps (called razor bumps) and ingrown hairs.

• Never shave in a hurry or use a dull blade. Haste and blunt blades are the most common causes of bloody, toilet-paper faces.

• Follow up the shave with a cold-water rinse. Then if you like, apply an ice-cold, wet washcloth to help close the pores and prevent rashes and ingrown hairs. If you enjoy aftershave, choose one without alcohol to avoid stings and dryness.

The Quest for the Perfect Shave

The perfect shave should leave your face smooth, clean, and free of nicks. The closest shave comes from a wet blade, but men with sensitive skin, acne, warts, or ingrown hairs, might prefer using an electric shaver, which reduces the likelihood of nicks, cuts, and irritation.

1 Ideally, take a shower before you shave to soften the hairs. Otherwise, drench your whiskers thoroughly with warm—not hot—water at the sink.

2 Use a shaving cream or gel to apply a lather. Don't be tempted to use soap, however, because it can dry out your skin over time.

3 Hold your skin firm ahead of the razor as you draw it along, and shave in the direction of the whiskers' growth. Start with your cheeks, then do your mustache, chin, and neck. Don't rush. For the closest shave possible, repeat the process.

4 Rinse with cold water, then apply an ice-cold, wet washcloth for about a minute. Dry your face and, if you want to, apply an aftershave, keeping in mind that aftershaves with alcohol sting and dry out the skin.

▶ *Want a smooth, nick-free shave? Always cut with the grain of the hair.*

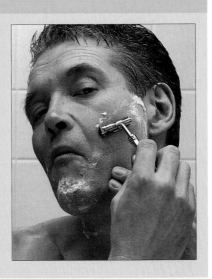

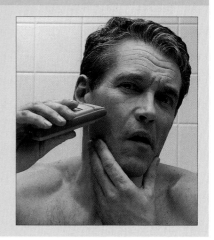
AVOIDING INGROWN HAIRS

Improperly shaving your neck, then putting on a stiff collar and snug tie often leads to painful ingrown hairs. Curly-headed men suffer most from ingrown hairs, especially men of

African descent. The hair starts off by growing curly in the follicle, and this makes it difficult to determine how to shave with the grain, says Los Angeles hair- and skin-care specialist Jan Turley.

If you suffer from chronic ingrown hairs and razor bumps, don't stretch your skin taut while scraping it with the blade. If the condition persists, consider growing a beard. If the ingrown hairs or skin infections continue to the point of severe pain, see a dermatologist.

Make Facial Hair Look Good

Some men should probably avoid facial hair altogether, especially if they have fine or thin hair that

sprouts sporadically after a few weeks' growth. If you've got a "sweet baby face," says Anaheim, California, barber Teresa Carter, leave it naked, though some authoritarian types—lawyers and professors, especially—try to mask their boyishness in facial hair. Beards have long been associated with distinguished men, and gray beards often connote wisdom.

If you're planning on growing a beard, realize that certain types of beards suit certain faces. A full beard and mustache, for example, look best on a narrow face. A lean beard and mustache are most suitable on a round face. Round or square faces look good with a goatee and mustache, while an unconnected beard

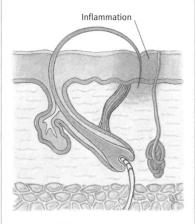

and moustache go well with a round face. A standard beard and moustache look best on an oval face.

MAINTENANCE

As one barber commented, "Beards are like hedges. The most beautiful are taken care of all the time." If you're going to grow a beard, plan on trimming it twice a week. This is best done when the hair is dry. Comb and untangle it before trimming. An electric beard trimmer can make the job easier.

At the end of the trim, you need to clean up the lines by shaving along them. Using the length attachment, trim the sides of the beard, a trimmer-width row at a time, from the bottom to the top.

Beards should be washed, conditioned, and brushed daily between visits to the barber or hair stylist. If you don't keep your beard clean, it can become cakey and white underneath, which is sure a sign that you have dandruff. If this happens, wash the beard with a good dandruff

shampoo until it becomes soft again, then return to your regular routine of daily shampoos and conditioning.

A barber or hair stylist can usually diagnose – and may be the cause of – what's called barber's itch, an infection in the beard area usually caused by using unclean or contaminated combs, scissors, razors, or clippers. Wash your beard equipment periodically in shampoo and avoid borrowing or lending it. The best way to avoid infection is to prevent it.

When to Skip Shaving

Most men prefer a close shave, one that leaves the face soft, and looking youthful and vibrant. But close shaving often irritates the skin, especially if you have curly hair or your hair grows in chaotic patterns. The reason: when you shave curly hair, it often curls back into the follicle, causing inflammation or ingrown hairs, an affliction common to men of African descent.

Skip shaving if your skin is nicked, cut, or irritated to the point of looking red

and raw, or you start to form rough or scaly patches. Resume when your skin has healed. Shaving over broken skin often leads to infection that might eventually require antibiotic treatment.

If you have to skip more shaving days than your employer allows, try giving yourself an electric rather than wet shave. If that doesn't work, you might have to think about electrolysis or a facial depilatory. Or grow a beard and avoid the problem altogether.

Other Facial Hair

For men over 40, hormonal changes increase hair production in the oddest places, in particular the ears and nose. Trim it back with a pair of sharp scissors. If you feel squeamish about it or have a history of drawing blood, leave it to your hair stylist.

Nose and ear hair can also be removed permanently with electrolysis, a perfectly safe technique that kills the hair follicle with a quick jolt of electricity.

Find the Best Beard Style

Your beard style should resemble your hair. If you have longer hair, choose a longer beard. Those with shorter hair should choose a more closely cropped look. Most barbers are hard-pressed to come up with names for the beard styles they cut, though many associate certain types of beards with the famous men who wore them.

The Vandyke
Named after the 17-century Flemish artist, the Vandyke is a longer, more pointed goatee than the Beatnik.

The Abraham Lincoln
This style has become less full and square than the more traditional beard worn by the American president.

The Elvis Presley
In his later, Las Vegas years, Elvis wore mutton-chop sideburns trimmed at

the jaw line, leaving his chin bare and giving the effect of a beard.

The ZZ Top
Near waist-length, flowing beards are the rock group's trademark – not exactly in sync with life in most offices.

The Beatnik
In fashion in the 1950s, the beatnik is similar to a goatee, a pointed tuft of hair on the end of the chin.

The Soul Patch
Actor Val Kilmer wore a soul patch, a small area of hair on the chin directly below the bottom lip, in his role as the frontiersman Doc Holliday in the film *Tombstone*.

The André Agassi
Popular among men in the sports and entertainment industries, this full beard looks like stubble or a five o'clock shadow; it conveys a sense of casualness.

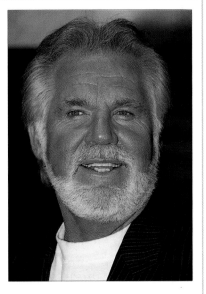

▲ *Kenny Rogers, superstar of country music, has made this full, close-cut beard style his trademark.*

Dress Sense for Men

Odds are you don't want to spend a lot of time thinking about your wardrobe. But you also don't want to commit an embarrassing fashion faux pas. How do you know whether today's hot fashion trend is tomorrow's Nehru jacket? Here's how to select clothes that will always keep you in style.

Where to Start?

So you wear whatever you find in your closet until it shreds or until someone makes a crack about your suit still living in the previous decade? At that point you realize you must go shopping.

Two fashion rules prevail, says Elena Hart, fashion marketing director of the New York–based Fashion Association, which provides consumers with information on fashion and trends.

• Rule number one: Never throw anything out. Wait long enough and it always comes back in style.

• Rule number two: Start with the basics. Then take your time building up a wardrobe piece by piece.

WHAT ARE THE BASICS?

This is what a basic wardrobe for a professional should include:
• A navy blazer
• A white shirt
• A striped shirt
• A gray, navy, or pinstripe suit (or all three if your work colleagues are in the habit of wearing suits to the office every day)
• A rep tie and a woven solid tie
• Khaki pants and blue jeans

Quest for the Perfect Jeans

Spend a lot of time in jeans? If so, it's worthwhile spending time finding a pair that fits well. That sounds obvious, but look around and you'll see streets full of men wearing jeans that are too loose, too tight, too short, or too long. The moral: Shop around.

Now comes the hard part. Start mixing and matching the basics to give yourself a unique look every day, sticking to these cardinal rules:

• Don't combine stripes and plaids, and make sure you match solids to patterns. This is what your parents probably taught you, and it's still good advice.

• Coordinate colors. Some colors go together well for all men, particularly combinations of burgundy or red with navy, using white or gold

Colors to Suit Your Complexion

Color is a powerful thing. To look your best, the color of your clothes should complement your natural skin tone and hair color. Color combinations that work for you will make you look more handsome, vibrant, and healthier, while ones that don't can make you look tired and sallow, accentuate blemishes, or simply overpower your face.

It's true that certain colors make most men look good, but if you want to look *great*, follow the do's and don'ts for your skin type below.

Irish or Ruddy Complexion
Stick to navy blue with a red-based tie and khaki pants. Try to create a contrast in your clothes to even out your skin tones.

Yellow Complexion
Stick with neutral colors, natural khakis, and greens. Stay away from black.

Olive Complexion
Stay away from olive drab or army khaki. Stick to natural colors, anything that doesn't have a lot of drab in it. You can use a splash of color in the tie or shirt for accent.

Black Complexion
Avoid extremely light pastels, grays, and navys, which might look drab. Stick to bold colors, black, and softer, deeper blues.

Blonde or Fair Complexion
Wear lighter-colored clothing, such as salmon, ivory, or light gray. Wear soft colors with bold ties.

Brown Complexion
Stay away from deep reds or deep colors. Stick to neutral, basic, or bold colors.

▶ *Fair-complexioned men should avoid very dark colors. A light-gray suit works well teamed with a light-blue shirt.*

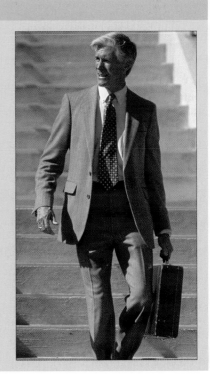

for highlights. Other good combinations include navy and khaki; light green and khaki; and natural colors or darker colors.

Buying Clothes

Some guys have a tendency to buy everything at once, getting it over and done with. Not a good idea. You'll always have second thoughts and wind up regularly wearing only 50 percent of your purchases. Instead, buy one or two pieces, then go home and see how they work with what's already in your closet. "Keep the basics and expand on them," says Hart. Here are some additional shopping tips.

• If you lack clothes confidence, shop with your partner or a trusted friend to get a second opinion.

• Though old rules dictated you had to stick to 100 percent natural fabrics, today's higher quality synthetics allow you to choose mixed fabrics, too. But, warns Hart, stick with a combination that has no less than 80 percent natural fibers.

• Spend as much as you can on suits and jackets. Go for high-quality fabrics that will last.

• Buy shirts with either button-down or loose collars, according to your preference, but be aware that button-down collars send the message that you're a prep school and country club sort of guy, Hart says.

• Make sure jackets and blazers don't strain across the chest.

A Style for Every Size and Shape

"Trendy is not for everyone," says Elena Hart, fashion marketing director for the New York–based Fashion Association. Dress according to what looks good on you, what complements your size and shape. When it comes to choosing the right clothes, "let the mirror be the judge," says Hart. Don't be swayed by trends or what you saw the night before on the Academy Awards or MTV. Trendy clothes on the wrong body type invariably become a fashion nightmare.

One way to avoid getting on the worst-dressed list is to get someone else's opinion when shopping. "Always bring along a friend or relative when you shop," Hart says, "someone you trust who will tell you honestly if what you want looks good on you."

Once you have a basic wardrobe—a navy blazer, a white shirt, a striped shirt, a gray, navy, or pinstripe suit, a rep tie, a woven solid tie, khaki pants, and blue jeans—"try experimenting," she adds.

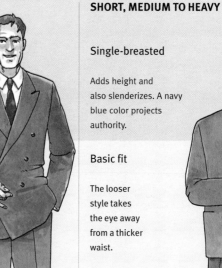
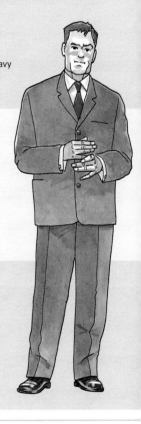

	TALL AND SLIM	SHORT, MEDIUM TO HEAVY
Suit Styles The four-button double-breasted suit is a classic look, while the six-button type conveys a "high-powered" feel. The classic single-breasted suit has two buttons; those with one, three, or four are more contemporary styles.	Single- or double-breasted Styles flatter height and build.	Single-breasted Adds height and also slenderizes. A navy blue color projects authority.
Shirt Styles Choose shirts that give a flattering fit and smart finish. The basic fit is loose through the waist; the athletic is wide in the shoulders, narrow at the waist; the loose is oversize and full through the body; and the European cut is a tapered, shaped dress shirt.	European cut or basic fit Both display a slender waist to good advantage.	Basic fit The looser style takes the eye away from a thicker waist.
Pants Styles Pants with pleats will make you look more slender, so they're a good choice for all shapes and sizes. A tight cut, currently becoming fashionable, will pick up any bulges around your buttocks and thighs, so avoid it if you're on the heavy side.	Pleated, tight, or regular cut Cuffs minimize height if physique is very skinny.	Pleated or regular cut; never tight Adds the illusion of height.

How to Pick the Best Fabrics

The old rule about never wearing man-made fibers no longer holds true. Blended fabrics with up to 20 percent synthetic materials often provide style, quality, and convenience. Linen, for example, wears less like an old rumpled laundry bag when there's a little non-natural fabric mixed in to stiffen it.

Look for fabrics that move with you, but avoid those with a high content of non-natural materials. Always touch the fabric first. If it feels scratchy, don't bother trying it on. Though you don't want to be a slave to labels, look for clothing made by reputable companies or by a high-quality department store's private stock. A company that's been around for a while is less likely to sell you clothes that fall apart. And they're more likely to take them back and give you a full refund if they do self-destruct after a few washings.

▶ *Good fabrics should move with you, feel comfortable, and still look good even after a full day's use.*

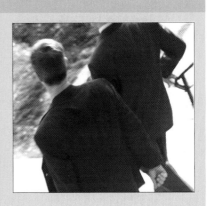

"Especially if you don't need to wear a suit every day. Put a navy jacket together with khaki pants one day, then combine the pants from your suit with the jacket the next."

When it comes to matching clothes to your own size and shape, certain fashion truisms prevail: Double-breasted suits look best on slender builds, since they add bulk. Pleated pants tend to make the wearer look more slender, but the trend these days is toward a slimmer cut, which isn't good news for heavier men.

And though a good-quality, five-pocket pair of jeans is essential to any wardrobe, Hart warns against wearing them in the office, even on popular "dress-down" Fridays. "Wear khakis and a blazer instead, that look relaxed and professional," she suggests.

The table below is designed to help you choose the best and most flattering style of office or formal clothing for your size and shape.

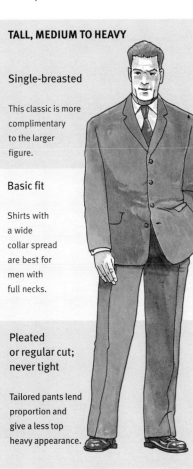

TALL, MEDIUM TO HEAVY

Single-breasted

This classic is more complimentary to the larger figure.

Basic fit

Shirts with a wide collar spread are best for men with full necks.

Pleated or regular cut; never tight

Tailored pants lend proportion and give a less top heavy appearance.

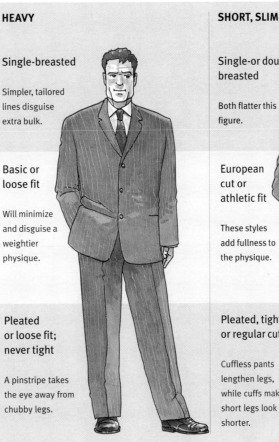

HEAVY

Single-breasted

Simpler, tailored lines disguise extra bulk.

Basic or loose fit

Will minimize and disguise a weightier physique.

Pleated or loose fit; never tight

A pinstripe takes the eye away from chubby legs.

SHORT, SLIM

Single- or double-breasted

Both flatter this figure.

European cut or athletic fit

These styles add fullness to the physique.

Pleated, tight, or regular cut

Cuffless pants lengthen legs, while cuffs make short legs look shorter.

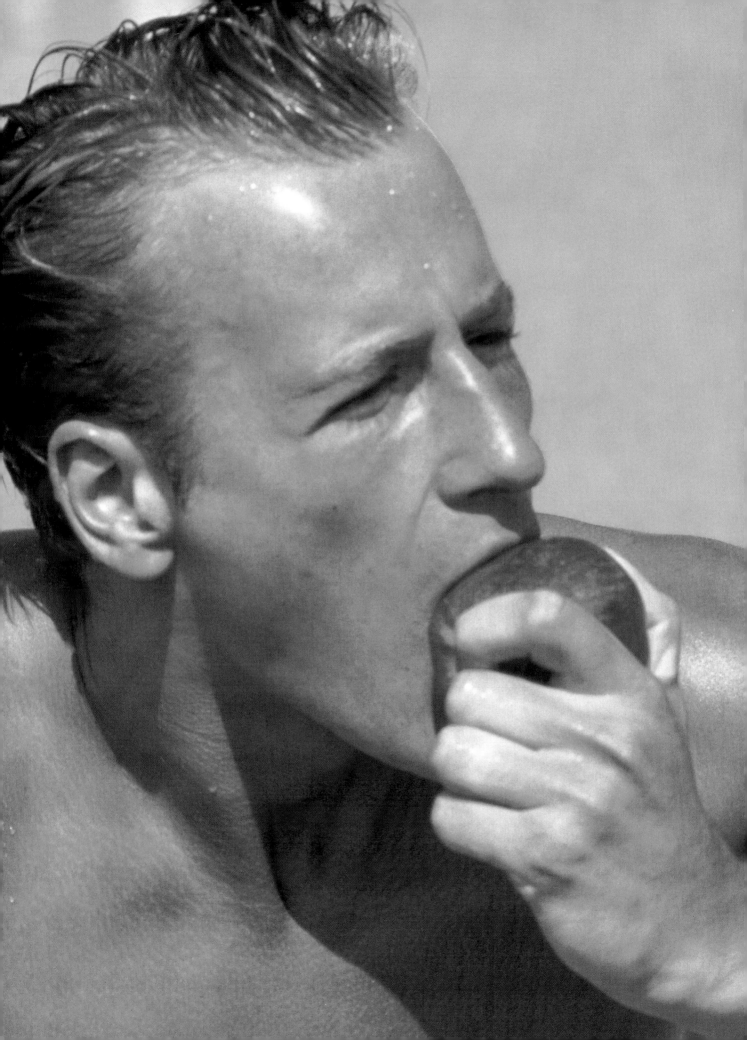

Healthy Eating

What a Man Needs to Eat

Your body may look solid, but consider this: One year ago, 98 percent of its atoms were not there. You build a new skeleton every three months and a new liver every six weeks; every four days your stomach lining is replaced. The building materials for all this construction come from nutrients in your food.

> "Your choice of diet can influence your long-term health prospects more than any other action you might take."
>
> C. Everett Koop, former U.S. Surgeon General

Why You Need Food

Food contains the raw materials you need to build your body as a child, and to maintain and repair it throughout life. A hub of constant activity, your body is ceaselessly tearing down and building up tissue. Eating (along with breathing and drinking) brings in a stream of atoms and molecules to renew cells, muscles, blood, and bones.

You also need food for energy. The food you put in your mouth is the fuel that runs your body. Everything you do—working, walking, digesting, making love, even sleeping or watching television—requires energy.

When we eat a meal, it enters our very own food processor—the digestive system—and is broken into usable components of amino acids, simple sugars, and fatty acids. The primary simple sugar (glucose) enters the circulatory system and is delivered along with oxygen to our cells. Glucose and oxygen are burned by the cells to produce the energy that powers our bodies.

The ongoing process of breaking down food substances to produce energy and build up body tissues and cells is known as metabolism.

What Is Food?

From a nutritionist's point of view, food is what provides the nutrients your body needs for survival and growth. You have to get six main types of nutrients from food. Your body either can't make these at all, or it just can't make enough of them. These heavy hitters include carbohydrates, protein, fat, vitamins, minerals, and water. Fiber—not really a nutrient—is so important we're going to put it into the lineup, too.

CARBOHYDRATES

Carbohydrates (the starches and sugars) are found mainly in vegetables, fruit, legumes, and grains. They are broken down primarily into glucose (blood sugar), the main fuel the body uses for energy.

There are two types of carbohydrate. Simple carbohydrates (sugars) break down rapidly when eaten and are quickly absorbed. Complex carbohydrates (starches) take longer to break down, so they are absorbed more slowly into your bloodstream.

What Happens to Your Food after You Eat?

Food goes through major changes before your body is able to burn it for energy or use the nutrients to rebuild your cells. Here's a quick rundown on what happens when you take a bite out of an apple.

Mouth
Your teeth and tongue cut, crush, mash, and mix the food, while chemicals in the saliva help break it down.

Throat and Esophagus
You swallow, and muscles in the esophagus propel the food into the stomach.

Stomach
Hydrochloric acid and other gastric juices attack the food. Powerful muscle contractions churn it, breaking it down to a soupy liquid.

Small Intestine
Juices pour in from the liver, pancreas, and gallbladder to complete digestion. Nutrients move through the intestine wall. From there, they go via the bloodstream and lymph highways to every cell in the body.

Large Intestine
Water and minerals are absorbed through the intestinal wall. The remaining material passes into the rectum as feces to be eliminated through the anus.

Eat According to Your Age

What was that? You say you can eat all you want and never gain weight; it just seems to burn right off? Well, if you're one of the lucky guys for whom this is true—yes, there are some of you out there—then just wait until you're 30. Around that time, our metabolism starts to slow down, and we burn calories less efficiently. What happens is that most of us just keep on eating about the same amount, but the result that we start to pile on the pounds.

From age 30 on, the average man can expect to put on between 1 and 1½ pounds every year.

The table below is designed to help you combat this insidious trend. Look up the weight closest to your own and read down to the calorie figure in your age group. That's the number of calories you can afford to eat without putting on weight.

To maintain your current weight, tailor your food consumption to your age. If you

need to lose weight, you'll have to cut down by about 500 calories a day and increase your level of exercise. We're not saying that you need to watch every calorie you consume; eating should be a pleasure, after all. The best way to lose weight is not by fanatic calorie-counting (although you've got to be aware of calories), but through regular exercise and a low-fat diet that is centered on fruit, vegetables, and grains.

	Body weight (lb.)										
Age	120	130	140	150	160	170	180	190	200	210	220
18–30	2,515	2,668	2,821	2,974	3,127	3,280	3,433	3,586	3,739	3,892	4,045
31–60	2,271	2,387	2,503	2,619	2,735	2,851	2,967	3,083	3,199	3,315	3,431

PROTEIN

The body's chief building material, protein makes up 15 to 20 percent of your weight. During digestion your body breaks down large protein molecules from food into amino acids, then puts these smaller molecules back together again as the main ingredients in skin, bones, muscles, hair, teeth, and so on.

FAT

Often perceived as the bad guy in the movie, fat sometimes wears a white hat, too. It's burned as energy and stored for future use in case other energy sources run low. Fat teams up with proteins to form the membrane around every cell. It insulates the body against heat loss, and cushions vital organs.

WATER

The most essential of all nutrients is water. You can live a long time without food or particular vitamins

and minerals, but only a few days without H_2O. It dissolves the other nutrients and transports them throughout the body. Water is indispensable in digestion, absorption, circulation, and elimination. Nearly all of the body's millions of chemical reactions are water-based.

FIBER

Strictly speaking not a nutrient, fiber is nevertheless vital for health. It's the stuff in plant foods—vegetables, fruit, grains, and legumes—that your body cannot digest. Fiber gives you a feeling of fullness without the excess calories, so it helps control weight, and it sweeps through the digestive tract, helping to keep it clean and functioning properly.

VITAMINS

Though used by the body in only tiny amounts, vitamins are key players in nutrition. They help regulate metabolism, are vital to growth,

reproduction, and digestion, and aid mental alertness, hormone production, vision, and immunity.

The water-soluble vitamins, which include vitamin C and all eight B vitamins, operate in the water-filled parts of cells. They're not stored for future use, but are flushed out in your urine by the kidneys. Other vitamins, such as vitamins A and E, are stored by the body in fatty tissue.

MINERALS

These inorganic substances are vital for a wide range of bodily structures, including the bones, teeth, and hair.

TRUE OR FALSE?

Eating a lot of protein foods helps make you strong.

False. High protein intake doesn't stimulate muscle growth. It does, however, provide the raw material if you are exercising enough to build muscles up.

They're involved in countless processes, from muscle movement to immune function and the transmission of nerve impulses. The so-called macrominerals—including calcium, magnesium, and potassium—make up 4 percent of your body weight, about 6 pounds in a 160-pound man. The other 50 or so—the trace minerals or microminerals—would barely fill a teaspoon.

You and Your Diet

Why is it important to know about carbohydrates, fat, protein, and the rest of them? It's not an academic exercise. It's important to know these facts because most of us have diets that are out of kilter with our body's needs: We eat too much fat, for instance, and not enough fiber. And we know now that diet plays an important role protecting the body against a range of diseases; the link between a low-fat diet and low rates of heart disease is perhaps the best-known example.

So if you become more aware of what you put into your mouth every day, you'll be in a better position to make well-informed choices about your diet. The payoff is better nutrition, improved day-to-day health, and probably a longer life.

Macro- and Micronutrients

As you've seen, your body manufactures thousands of chemical compounds every day: proteins to build new cells and repair damaged ones; hormones to regulate everything from metabolism to sex drive; sugars to fuel the whole shebang. To accomplish all this, your body needs raw materials in the form of nutrients.

The tables below and on the following pages list these vital nutrients, their role in your continued good health, the foods they're found in, and the required daily amounts.

There are two basic groups of nutrient. Macronutrients are needed in large quantities, and include proteins, carbohydrates, fat, and water, as well as a few minerals. The micronutrients are needed in very small quantities, which are measured in milligrams (mg.) and micrograms (mcg.). They include vitamins and the majority of minerals.

Macronutrients

Nutrient	Role in Health	Best Sources	Requirement
Carbohydrates	Primarily burned for energy. Help break down fat and keep skin, bones, and nails healthy.	Complex carbohydrates (starches): vegetables, fruit, legumes, whole grains. Simple carbohydrates (sugars): refined sugar, honey, molasses.	Complex carbohydrates should make up 55 to 65 percent of your daily diet. Minimize simple carbohydrates.
Protein	Growth and repair of cells, muscles, skin, hemoglobin. Production of hormones and digestive enzymes.	Poultry, fish, eggs, beans, whole grains, nuts, dairy products.	About ⅓ g. per pound of body weight (around 56 g. or 2 oz. for a 165-lb. man). Most American men eat much more.
Fat	Forms the outer membrane of every cell. Important for nerves, some hormones, and for hair and skin. Insulates against heat loss. Burned for energy and stored for future energy needs.	Monounsaturated oils (such as olive and canola) and polyunsaturated oils (corn, sunflower, safflower). Avoid saturated fats (meat, dairy, and palm and coconut oils).	We require only 2 to 5 percent of calories from fat. Standard recommendation is 30 percent; more and more experts urge a maximum of 25 percent.
Water	Cools and lubricates the body; transports all other nutrients through the circulatory system, flushes out waste matter and toxins. The major component of all bodily fluids. Every chemical reaction in the body's cells depends on water.	Water, juices, fruit, vegetables.	The body requires 2–3 qt. a day, but about half typically comes from food. Drink six to eight eight-ounce glasses, more if you're physically very active.

Water-Soluble Vitamins

Nutrient	Role in Health	Best Sources	Requirement
Vitamin C	An antioxidant. Necessary for bone-building, formation of neuro-transmitters (such as serotonin), and detoxifying processes in the liver. Boosts immunity and may help prevent colds, cancer, and heart disease. Promotes healthy gums.	Oranges, grapefruit, cantaloupes, sweet red peppers, raw spinach, broccoli, Brussels sprouts, cauliflower, mangoes, papayas, strawberries, potatoes.	60 mg. Optimal dose is hotly debated. Many experts advise from 250–1,000 mg. per day.
Thiamin (vitamin B$_1$)	Involved in converting carbohydrates to energy; deficiency may cause depression, fatigue, appetite loss.	Peas, beans, whole grains, pork, fortified breads.	1.5 mg.
Riboflavin (vitamin B$_2$)	Helps create energy from carbohydrates, fat, and protein. Vital in formation of red blood cells and hormones. Helps maintain tissues.	Milk products, whole grains, fortified breads, broccoli, asparagus, peas, potatoes, oranges/orange juice, eggs, liver.	1.7 mg.
Niacin (vitamin B$_3$)	Helps convert carbohydrates, amino acids, and fat into energy.	Grains, cereals, baked goods, meat, poultry, fish, soybeans, peanuts, beer.	20 mg.
Pantothenic acid (vitamin B$_5$)	Helps metabolize proteins, carbohydrates, and fat, and to produce important hormones and neurotransmitters.	Found in all animal and vegetable tissue; high levels in avocados, broccoli, bran, organ meats, eggs.	10 mg.
Vitamin B$_6$	Helps regulate nervous system. Important in breaking down protein and amino acids and converting them to energy. Also helps in metabolism of glucose and fatty acids, and helps build red blood cells.	Whole grains, potatoes, chicken, fish, egg yolks, bananas, avocados.	2 mg. If you eat large amounts of protein, you may need more than this.
Vitamin B$_{12}$	Essential for DNA synthesis and cell division. Red blood cell production depends on vitamin B$_{12}$; deficiency results in pernicious anemia.	Liver, oysters, beef, pork, whole-milk dairy products, eggs.	6 mcg. Vegetarians who eat no dairy products or eggs cannot get enough vitamin B$_{12}$ without supplementation.
Folic acid	Required for the growth and division of cells and formation of hemoglobin.	Beans such as pinto and navy, cereals, spinach, asparagus, broccoli, okra, various seeds, liver.	400 mcg.
Biotin	Helps immune system function. Vital in metabolism of protein, fat, and carbohydrates, and formation of new proteins, hormones, neurotransmitters.	Peanut butter, legumes, nuts, grains, egg yolks, organ meats such as liver and kidney, yeast, cauliflower.	300 mcg.

(continued)

Fat-Soluble Vitamins

Nutrient	Role in Health	Best Sources	Requirement
Vitamin A	Required for normal vision, reproduction, cell development, growth, immunity. Maintains the health of the skin and mucous membranes. Beta-carotene, which converts to vitamin A in the body, is an antioxidant.	Cantaloupes, peaches, apricots, mangoes, papayas, carrots, spinach, broccoli, tomatoes, lettuce, green peas, green beans, sweet potatoes, yellow squash, fish, liver, egg yolks, whole milk.	1,000 mcg. (5,000 IU). Be cautious with supplements: Vitamin A is toxic in high doses.
Vitamin D	Vital for absorption of calcium. Key to bone-building, healthy teeth, and nerve–muscle interaction.	Sunshine (helps the body produce its own vitamin D); canned sardines, salmon, and herring; vitamin D–fortified dairy products.	10 mcg. (400 IU)
Vitamin E	An antioxidant, it protects cells and tissues from oxidation damage by free radicals. May prevent heart disease. Lowers cholesterol and helps prevent buildup of plaque in arteries. Boosts immunity. Helps prevent cataracts.	Nuts (such as almonds, peanuts, and pecans), pumpkin and sunflower seeds, kale and other green leafy vegetables, wheat germ, whole grains.	20 mg. (30 IU) This is the recommended Daily Value. Many experts suggest supplementation of 100–400 IU for antioxidant effect.
Vitamin K	Helps regulate clotting of the blood.	Green leafy vegetables, fruit, seeds, eggs, dairy products, meat.	80 mcg.

Macrominerals

Nutrient	Role in Health	Best Sources	Requirement
Calcium	Builds bones and teeth. Important in blood clotting, the structure of cell membranes, and transmission of nerve impulses. Helps prevent brittle bones. May protect against high blood pressure and colon cancer. Vital for normal growth in children.	Dairy products, such as milk, cheese, yogurt. Also, sardines, almonds, sesame seeds, broccoli, soybeans, green leafy vegetables.	1,000 mg.
Chloride	Vital for nervous system and maintaining fluid balance.	Table salt is sodium chloride: It's found everywhere both in nature and in packaged foods.	3,400 mg.
Magnesium	Bone-builder; helps regulate the heart and protect against heart disease; important in enzyme activity, and in metabolism, converting protein, fat, and sugars to energy.	Green leafy vegetables, legumes, seafood, nuts, soybeans, eggs, whole grains, dairy products.	400 mg.
Phosphorus	Vital for bone-building. Helps maintain acid–alkaline balance and is important in metabolism.	Dairy products, meat, fish, grains, nuts, beans.	1,000 mg.

Macrominerals—Continued

Nutrient	Role in Health	Best Sources	Requirement
Potassium	Regulates blood pressure and heart function. Vital for muscle contraction and transmission of nerve impulses. Important in nucleic-acid production.	Citrus fruit, bananas, tomatoes, most other fruit and vegetables, seafood.	3,500 mg.
Sodium	Important in transmission of nerve impulses. Helps regulate blood pressure. Involved in metabolism of protein and carbohydrates.	Found naturally in almost all foods, and added to canned and frozen vegetables, baked goods, cereals, as well as potato and corn chips, etc.	2,400 mg. (max.)

Microminerals

Nutrient	Role in Health	Best Sources	Requirement
Chromium	Helps reduce risk of diabetes and heart disease by regulating blood sugar and insulin levels and lowering cholesterol in the blood.	Brewer's yeast, wheat germ, and whole-wheat bread, meats, cheese, wine, beer.	120 mcg.
Copper	Assists T-cells in the immune system. Involved in hormone production. Essential for maintaining healthy bones, hair, and skin. Present in many antioxidant enzymes.	Shellfish, nuts, cocoa, mushrooms, whole grains, peas, dried beans, green vegetables, liver.	2 mg.
Iron	Vital for formation of red blood cells and transport of oxygen throughout the body. Essential for combustion of protein, fat, and carbohydrates to produce energy.	Red meat, poultry, fish, nuts, whole grains, apricots, kidney beans, peas, parsley, egg yolk, spinach and other green leafy vegetables.	10 mg. Be cautious with supplements: Excess iron may form free radicals leading to cancer and heart disease.
Manganese	Involved in glucose metabolism and bone-building. An important antioxidant. Necessary for synthesis of dopamine, a key brain neurotransmitter.	Whole grains, nuts, fruit, seeds, eggs, green vegetables, meat, shellfish, milk products.	2 mg.
Selenium	A powerful antioxidant; combines with vitamin E to protect cell membranes against free radicals in the heart, liver, kidneys, and lungs. Vital for cell growth and fighting infections.	Fish, meat, whole grains (especially wheat), dairy products, eggs, nuts, broccoli, cucumbers, onions, garlic, radishes, mushrooms.	70 mcg.
Zinc	Promotes growth. Vital for sex drive and fertility. Important for immunity and healing of infections and wounds. An important antioxidant.	Seafood, beef, turkey, oatmeal and other whole grains, yeast, beans, wheat germ, nuts, milk, eggs.	15 mg.

The Essentials of Good Nutrition

Most of us live on the run, paying too little attention to what we eat. But food is too important to leave to chance. By learning the essentials of good nutrition—what foods you need, what supplements might be helpful, and what to avoid—you can greatly improve your odds for lifelong good health.

Learn Your Needs

Every man's need for nutrients is unique and depends on many factors, including heredity, lifestyle, body type, and general health. Although there are broad guidelines all of us would be wise to follow—eat lots of fruit, vegetables, and whole grains, minimize fat, drink enough water—each of us has to assess his current diet and find his own way to a tailor-made eating plan.

To make sure your diet contains everything you need, consult the U.S. Department of Agriculture Food Guide Pyramid (see "Secrets of the Pyramid"). It's an indispensable visual reference. In basic terms, the Food Guide Pyramid says this:
• Eat a variety of foods every day to get all the nutrients you need.
• Eat lots of grains, fruit, and vegetables: Make these the central part of each meal.
• Eat animal-derived foods in moderation only: They're usually high in saturated fats.

• Eat oils, fat, and sugary foods sparingly: Need we say why?

MAKE A PLAN

Sorry, but simply reading about it won't be enough. The chances are that you won't make significant dietary changes unless you take charge of the situation. Healthy eating should be pleasurable, but it doesn't happen by itself; it requires thought, decisions, and vigilance.

Learn your nutritional needs, then give some thought to what changes you should make to your existing diet. It's a good idea to write down these changes.

Make direct and simple statements that you can act on: "I want to eat less sugar, more complex carbohydrates;" "I want to eat less saturated fat." Also write down why you want to make these changes ("have more sustained energy"; "cut my risk of heart disease"). Finally, set specific goals, writing down what you want to accomplish: two or three more servings of vegetables each day; more whole grains; no more full-fat dairy products; fish instead of steak twice a week, and so on.

Chart your progress and reward yourself for success.

Goodbye to All That

If you decide to follow the food pyramid—and you should—you'll probably have to cut down drastically on some dearly loved favorites.

Top 10 Nutrition Tips

1 Cut your risk of heart disease, cancer, and diabetes by limiting consumption of red meat, whole-milk products, and fried foods.

2 For vitamins, minerals, and fiber eat your fruit and vegetables.

3 Complex carbohydrates (found in whole grains, vegetables, and fruit) are your best energy source.

4 Eat a wide variety of foods.

5 Be sure to get the recommended Daily Values of vitamins and minerals.

6 Limit alcohol consumption. More than two drinks per day can lead to accidents, illness, and addiction.

7 Eat more fiber. Dietary fiber (from whole grains, fruit, vegetables, and legumes) helps lower cholesterol and may reduce the risk of colon cancer.

8 Switch to fish. You'll get as much protein from fish as you would from red meat—but without the saturated fats red meat contains.

9 Everyone needs six to eight glasses of water a day.

10 Avoid diets; they don't work.

The majority of fatty and sugary foods—and those delicious desserts that combine the two—need to be on your "No" or "Well, maybe just a little" lists. Sweets are simple sugars, often called "empty calories" as they provide no nutrition. Fat tends to accumulate in places we don't really want it; in addition to extra bulges, it may clog our arteries and lead to life-threatening heart disease.

Here are some of your favorite foods you'd be better off avoiding or at least eating in moderation.
• Beef products, including steaks, hamburgers, roast beef, and organ meats (very high in saturated fat)

Secrets of the Pyramid

For many men, the U.S. Department of Agriculture Food Guide Pyramid has a musty, schoolbook feel about it that provokes yawns and drooping eyelids. Well, drop those preconceptions for a moment and take another look. Believe it or not, the pyramid holds the key to your continued good health.

It's showing you three fundamental things. You should:
- Eat a variety of foods every day.
- Eat the recommended proportions (more of the bottom two tiers).
- Eat certain foods (the top two levels) in moderation.

As the long base of the pyramid suggests, the lower two tiers—the grains, fruit, and vegetables—should form the basis of your diet. The mainly animal-derived foods in the next tier—which are to be eaten in moderate amounts—are loaded with saturated fat;

beans, legumes, and tofu may be substituted for meat. The foods at the very tip of the pyramid (butter, oils, sweets, and so on) should be used only sparingly.

The pyramid also gives you recommended servings, which are for both men and women. Men should gravitate toward the larger number of servings, especially if they're active. If meeting these recommendations seems a little daunting, consider this: For the grains, if you eat a bowl of cereal with a slice of toast for breakfast, a sandwich for lunch, and a man-size portion of pasta (let's say, double the ½ cup baseline) for supper, you're up to six servings already.

Most men who adapt their diets to fit the pyramid will find that they increase their intake of complex carbohydrates and cut down on fat—especially the saturated variety—and sugar.

What's in a Serving?

Grains: 1 slice of bread, 1 ounce of cold cereal or ½ cup of either cooked cereal, rice or pasta

Vegetables: 1 cup of raw, leafy veggies; ½ cup of other vegetables, cooked or chopped raw; ¾ cup of vegetable juice

Fruit: 1 medium apple, banana, or orange; ½ cup of chopped, cooked, or canned fruit; ¾ cup of fruit juice

Dairy: 1 cup of milk or yogurt; 1½ ounces of cheese

Meat, poultry, fish, dry beans, eggs, nuts: 2–3 ounces of meat; equivalent servings include ½ cup cooked dried beans; 1 egg; 2 tablespoons of peanut butter

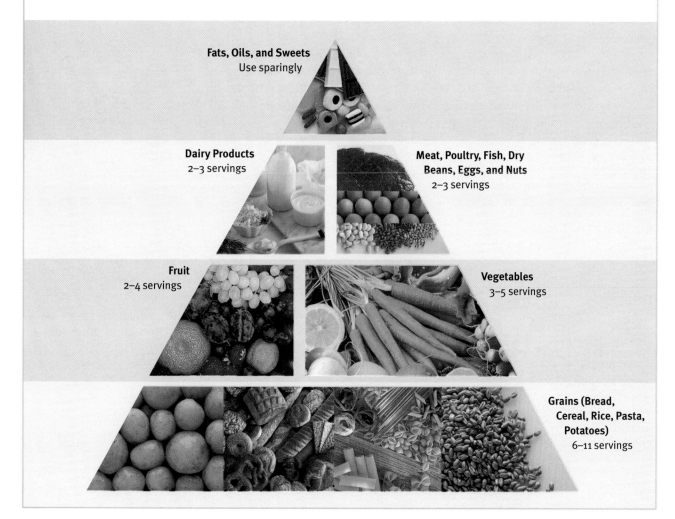

Fats, Oils, and Sweets
Use sparingly

Dairy Products
2–3 servings

Meat, Poultry, Fish, Dry Beans, Eggs, and Nuts
2–3 servings

Fruit
2–4 servings

Vegetables
3–5 servings

Grains (Bread, Cereal, Rice, Pasta, Potatoes)
6–11 servings

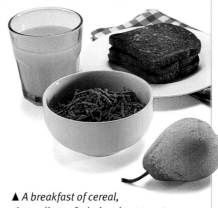
- Chicken or turkey cooked with the skin (high in saturated fat)
- Chocolate chip and most other cookies (high in fat and sugar)
- Coconut and palm oil (very high in saturated fat)
- Deli meats (high in saturated fat and sodium)
- Doughnuts (high in fat and sugar)

The Underrated Breakfast

It's been estimated that nearly half of us skip breakfast, running on an empty tank until we refuel at lunch (or at mid-morning with a high-fat, sugary snack). Breakfast is important: Research shows that by late morning those who eat breakfast are performing better both physically and mentally than people who chose to skip the meal.

But don't go for the old standbys. Bacon, ham, and sausages are loaded with artery-clogging saturated fat. Instead, try a bowl of fiber-rich cereal with skim milk and fruit. The protein in the milk will invigorate your brain; the complex carbohydrates in the cereal and fruit will give you sustained energy until midday. Some tasty alternatives include low-fat cottage cheese or nonfat yogurt, whole-wheat bread, or a bagel with jam or jelly.

- Egg yolks (very high in cholesterol)
- Hydrogenated vegetable oils (these produce free radicals; may be worse for you than saturated fats)
- Mayonnaise (very high in cholesterol and fat)
- Chocolate (high in fat and sugar)
- Peanut butter (high in fat)
- Pork products, such as sausages, bacon, ham (high in saturated fat, usually high in sodium)
- Whole-dairy products (very high in saturated fat)

If you can't live without some of these old friends, do your best to eat a moderate amount, or search out low-fat alternatives. If you choose to eat beef or pork, take care to select the leanest cut available.

IT'S OKAY TO EAT SNACKS!

Doughnuts, cookies, and chocolate bars—three much-loved snacks that we've just advised you to drop. Are *all* snacks bad?

The answer, we're pleased to tell you, is a resounding no. Snacks are helpful not only to keep up energy levels and mental clarity, but also, believe it or not, for weight control. Why? If you put off eating for too long, chances are you'll stuff yourself when you finally get around to it. But

it's also important to avoid impulse-buying of chocolate bars, doughnuts, cookies, and the others—healthy snacks are low in fat and sweeteners, and are eaten only in modest amounts.

Good, nutritious choices for between-meal snacks include fruit or fruit juice; vegetable sticks; a cup of soup with a slice of whole-grain bread; whole-grain crackers or pretzels; and plain, air-popped popcorn (without butter).

It's All in the Timing

Another thing to keep in mind if you're reassessing your diet is the timing of meals. Nutritionists say that *when* you eat is more important than most people might think.

For one thing, it's been shown that if you don't eat for more than four to five hours, your blood sugar dips, possibly leading to irritability, fuzzy thinking, tension, and tiredness.

Eating too late at night may cause insomnia, as well as heartburn and indigestion. It also tends to encourage weight gain because metabolism slows down then.

Nutritionists advise eating regular meals, starting with a good, filling breakfast. They say you should have your largest meal around the middle of the day. For supper have a small, light meal, leaving the stomach relatively empty when you go to sleep.

Don't Forget the Fiber

Fiber, the part of plant foods that the body cannot absorb or digest, passes through your digestive system pretty much intact. But it's not just a waste product; it is, in fact, an essential part of a healthy diet. Just consider the following:

• Fiber makes for softer, bulkier stools, so it helps prevent constipation and irregularity.

• Research has shown that a diet high in fiber may protect you from colon cancer.

• Fiber (of the kind found in oat bran, barley, apples, and legumes) helps lower your cholesterol levels, thus reducing your risk of heart disease.

The experts recommend that you consume 20 to 30 grams of fiber every day. To accomplish this, you'll need about five servings of fruit and vegetables, as well as half a dozen servings of grains. (See "Your Fiber

Food Combining: Myth or Fact?

Is it all a lot of hot air? Some people say combining certain foods, such as fruit and grains, produces toxins in the stomach, resulting in a lot of gas. Others claim you shouldn't eat proteins and carbohydrates together.

Most nutrition experts reject these notions, pointing out that our digestive system routinely handles complex combinations, even in the simplest foods. Beans contain carbohydrates, fiber, and protein; milk comprises protein, carbohydrates, and fat. "The overwhelming evidence is on the side of a varied, balanced diet, with foods eaten in nutritious, appetizing combinations," says the *Wellness Letter* of the University of California at Berkeley School of Public Health.

When Do You Need Vitamin Supplements?

"A poor diet plus vitamins is still a poor diet," says health educator Art Ulene, M.D. Eating the right foods is the best way to get the nutrients you need. And we know you want to eat all the right foods. But just in case... it wouldn't hurt to have a little nutritional insurance in the form of a high-quality supplement of vitamins, minerals, and antioxidants such as beta-carotene.

If you're healthy, taking supplements may help enhance your immune system. If you smoke, drink a lot of alcohol, or if you've been sick or dieting for a while, or if you follow a strict vegetarian diet, supplements may be important. Look for a formula that contains about 100 percent of the Daily Values for all 13 vitamins, as well as zinc, selenium and, if possible, copper.

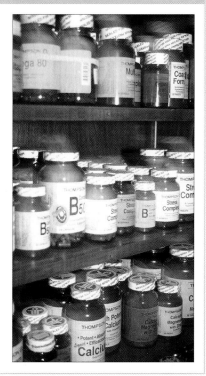

▶ *Supplements like these may enhance your immune system, but they can't turn a poor diet into a good one.*

Options" for a listing of fiber-rich foods.) That dovetails neatly with the Food Guide Pyramid, which gives star billing to these food groups.

Cut Your Cholesterol

Do you figure you're young and active enough not to worry about cholesterol? Well, then you better think again. If you eat a typical American diet, high in the saturated fats the body converts into cholesterol, you may be on the road to serious health problems.

Cholesterol is a thick, sticky gunk that gradually builds up on the lining of your arteries and obstructs the flow of blood. When the blood supply to your heart is sufficiently blocked, you may have a heart attack; if the blockage is to the brain, you may have a stroke.

The culprit is fatty food, especially animal fat, such as red meat and full-fat dairy, and fried foods. Does that sound familiar? In the words of William Castelli, M.D., the director

of the Framingham Heart Study, "When you see the Golden Arches, you are probably on the road to the pearly gates."

To lower cholesterol, strictly limit foods high in saturated fat, including red meat, pork, dairy products made from whole milk (cheese, butter, yogurt, ice cream, sour cream), coconut and palm oil, and fried foods. Instead, favor fiber, including whole grains (such as wheat, oats, and barley), vegetables, fruit, and all types of beans. And increase your daily amount of exercise.

The cholesterol content of what you eat is not as crucial in raising blood cholesterol as are the levels of saturated fat. Even so, to be on the safe side it's best to go easy with such high-cholesterol foods as eggs and shrimp.

Some people have a genetically determined tendency toward high cholesterol levels. If you're in that boat, you need to be extra-vigilant to stick to the dietary guidelines.

What's in the Food You Eat?

Always wanted to know how much pantothenic acid there is in a baked potato? Here's your big chance! The following table lists the nutritional values—protein, carbohydrates, fat, and the most important vitamins and minerals—of 45 common foods. Use it in conjunction with the table of nutrients on pages 50–53 to find out if you're getting enough nutrients from your diet.

Key
t = trace
u = unknown

	Calories	Protein (g.)	Fat (g.)	Carbohydrates (g.)	Calcium (mg.)	Phosphorus (mg.)	Magnesium (mg.)	Sodium (mg.)	Potassium (mg.)	Zinc (mg.)	Iron (mg.)	Vitamin A (mcg.)	Thiamin (mg.)	Riboflavin (mg.)	Niacin (mg.)	Vitamin B$_6$ (mg.)	Pantothenic acid (mg.)	Folic acid (mcg.)	Vitamin C (mg.)
Beverage																			
Beer (12 oz.)	150	0.9	0	13	15	50	35	18	115	0.2	0.1	0	0	t	1.8	0.2	0.2	20	0
Cola (12 oz.)	140	0	0	38	10	60	4	10	6	0.02	0.2	0	0	0	0	0	0	0	0
Juice, orange (1 cup)	110	1.7	0.5	26	25	40	25	2	495	0.1	0.5	50	0.22	0.07	1	0.1	0.5	110	125
Breads																			
Bagel	175	6.5	1.5	34	25	40	12	215	45	0.3	1.6	0	0.2	0.2	2.1	0.03	0.2	14	0
White, enriched (1 slice)	65	2.1	1.0	12	30	25	5	125	30	0.2	0.7	t	0.1	0.08	0.9	0.01	0.1	9	t
Whole-wheat (1 slice)	60	2.4	1.1	11	20	65	25	160	45	0.4	0.9	t	0.09	0.05	1.0	0.05	0.2	14	t
Cereal																			
Corn Flakes (1 oz.)	110	2	0.1	24	1	20	3	350	25	0.08	1.8	0	0.3	0.4	3	0.02	0.05	3	0
Oatmeal (1 cup)	145	6	2.4	25	20	180	55	380	130	1.2	1.6	4	0.26	0.05	0.3	0.05	0.5	7	0
Dairy																			
Cheese, Cheddar (1 oz.)	115	7	9.5	0.4	205	145	8	175	30	0.9	0.2	85	0.01	0.1	t	0.02	0.1	5	0
Milk, whole (1 cup)	150	8	8.2	11	290	225	30	120	370	1	0.1	75	0.09	0.4	0.4	0.1	0.8	10	2
Milk, skim (1 cup)	90	8.5	0.4	12	300	245	30	125	400	1	0.1	140	0.09	0.4	0.2	0.1	0.8	15	2
Desserts and Sweets																			
Chocolate, bar (4 oz.)	600	8.8	36	64	260	260	80	100	440	0.4	1.28	0	0.08	0.4	0.4	t	0.12	8	0
Doughnut	170	2	9	20	15	90	10	225	40	0.2	0.6	7	0.1	0.08	0.7	0.01	0.2	3	3
Ice cream	175	2	12	16	75	60	8	50	110	0.6	0.05	105	0.02	0.15	0.05	0.03	0.3	1	0
Pie, apple (1 slice)	400	3.5	17.5	60	15	35	5	475	125	0.1	0.5	5	0.03	0.03	0.6	0.06	0.2	8	2
Fast Foods																			
Big Mac	560	26	32	40	160	190	30	1,060	u	u	3.8	40	0.85	0.6	6.5	0.2	u	30	5
Pizza, cheese (1 slice)	150	8	5.5	18	145	125	20	455	85	0.8	0.7	100	0.04	0.1	0.7	u	u	24	5
Fruit																			
Apple	80	0.3	0.5	20	10	10	6	1	159	0.05	0.3	7	0.02	0.02	0.1	0.07	0.1	75	8
Banana	105	1.2	0.6	27	10	20	35	1	450	0.2	0.4	9	0.05	0.1	0.6	0.7	0.3	22	10
Cantaloupe (½)	60	1.4	0.4	13	20	25	15	15	495	0.2	0.3	510	0.06	0.3	0.9	0.18	0.2	27	65
Raisins (¼ cup)	105	1	0.2	28	15	35	10	4	265	0.1	0.7	t	t	t	0.3	0.08	t	1	1

Meat, Fish, Poultry	Calories	Protein (g.)	Fat (g.)	Carbohydrates (g.)	Calcium (mg.)	Phosphorus (mg.)	Magnesium (mg.)	Sodium (mg.)	Potassium (mg.)	Zinc (mg.)	Iron (mg.)	Vitamin A (mcg.)	Thiamin (mg.)	Riboflavin (mg.)	Niacin (mg.)	Vitamin B_6 (mg.)	Pantothenic acid (mg.)	Folic acid (mcg.)	Vitamin C (mg.)
Hamburger, lean (4 oz.)	240	20	16.5	0	10	160	20	50	220	3.7	2.6	10	0.07	0.2	4.5	0.4	0.3	3	0
Steak, sirloin (3 oz.)	330	20	27	0	10	160	20	50	220	3.7	2.5	15	0.05	0.2	4	0.3	0.4	3	0
Salmon steak, broiled (7 oz.)	230	35	9	0	u	530	60	150	565	2.4	1.5	60	0.2	0.08	12.5	1	1.9	30	0
Shrimp, boiled (3 oz.)	100	20.5	0.9	0.6	100	225	45	835	105	1.8	2.7	t	0.01	0.03	1.5	0.05	0.2	10	0
Tuna, canned in water (½ cup)	130	28	0.8	0	15	190	25	865	275	u	1.6	25	0.05	0.1	13	0.4	0.3	15	0
Chicken, fried (½ breast)	220	315	2	16	230	29	75	255	1.1	0.1	15	0.08	0.1	13.5	0	0.6	1	4	0
Chicken, roasted (5 oz.)	240	43.5	6	0	21	300	40	110	345	1.7	1.5	12	0.09	0.2	17.4	0.8	1.4	5	0
Bacon (2 strips)	140	6.5	12.5	1	3	55	5	245	60	1.2	0.8	0	0.1	0.08	1	0.03	0.08	0.5	0
Frankfurter	145	5	13	1	5	40	5	505	75	0.8	0.5	0	0.09	0.05	1.2	0.06	0.2	2	12
Sausage, pork (3 links)	185	11	15	1	15	80	10	720	160	1.4	0.6	0	0.3	0.1	2.2	0.2	0.4	7	t
Pasta																			
Spaghetti, plain (1 cup)	190	6.5	0.7	40	15	85	25	1	105	0.6	0.7	0	0.03	0.03	0.5	0.03	0.2	5	0
Spaghetti and meatballs (1 cup)	330	18.5	11.5	40	125	235	40	1,010	665	3.5	3.7	300	0.2	0.3	4	0.4	0.5	15	20
Vegetables and Legumes																			
Baked beans with pork (½ cup)	160	8	3.5	25	70	115	35	590	270	1	2.3	15	0.1	0.04	0.8	0.4	0.1	30	3
Broccoli (½ cup)	25	2.4	0.2	4	45	45	14	2	190	0.2	0.7	170	0.04	0.09	0.4	0.11	0.2	50	50
Peas (½ cup)	65	4	0.4	11	20	70	20	80	120	0.6	1.2	55	0.2	0.1	0.1	0.1	u	70	8
Potato, baked (1 large)	140	4	0.2	35	15	100	45	5	780	0	0	30	1	10	t	0	20	0	2
Rice, white (enriched) (⅔ cup)	150	3	0.1	35	15	85	10	515	40	0.5	1.2	0	0.2	0.01	1.4	0.05	0.3	12	0
Swiss chard (½ cup)	15	1.5	0.2	2	55	20	45	60	230	u	1.3	390	0.03	0.08	0.3	u	0.1	u	0
Miscellaneous																			
Butter, salted (1 tsp.)	35	t	4	t	1	1	t	40	1	t	t	40	t	t	t	0	0	0	0
Margarine (1 tsp.)	35	t	4	t	1	1	t	50	1	0.01	0	5	0	0	0	0	0	0	0
Eggs, scrambled, with milk (2 eggs)	190	12	14	3	95	195	15	310	170	1.4	1.9	160	0.07	0.3	0.1	0.1	1.8	50	t
Mayonnaise (1 Tbsp.)	100	0.2	11	0.3	3	4	t	80	5	0.02	0.1	10	t	0.01	t	u	0.02	0	0
Peanut butter (1 Tbsp.)	95	4	8	3	10	60	25	95	100	0.4	0.3	0	0.02	0.02	2.4	0.05	0.3	3	0
Tofu (4 oz.)	85	9.5	5	3	155	150	130	10	50	u	2.3	0	0.07	0.04	0.1	u	u	u	0

Are You Overweight?

About 35 percent of Americans tip the scales beyond their optimal level for good health. Our high-fat diet and sedentary lifestyle make it easy to put on the pounds, and difficult to take them off. But getting to a healthy weight is one of the most important things you can do to avoid serious illness.

Why Weight Matters

We don't want to scare you, but the health risks of carting around excess poundage are real. If you're only a few pounds or so overweight, your increased risks are minor, but if you're truly obese—defined as more than 20 percent above your optimal weight or wearing more than 25 percent body fat—these are some of the dangers you're looking at.

• At least twice the risk for high blood pressure; almost six times the risk if you're under 45

• Likelihood of high cholesterol, leading toward clogged arteries

• Higher chances of stroke

• Increased risk of heart disease and heart attack

• Increased risk of colon cancer and prostate cancer

• Increased risk of developing adult-onset diabetes

• Greater likelihood of sleep apnea, gallbladder disease, osteoarthritis, and sexual problems

Here's the case in a nutshell. According to Morton H. Shaevitz, Ph.D., the director of the Eating Disorders Program at Scripps Clinic and Research Foundation, "Fat men die young."

THE PSYCHOLOGICAL DIMENSION

If that's not enough to get you on a healthy diet, think about this: Experts at the National Institutes of Health point to the psychological toll of being overweight—anxiety about health, feelings of shame, self-consciousness.

It's not only women in Western countries who have a negative self-image from comparing themselves to the sculpted forms of fashion supermodels. Millions of men, trying to rebuild deflated self-esteem, are spending a fortune on diets that don't work, fueling the diet industry, worth billion of dollars.

Do You Weigh Too Much?

Obesity is a reality for many of us. But do *you* really have to worry? Research shows that although only about one-third of men are truly overweight, many more than that think they are.

Why are so many of us convinced we're fat? A lot of it has to do with cultural stereotypes: Lean is good, pure and simple. Many international observers are amazed and amused by the American obsession with leanness. We're not saying, "You're only fat if you think you are." On the other hand, the range of healthy, acceptable body shapes and sizes is far greater than certain sections of the media might have us believe.

It comes down to this: Get things in perspective, take a realistic view

Love That Body

The quest for the perfect body. . . If it motivates you to work out regularly and eat a healthy diet, it's a blessing. But it can be insidious. The number of American men dissatisfied with their bodies has risen dramatically. Most of us feel some insecurity and self-doubt when we compare our builds to the hard bodies of actors and athletes.

What can you do about it? First, accept who you are. Your body type is yours for life, and there's only so much you can put on a lean frame or take off a heavy-set one. Get a handle on how much your discomfort may stem from media images most of us will never live up to. You're an individual with your own assets. Appreciate yourself.

▶ *Media images of the "perfect" body make some men feel insecure about their appearance.*

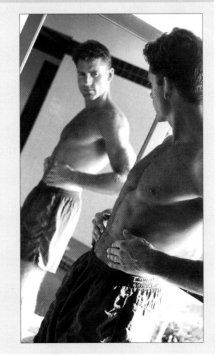

of your body, and don't get fanatical about your weight, or torment yourself with guilt about it.

So it's important to take a realistic line on your weight. How do you do that? As a first step, work out your optimal weight by using the methods that are detailed in "What's Your Optimal Weight?"

It's also important to know the proportion of fat to muscle in your body. If you're a trained athlete or work out a lot, you may have a high percentage of lean muscle mass. Muscle weighs more than fat. Compare a couch potato with a guy who actually uses his health club membership to work out regularly. Both may be the same height and have the same body type—they may even

weigh the same—yet one will be trim and healthy, the other chubby and at risk. Nutritionists say that a body-fat percentage of between 15 and 20 is healthy. Find out how you rate by looking at "How Much Fat Are You Carrying?" on page 62.

You've also got to take into account another factor: your age. Once a man turns 30, his metabolic rate starts to slow down, resulting in an average weight gain of 1 to 1½ pounds per year (unless, that is, calorie intake is reduced and exercise levels increased).

Until recently this was considered bad, period. But some experts say that maybe Mother Nature's not so crazy after all, and that a little weight gain as we go along is okay,

Take the Pinch Test

No, we don't want to know whether you're awake or dreaming. But we do want you to check for a potentially serious risk factor for heart disease and adult-onset diabetes.

For reasons that are not yet fully clear, flab on the hips and buttocks is less of a health risk than a spare tire around the middle. But even more serious is fat you can't see at all. Known as visceral fat, this excess lard lies hidden in the abdominal cavity. If you have an expanded waistline but a hard belly so that you can't grab much flab when you pinch the skin, it might be wise to talk to your doctor.

Subcutaneous fat—the kind you can grab hold of—may not be pretty but it's less of a risk.

What's Your Optimal Weight?

Experts define "overweight" and "underweight" as 10 to 20 percent more or less than your optimal weight. So, what's your optimal weight? Here are two ways to find out.

Since a healthy weight depends on your build, you first need to measure your frame. Use a tape measure (or a piece of string that you can lay against a ruler) and measure the circumference of your wrist, in front of the wrist bones

where the wrist bends. Small-framed men have a circumference less than 6¼ inches, men with medium-size frames are 6¼ – 7 inches, and large-framed men are over 7 inches. Use this frame size in conjunction with the weight tables below to find your optimal weight.

Another method is to determine your Body Mass Index (BMI). You do this by dividing your weight (in pounds) by your height (in inches) squared, and

multiplying the resulting number by 705. You should come out with a BMI between 19 and 30. For example, Ted weighs 160 pounds and is 5 foot 9 (that is, 69 inches). Multiply 69 by 69 to get his height in inches squared, then divide 160 by that number (4,761), giving 0.0336. Multiply that by 705. The result is 23.69. A BMI between 22 and 24 is the healthiest (so Ted makes the cut). You are considered overweight if your BMI is 25 or above.

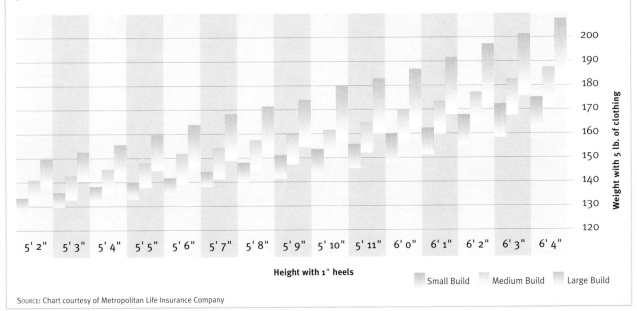

200
190
180
170
160
150
140
130
120

Weight with 5 lb. of clothing

5' 2" 5' 3" 5' 4" 5' 5" 5' 6" 5' 7" 5' 8" 5' 9" 5' 10" 5' 11" 6' 0" 6' 1" 6' 2" 6' 3" 6' 4"

Height with 1" heels

Small Build   Medium Build   Large Build

SOURCE: Chart courtesy of Metropolitan Life Insurance Company

How Much Fat Are You Carrying?

Most men's bodies are roughly 60 percent water and 5 to 6.5 percent minerals, with the remainder divided about equally between fat and protein. From 15 to 20 percent fat is considered healthy, though a trained athlete might have as little as 7 percent, with the rest high-protein muscle.

The diagram below allows you to determine your own body-fat percentage. First, measure your waist, then draw a line from your weight on the left-hand scale to your waist size. The point where the line intersects the diagonal scale (center) will give you a rough estimate.

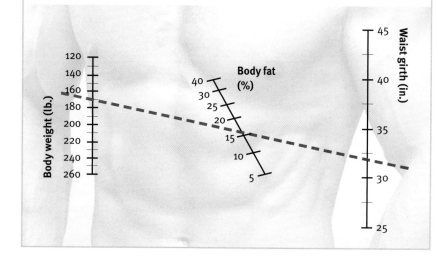

even healthy. The jury's still out on this new point of view. But before you head for the frozen dessert case, keep in mind that this weight gain will happen if you continue to eat just as you are now. Don't go looking for trouble.

Why We Weigh Too Much

If you made a pie chart called "Why we are overweight," one slice might be called "Family: genes and habits." The rest of the pie would be divided into slices labeled "Eat too much," "Don't exercise enough," and "High-fat diet." The problem is that too many of us don't take only one slice, we eat the whole pie! Let's look at these in turn.

FAMILY INHERITANCE

Well, it's not exactly *all* your parents' fault, but nutritional researchers now believe that human beings may be genetically programmed to carry different weights and also different

amounts of body fat. Each one of us may have a biologically determined "setpoint" for fatness, a specific amount of fat our body "wants" to carry, so that no matter how much we diet, it will keep trying to get back to that setpoint.

In other words, what is normal for one person may be high—or low—for someone else. That makes a lot of sense, considering that all sorts of other characteristics, such as height, hair color, body type, and build, run in families.

Genetically, you may inherit from your parents a large body frame, a slow metabolism, and a large number of fat cells. If you get this package, you'll have to work very hard to maintain a healthy weight.

TOO MUCH FOOD, TOO MUCH FAT

Most of us simply eat too much food, more than we need to sustain all the body's activities. If you take in more calories than you burn, the excess

gets converted into fat and stored in fat cells for future use. Little by little the bulges build up.

We also don't get the balance right. Men get 35 to 40 percent of their calories from fat; it should be 25 to 30 percent. Pound for pound and gram for gram, fat is more fattening than other foods. Protein and carbohydrates contain four calories per gram, a gram of fat nine calories. That means you can eat twice as much protein or carbohydrate as fat and still not take in as many calories. Also, fatty foods are readily converted into fat cells; complex carbohydrates and protein, on the other hand, are not.

SEDENTARY LIFESTYLE

How many times have you been reminded of the importance of exercise, and vowed to do more? Yet we'd have pretty good odds if we bet that you didn't do much.

Only 10 to 15 percent of Americans exercise regularly, and vast numbers of us don't get any exercise at all. If you keep stuffing your face and don't burn those calories off, they're going to be staring you in the face from your mirror.

The Curse of the Fat Genes

We all know that heredity plays an important role in determining how much weight we carry. But here's the catch. Genes don't determine what you're going to eat for dinner, or how much you're going to exercise. That part is up to you. A genetic predisposition toward overweight is no more than that: It's not a life sentence. The way you live, and the decisions you make, will ultimately determine whether you get fat.

If you have that genetic tendency, you'll have to work harder—and smarter—to eat foods that are high in fiber and low in fat, foods that fill you up without filling you out.

What Is Fat?

The smell of roasting meat, the taste of sour cream on a baked potato or gobs of butter on fresh warm bread, the smooth, rich feel of ice cream on the tongue—fatty foods have an undoubted allure. We eat far too much of this seductive stuff, though, and for our good health we have to learn to resist its siren song.

What Fat's For

We need fat. It helps maintain our cell membranes and blood vessels, keeps our hair and skin healthy, cushions and insulates our bodies, and it's vital in producing many hormones.

Fat is also the cleanup hitter in your body's energy line-up. Your most concentrated form of energy, it packs nine calories per gram as compared to four calories per gram in both protein and carbohydrates.

This high energy concentration makes fat great for storage. When you consume more food than you need for immediate energy, body-building, or repair, the body converts all the remaining protein and carbohydrate into fat and socks it away (along with fat from the food you eat) for future use.

The fat is stored in billions of cells. These fat cells can shrink way down when they're not needed, but they don't go away. Ever. As they swell up with fat—each one becoming up to a thousand times bigger—so do you.

Later on, if we take in less food than our bodies need, the energy reserves in the fat cells are mobilized for action and burned as fuel. In the course of human evolution this brilliant plan has sustained countless lives through periods of famine, but in affluent societies it has just one result: unhealthy weight gain.

We Eat Too Much Fat

If you aim to be a lard bucket, eating fatty foods is your path to success, as fat has more than twice the calories as carbohydrates and protein. And dietary fat is your body's food of choice for conversion into blubber. While dietary protein and carbohydrates tend to get used up for energy and cell rebuilding, fat quickly becomes part of your spare tire.

Official guidelines say that men should get no more than 30 percent of their daily calories from fat, although more and more experts urge a maximum of 25 percent. For a man consuming 2,500 calories, this would be 69 grams of fat per day.

We Eat the Wrong Fat

As well as eating too much fat, we eat the wrong kind. Butter, hard cheese, french fries, and red meat are but a few of our favorite foods that have high levels of saturated fat, the type that increases blood cholesterol and blocks arteries.

In China, where the daily diet consists essentially of vegetables and rice, the average cholesterol level is 127. In the United States, over half of us have levels over 200. Enough said?

Good Fat, Bad Fat

The fat you eat comes in four varieties: monounsaturated, polyunsaturated, saturated, and hydrogenated. While all dietary fats are rich in calories and tend to add to your bulk, some are better for you than others.

Monounsaturated
These are common in vegetable and nut oils such as olive, canola, and peanut. They raise total cholesterol to a lesser degree than saturated fats, and do not suppress the helpful HDL cholesterol.

Polyunsaturated
This type comes from plants such as sunflowers and safflowers. Although they also raise cholesterol less than saturated fats, they lower the level of HDL and may aid in the development of cancer and suppress the immune system. Use them sparingly.

Saturated
These are numero uno on the no-no list. Found in all animal foods, including meat and dairy products, saturates, which are solid at room temperature, pose the highest risk for heart disease. They are easily converted by your liver into LDL (bad) cholesterol, and can clog up your arteries. They have also been implicated in colon cancer and prostate cancer. Three vegetable oils—coconut, palm, and palm kernel—are also highly saturated and should be avoided.

Hydrogenated
Also called trans-fatty acids, hydrogenated fats are liquid oils that have been chemically altered to make them more solid. Used in margarine and vegetable shortening, they lower HDL cholesterol, clog coronary arteries, and are no better for you than saturated fat.

Getting Back to Lean

If you're tired of your excess flab but discouraged about diets, confused by inconclusive scientific theories, and daunted by "calories from fat" calculations, we have good news for you. Real, lasting, healthful weight loss is possible, and the way to achieve it is really quite simple.

Why Crash Diets Don't Work

We've all seen the advertisements for those miraculous-sounding diet plans: "Lose 30 pounds in two weeks." Sounds very tempting if you happen to be carrying some extra weight. But don't bother; crash diets simply don't work.

Although many people on these diets do lose weight in a short space of time, research shows that most of them—well over 90 percent—eventually regain the weight they lost. That's partly because of a metabolic reaction that kicks in when you stop eating an adequate amount of food.

Basically, your body switches into survival mode and slows itself down to make sure that it won't burn up all its fat stores. When eventually you start eating normally again your metabolism is still slow, so any pounds you may have managed to shuck quickly grow back.

The failure of crash diets also has a lot to do with the fact that they take the pleasure out of eating. Who's going to stick with a daily diet of an apple, carrots, and boiled rice? It's boring! Eating should be a pleasure, and healthy eating is about enjoying a variety of nutritious foods.

Fat-Fighting Tips

Maintaining your weight in a healthy range requires a lifelong program of regular exercise and smart eating. Here are some effective strategies to help you succeed.

• At home, take smaller portions. Use a smaller plate.

• Don't get fanatical. If you push too hard to curtail fat, you'll just spring back. Allow yourself some leeway. Eat ice cream once a week instead of every day—and a cupful rather than a pint!

• Brown bag it. Bring your own low-fat lunch to work. Include fruit, and maybe a lean chicken sandwich.

• Don't eat fatty foods at night. Your digestive capability drops by 20 to 40 percent, and you're not exercising to burn it off.

How to Cut Fat from Your Diet

Most men still get 35 to 40 percent of their daily calories from fat. This is not just unhealthy for your heart; it also makes weight loss difficult, if not impossible. To get back to lean, try to limit yourself to 20 or 25 percent. It's easier than you think, if you follow these guidelines.

• If you eat red meat, use only lean cuts in small portions; better still, switch to fish, and white-meat poultry without the skin.

• Use only nonfat or low-fat dairy products. That means no butter, no sour cream, no ice cream, and no cheese other than low-fat varieties.

• Try no-oil salad dressings, such as plain lemon juice.

• Get out of the habit of adding butter or oil to your food.

• Avoid fried foods. Broil, bake, poach, sauté (in wine or a low-fat broth), or steam rather than fry your food.

• Cook vegetables in broth or water and herbs instead of sautéing them in butter or oil.

• If you eat canned tuna, choose the kind packed in water rather than oil.

• Avoid pastries and rich desserts such as cheesecake.

• Check labels of packaged foods for fat content and reject unhealthy high-fat products.

These are guidelines, not rigid rules. If you have to have a slice of cheese or some ice cream now and then it's no big deal, but make an effort to compensate by cutting down on something else either that day or the next.

Shedding those pounds will take some work, but if you have the long-term commitment, all you need do is follow three simple principles.
• Burn up more calories than you take in.
• Lose weight gradually.
• Make some lifestyle changes.

CALORIES: SLASH AND BURN
"Don't spend more than you earn." Good advice for managing your money, no doubt. But when it comes to weight, forget it. In fact, reverse it.

The only way to melt excess blubber is to burn more calories than you consume—to increase caloric spending while decreasing caloric income—not just today or this week, but for the rest of your life. That's why you need long-term strategies like walking or riding a bicycle to work instead of driving, or switching to nonfat instead of full-fat dairy products, or to fish instead of beef. For most men, simple changes like trimming some fat from the diet and getting a sensible amount of aerobic exercise will be enough.

SLOW AND STEADY WEIGHT LOSS
Maintaining a desirable weight over your lifetime requires more than the intense focus of a quick weight loss. It needs the sustained care of a healthy lifestyle.

It's like the difference between a passionate love affair and a successful marriage. Can you drop 20 pounds in the next six months? Sure. You may even enjoy the challenge. But then what? Once success is gained, most men relax their efforts. Little by little the old eating patterns and sedentary habits—which originally packed on the padding—creep back in. For long-term success, you need a long-term strategy for gradual weight loss.

CHANGE THE WAY YOU LIVE
High-fat eating habits and a sedentary lifestyle have almost certainly brought you to the point you're at now. To reverse the situation, and lose weight permanently, you need to change that lifestyle. That comes down to making consistent changes in your day-to-day living that will improve your diet and increase your physical activity.

We're not saying you have to turn your entire life upside down, either; straightforward changes to diet and exercise will do the trick.

How to Refocus Your Diet

Serious about changing your diet? First of all you need a healthy, varied diet, full of tasty foods that you'll look forward to eating. Swear off the junk, and head for the fresh food in the produce section. Instead of packaged food, sweets, and greasy fast food, fill up with vegetables, fruit,

Tasty Substitutes for High-Fat Favorites

We know you love those luscious high-fat foods and treats. But it is possible to learn to live without them and still enjoy delicious, satisfying meals and snacks. As much as you can, substitute low fat for high fat.

High-Fat Food	Low-Fat Substitute
Whole-milk products, including milk, yogurt, full-fat cheeses	Nonfat or low-fat milk, yogurt, cottage cheese, reduced-fat cheeses
Sour cream	Nonfat or low-fat yogurt
Ice cream	Frozen nonfat yogurt, sorbet
Ground beef	Ground chicken or turkey
Fish canned in oil	Fish canned in water
Mayonnaise	Nonfat mayonnaise
Salad dressing with oil	Oil-free dressings
Cream-based soups	Broth-based soups
Chocolate-chip cookies	Fig bars, ginger snaps
Doughnuts	Bagels with jelly
Potato or nacho chips	Pretzels, bread sticks, air-popped popcorn
Roasted peanuts	Raisins, dried apricots

What Difference Does it Make?

Not convinced about the benefits of low-fat eating? The chart below might change your mind. It compares the calorie and fat content of a variety of snacks, both good (low fat, low calorie) and bad (high fat, high calorie). See the difference?

Calories	Snack	Fat
840	Roasted nuts (1 cup)	71 g.
435	Raisins (1 cup)	1 g.
350	Premium vanilla ice cream (1 cup)	24 g.
173	Vanilla frozen yogurt (1 cup)	1 g.
210	Potato chips (20)	14 g.
108	Air-popped popcorn (1 oz.)	1 g.
289	Jelly doughnut	16 g.
204	Bagel with jelly	2 g.

which is high in saturated fats, or at least buy the leanest cuts. As a substitute, eat more fish and poultry.

LIGHTEN UP ON DESSERT

When you crave something sweet at the end of a meal, look for something light and nonfatty. Do as many Europeans do: Have a piece of fruit. Chewing on a juicy, crunchy apple will satisfy the craving with no fat and very few calories. Or just get up from the table and brush your teeth. Many times that clean, minty feeling will completely satisfy your desire to eat something sweet.

ALCOHOL AND WEIGHT

Alcohol in moderation may be good for your heart, but it won't make things easier if you are trying to lose weight. Drinking two 12-ounce cans of beer a day for a month adds up to about the same number of calories as 65 filet mignons!

Also, since your body can't store alcohol, it has to burn it up right away. While you're burning alcohol, you're not burning fat. Finally, alcohol is an appetite stimulant that's usually not served with carrot sticks and salads, but with high-fat cheese, meat, chips, and dips. If you really want to lose weight, cutting back on the booze is almost a necessity.

legumes, whole-grain breads, and cereals. These foods contain a lot of complex carbohydrates, which are not only packed with vitamins and minerals, but are fat-burners—your body has to work hard to digest them. To transform 100 calories of complex carbohydrates into body fat, the body uses 23 calories. Only 3 calories are needed to convert 100 calories of dietary fat into body fat.

Complex carbohydrates are also good sources of fiber. Vegetables, fruit, whole grains, and legumes are not only low in calories and extremely low in fat, they're also more filling and take longer to chew, so you're likely to eat less.

To increase your daily intake of complex carbohydrates:
• Eat more legumes such as lentils, kidney beans, pinto beans, and navy beans.
• Increase your intake of salads and cooked vegetables.
• Use whole-grain bread rather than white bread.
• Eat more potatoes, either baked or boiled, never fried.
• Choose whole-grain cereals, such as oatmeal.

Of course, you need more than just extra carbohydrates. You've still got to cut a lot of the fatty and other waistline-expanding items from the old days and replace them with low-fat alternatives you'll enjoy eating.

DOWN WITH FAT

Cutting fat from your diet is the key to your weight-loss program, along with regular exercise. The textbooks say that you should get about 30 percent of your daily calories from fat, but to lose weight, you'll probably have to cut down to 20 to 25 percent or even less.

Follow the guidelines in the Food Guide Pyramid (see "Secrets of the Pyramid" on page 55), in particular, eating fatty foods, oils, and sweets sparingly. Cut down on red meat,

How to Use Food Labels to Spot Fat

The "Nutrition Facts" panel required by the government on all packaged food gives you a pretty complete picture of what you're about to eat. For example, it tells you exactly how many grams of fat per serving, how much is saturated fat, and how many of the calories come from fat. There are also rules for product labeling.

• Fat free: less than ½ gram of fat per serving

• Low fat: 3 grams of fat or less per serving

• Reduced fat: at least 25 percent less fat than the regular product

• Light: One-third the calories or half the fat has been eliminated

• Lean (meat): fewer than 10 grams of fat per 100-gram serving

• Extra lean (meat): fewer than 5 grams of fat per 100 grams

Make sure that you check the serving size (also given on the label) and compare it to the amount you're actually going to eat.

Slow Down to Savor the Flavor

The faster you wolf down your food, the more you can devour in one meal. So if you want to eat less, slow down. It takes about 20 minutes for your body's internal feedback loop to let you know you've eaten enough. If you eat too quickly, you're likely to eat more than you need without realizing it. To help you slow down:

• Sit down to eat in a calm and settled atmosphere.

• At the start of the meal, take a moment to relax. Sit quietly and close your eyes. Take a few deep breaths and let tension melt away.

• Put your fork down after each mouthful. Chew and swallow all the food from one mouthful before loading up your fork again.

• Take time to really savor the taste and texture of your food.

The Importance of Exercise

Another reason diet plans fail is that many of them concentrate only on cutting back on fattening foods. Exercise is missing from the equation. Regular exercise goes hand-in-hand with a sensible, low-fat diet.

Aerobic exercise—sustained, rhythmic exercise using the large muscles of the body—helps you lose weight by stepping up the rate at which your body burns fuel, not just while you're exercising but for several hours after you stop.

Jogging, swimming, cycling, skiing, as well as action sports like basketball or tennis, are excellent ways to get your blood going and your fat burning. Three or four weekly workouts of 30 minutes each should be about right.

Getting more exercise doesn't necessarily mean health-club memberships, special clothing, or expensive equipment. It just means increasing your daily physical activity. Do more chores around the house. Take a half-hour walk every day, in the early morning, at your lunch break, or when you get home. Park your car a mile or so from work and walk the rest of the way. Ride a bicycle to work, or do errands or minor shopping by bike or on foot.

WHY YOU NEED MUSCLES

Besides aerobic fitness, you must also maintain muscle mass. From about age 30, unless you work to prevent it, you start losing a pound or so of muscle a year and trading it in for fat as your body's metabolism slows. "To wage war most effectively against fat, you need to be a good calorie-burning machine 24 hours a day, and having adequate muscle tissue is the only way to do that," says Bryant A. Stamford, Ph.D., former director of the Exercise Physiology Laboratory at the University of Louisville, Kentucky and co-author of *Fitness without Exercise*. That's because muscles burn more calories than fat. You'll burn 30 to 50 more calories a day, awake or asleep, for each additional pound of muscle.

To keep muscles toned or to build them up a little, you don't have to become a body-builder. Household jobs like raking and sweeping can accomplish all you need. If you prefer, a few minutes of weight training or even working out with a pair of five-pound dumbbells twice a week can build muscle mass and contribute toward a healthier weight.

Now's the Time to Break Sedentary Habits

Overweight? Do you spend most of your life sitting? Think there might be a connection? Just getting off your butt for a few minutes several times a day will help shed those pounds.

At Home
• If you're set up for it, go out and shoot some baskets.

• Pedal an exercise bike while watching television or while you're on the phone.

• While talking on the phone, walk around instead of sitting.

• Make chores part of your fitness plan. Rake leaves, shovel snow, sweep the sidewalk or driveway.

At Work
• Walk at least five minutes away to eat your lunch.

• Use all or part of your break time to take a short walk.

• Pass up the elevator and take the stairs. It burns calories and revs up your metabolism.

At the Mall
• Park far away from the shop you want to visit.

• Use the stairs instead of the escalator, or walk up the escalator.

▶ *Break those old habits. At lunch, get away from your desk and go for a walk.*

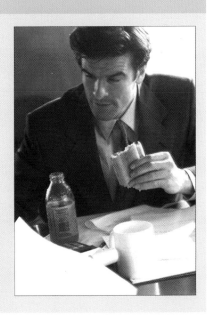

Guilt-Free, Damage-Free Drinking

Is alcohol good for you? The answer is an enthusiastic yes, if—and only if—you keep your drinking under control. Studies show that moderate drinkers have healthier hearts and live longer than either heavy drinkers or abstainers. The problem is that not everybody can call it quits after a couple of drinks.

The Benefits of Booze

If you are among the 115 million Americans who take a wee drop now and then, chances are you don't do it for health reasons, but because a little alcohol in your blood makes you feel good. Tension, stress, and inhibitions drop away. You feel relaxed, and you're likely to have a sense of well-being, even mild euphoria. And drinking is central to the social lives of many people.

Now we also know that downing a couple of drinks a day increases the level of HDL cholesterol, which helps carry away the artery-clogging "bad" LDL cholesterol. Harvard researchers found an average HDL increase of 17 percent; that translates into a 40 percent reduction in heart disease risk. It's also been found that alcohol decreases the blood's ability to form clots, which block blood vessels and cause heart attacks and stroke.

Alcohol and You

The effects of alcoholic drinks differ dramatically from person to person. Some men feel sleepy or get a headache from just a few sips, and may show definite signs of impaired judgment and perception after just one drink. Many men think they can handle a lot more—and some apparently can, though in the long run they will have a price to pay.

Here are some effects of drinking, divided into three categories. Note that many of the effects are in the gray area between moderate and excessive use, depending on the individual.

Moderate Drinking

• Accelerated heart rate

• Feelings of relaxation

• Feelings of exhilaration or joy

• Reduced risk of heart disease

• Mood swings

• Increased sexual desire; likelihood of decreased performance

Moderate to Heavy Drinking

• Headaches and hangovers

• Disruption of normal sleep patterns

• Slurred speech

• Memory lapses

• Impaired judgment, perception, and/or coordination

Heavy Drinking

• Feelings of depression and despondency

• Greater risk of heart disease

• Damaged heart muscle

• Stomach irritation and ulcers

• Liver disease

• Pancreas disorders

• High blood pressure

• Overweight

• Impotence

• Violent and/or erratic behavior

RED OR WHITE?
Is red wine better for you than white? Does it really matter what type of drink you have? A 1992 book, *The French Paradox*, argued that the consumption of red wine was behind the low rate of heart disease in France, a country with a notoriously high-fat cuisine.

But that wasn't the end of the story. A large study (some 81,000 drinkers) at Kaiser Permanente Medical Center in Oakland, California, found that those who drank *white* wine had the least heart disease.

Finally, Harvard Medical School put an end to the confusion. It reported that moderate drinking—whether it is beer, wine, or hard liquor—cuts heart attack risk. The magic elixir, then, seems to be the alcohol itself, not the form it's in.

MODERATION IS THE KEY

The benefits of alcohol depend on moderation. For most men, one or two drinks a day is considered to be moderate; anything greater than two is too much. A drink is defined as a ½ ounce of alcohol, in whatever form you like it: 5 ounces of wine, 12 ounces of beer, or 1½ ounces of 80-proof liquor. If you have a large frame, you may be able to handle a little more.

And Now, the Bad News

Medical research has shown that if you cross the line from moderate drinking, all the positives go down the tube. Instead of preventing heart disease, drinking can actually cause it, raising the risk of heart attack and stroke by damaging heart muscles and raising blood pressure. And there's more...

The consequences of heavy drinking cannot be exaggerated. Chronic alcohol abuse can seriously damage just about every organ in your body. The following is a short list:

Take Control of Your Drinking

• Set a limit and stick to it. Unless you have a large, muscular frame, your limit should be two drinks.

• Eat something first. Food in the belly slows absorption and reduces the severity of hangovers.

• Drink slowly. Limit yourself to one drink per hour.

• Don't drink every day. You may build up a tolerance and start drinking more. Take an occasional day off.

• Don't drink to elevate your mood. It won't work. Despite initial euphoria, alcohol is a depressant.

• Alternate alcoholic with nonalcoholic drinks. Have a plain soda or mineral water between drinks.

• Just say "no." The social pressure you feel may be all in your head.

• Skip the bubbly stuff. Champagne or drinks mixed with carbonated water are absorbed faster.

• Brain cells are destroyed; also, CT scans show that the brain itself actually shrinks.

• Nerve damage can lead to impotence; alcohol's toxic effects on sperm can cause infertility.

• A variety of liver diseases may develop, including liver cancer and potentially fatal cirrhosis.

• Digestion is impaired; the stomach and large and small intestines may become inflamed, and the pancreas damaged.

As well as the physiological damage, alcohol abuse gives rise to a range of social problems, including violent behavior, accidents of all kinds, job loss, family disruption and disharmony. Half of all traffic deaths and at least a quarter of murders and suicides are alcohol-related.

The bottom line is this: Enjoy the pleasures and benefits of moderate drinking, but be careful not to risk the dangers of excess. They're pretty grim. Set limits and stick to them.

How Much Alcohol Is in Your Blood?

Experts say up to two drinks a day will keep you not only in the safety zone, but will reap the rewards of alcohol as a preventer of heart disease and stroke. If you're thinking of going beyond this, this chart will tell you what you're getting into. When using the chart, subtract 0.015 for every hour you've been drinking, since alcohol leaves the bloodstream with time.

Keep in mind that at a blood level of 0.05 percent, alcohol is your friend (so long as you don't try to drive). At 0.10 you're legally drunk; at 0.20 you're likely to pass out; around 0.32, you're endangering your life. Most states will take away your license for driving with a blood alcohol content of 0.08 percent, some at 0.10.

One drink is equal to 1¹/2 ounces of 80-proof liquor, 12 ounces of beer, or 5 ounces of wine.

Number of drinks	Body weight (lb.)							
	100	120	140	160	180	200	220	240
1	0.04	0.04	0.03	0.03	0.02	0.02	0.02	0.02
2	0.09	0.07	0.06	0.06	0.05	0.04	0.04	0.04
3	0.13	0.11	0.09	0.08	0.07	0.07	0.06	0.06
4	0.18	0.15	0.13	0.11	0.10	0.09	0.08	0.07
5	0.22	0.18	0.16	0.14	0.12	0.11	0.10	0.09
6	0.26	0.22	0.19	0.17	0.15	0.13	0.12	0.11
7	0.31	0.26	0.22	0.19	0.17	0.15	0.14	0.13
8	0.35	0.29	0.25	0.22	0.20	0.18	0.16	0.15
9	0.40	0.33	0.28	0.25	0.22	0.20	0.18	0.17
10	0.44	0.37	0.31	0.28	0.24	0.22	0.20	0.18

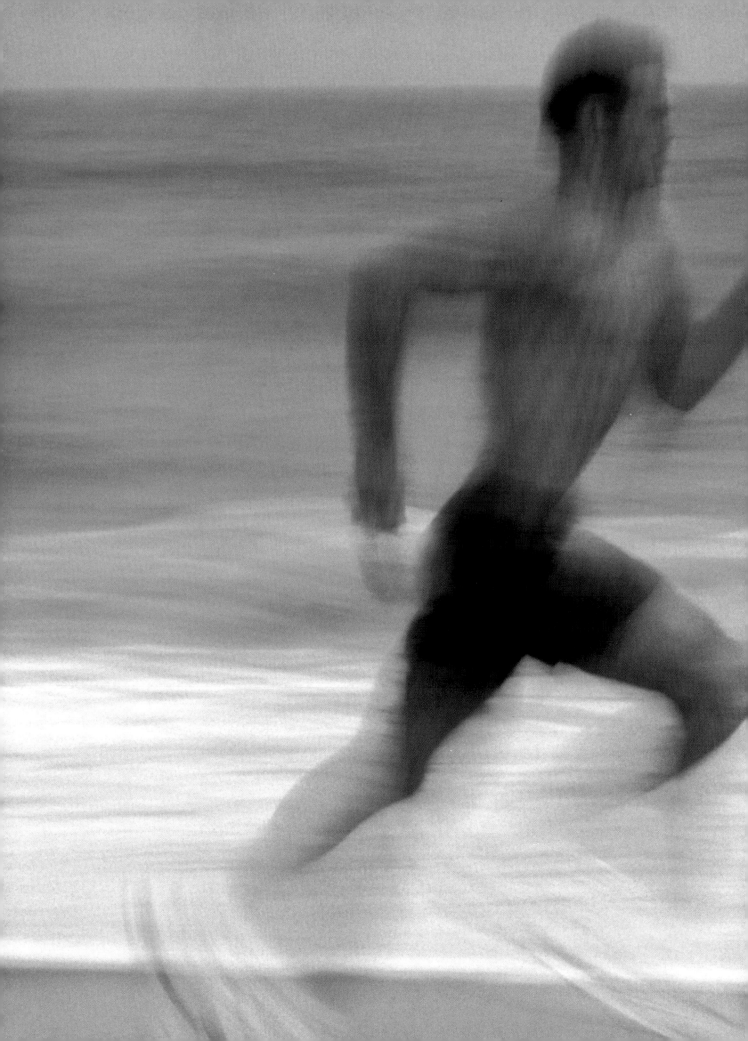

Exercise
and Health

The Value of Exercise

You're busy, you're tired, you've got better things to do. So why exercise? Not so long ago, men didn't ask that question because exercise was what we did all day long in the course of manual labor. That's largely not true anymore. And that's why we need exercise: Our bodies are designed for it.

The Physical Benefits

The consequences of not exercising are evident in the man who is seriously overweight, wheezes when climbing a flight of stairs, can't get near to touching his toes, and suffers from minor muscular aches and pains, or certain forms of diabetes.

The physical benefits of exercise are likewise easy to see—and feel. As fitness improves, the body composition moves from fat to muscle, producing a leaner, more limber, and more classically chiseled you.

Let's look at the three components of exercise: strength, endurance, and flexibility. Together, they add up to a body that is simply more elegant and attractive.

STRENGTH

Strength training fortifies an inherently masculine trait: possessing large, powerful muscles that enable you to lift heavy objects, as well as effortlessly accomplish mundane yet important tasks such as prying loose a nail, or suavely opening a bottle of champagne while soft music plays.

ENDURANCE

Endurance (also known as cardiovascular or aerobic) training enables the muscles, lungs, and heart to generate energy efficiently during sustained, vigorous activity, whether it's running, hiking, mountain biking, or skiing—or meeting everyday demands such as running for a train.

Do You Need a Physical?

Maybe you'd take a new car on a long journey, but as the miles pile up, it's increasingly wise to look under the hood first. For men, a checkup becomes mandatory if:

• You're over 40. You may be in fine shape overall, but it's natural for a few glitches to start showing up. At minimum, a thorough medical exam at this age provides a benchmark for what happens in the future.

• You're at risk for cardiovascular disease. Danger signs include a family history of heart disease; a total cholesterol level of 200 or more, or a total-to-HDL cholesterol ratio of 3 or more; high blood pressure; a pronounced pot belly; bruises that heal slowly, frequent infections, or tingling or numbness in the hands and feet; and smoking.

FLEXIBILITY

Often treated by men as an afterthought, flexibility exercises can help prevent problems caused by tight muscles, such as soreness and,

---

Keep Fit to Feel Younger

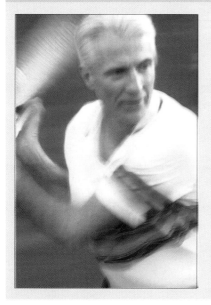

Exercise can lengthen your life and—more importantly—your years of good health. Among experts on aging, it's a truism that most of the changes we think inevitably result from growing older are actually due to de-conditioning, which is not only preventable, it's reversible. Studies have found, for example, that nine months of aerobic training can improve cardiovascular performance by 25 percent even in men age 60 to 72.

Age-related decline certainly takes place. Starting around age 30, overall physiologic function drops at the rate of about 1 percent a year. The fitter you are,

◄ *Keep fit through regular exercise and you'll extend your youth.*

however, the higher you'll be on the physical capacity chart as decline occurs. For that reason, it's possible for fit older men to have the strength and aerobic capacity of sedentary men half their age. Put another way, by age 70, a lean man who has long performed three hours of aerobic exercise weekly stands to be twice as fit than a sedentary man of the same age.

Exercise (combined with a proper diet) will stave off midriff padding, maintain suppleness, keep the heart healthy, retard bone loss, and make you less vulnerable to injury. Just make sure you keep your choices of activities appropriate to your age. For more information see page 78.

especially, lower-back pain. Good flexibility also helps keep you strong because your muscles become more powerful only within the range of motion through which they're put, so the more muscles you move, the suppler you will become.

The Mental Benefits

The psychological payoffs from regular exercise are less tangible than the physical ones. But they are very real nonetheless.

Stress, for example, has always been a part of modern life. It's the basic fight-or-flight instinct, a primer for physiological action triggered in the brain. Yet, in modern life (as we sit at a computer or behind the wheel of a car at high speed or stuck in a traffic jam), mental stress has no physical release. Exercise provides this and more, giving a sense of well-being, boosting problem-solving ability, offsetting anxiety, minimizing depression, and promoting good sleep.

The Overall Health Benefits

The combined mind-and-body benefits of exercise produce dramatic effects on total health. A body that is less stressed, has less fat, contains more muscle, and is cardiovascularly fit is less prone to heart disease and certain forms of cancer, has stronger bones, is better able to sustain sexual vitality, and possesses a more highly charged immune system. That translates to a longer life and better health to the end.

How Fit Are You?

Every exercise program needs benchmarks. The simple exercises below provide baselines for several fundamental measures of fitness. At intervals after starting a fitness program, check your progress by repeating the tests.

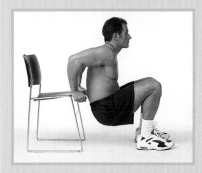

Upper Body Strength

Exercise: Chair dips.

Method: Sit on the edge of a chair. Place your hands on the chair's front edge and inch your butt off and away from the chair while supported by your hands. Keep your back straight. Slowly lower yourself until your upper arms are parallel with the floor, then lift back up. Do as many as you can.

Good result: 10 dips.

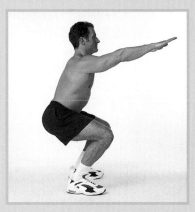

Lower Body Strength

Exercise: Slow squat.

Method: Stand with feet flat on the floor, shoulder-width apart. Time yourself while, moving as slowly as you can, you bend your knees until your thighs are parallel with the floor, then slowly raise yourself back up. (Balance yourself with outstretched arms.) Take as long as you can; even if you tire, complete the entire move.

Good result: 60 seconds.

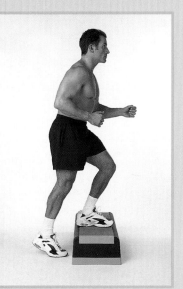

Aerobic Fitness

Exercise: Step test.

Method: Step up with one foot, then the other, then step down with one foot, then the other. Each up-up, down-down cycle is one count. Do about 20 counts per minute for 3 minutes. Take your pulse, counting for 15 seconds, then multiplying by 4.

Good result: 95 or below if you're already moderately active and in your thirties or forties.

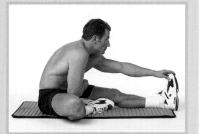

Flexibility

Exercise: Toe touch.

Method: Sit with your left leg straight in front of you, right foot tucked against your left thigh. Reach your left arm as far as you can toward your toes.

Good result: Wrist to toe.

Exercise Choices

Deciding what exercises you should do and at what intensity involves a range of factors that vary from person to person. These include your age, your current physical condition, your body type, and your goals, not to mention your definition of fun. The basic question, however, is where to start.

Body Under Construction

You probably tend to think in terms of "building up" the body. The truth is that becoming fitter is as much a process of tearing down as it is of building up.

The only kind of exercise that will produce gains in strength or endurance is the kind that calls on muscles to go beyond their usual level of exertion. Physiologists call it the overload principle: If you repeatedly tax muscles, they'll adapt to the new demands. This occurs as a kind of reconstruction project, in which exercise first tears muscles down—exhausting them, making them weak, and causing microscopic areas of damage. The body then rebuilds the damaged muscles, but fortifies them to better withstand similar abuse. The muscles are made larger, more powerful, and more efficient.

To keep this process of tearing down and building up going, however, requires a bit of balance. You want to tear down enough to make your body respond and improve, but not so much that soreness or injury hobbles your efforts or saps your motivation.

For this reason, it's important to start exercising at a level that's appropriate to your condition. From there, you can gradually add demands to your body—lifting more weight, running more miles, swimming more laps, increasing the intensity or duration of exercise.

Body Type and Exercise

Are you tall with lots of muscle? Or narrow-shouldered and weedy? A bit pudgy? The way you are built comes about partly through the characteristics of your muscles.

One type of muscle contracts rapidly and expends energy in short bursts. Called fast-twitch fiber, it's ideally suited to activities requiring quick bursts of force, such as sprinting and power lifting. Another type of muscle contracts less rapidly and expends energy more gradually. Called slow-twitch fiber, it's ideally suited to endurance activities such as cycling and running.

Your body is a mix of both types of muscle, but one type usually predominates. Knowing which it is can help you decide what exercises best suit you. How do you find this out? Look in the mirror. If you're long and thin with little fat (an ectomorph), your muscles are mostly slow-twitch and you'll probably have

> **"It's difficult to have optimal levels of everything at once, because different types of conditioning require different types of training. You have to decide what you want from training in order to design a program that will achieve satisfying results."**
>
> Alan Mikesky, Ph.D., director, Human Performance Laboratory, Indiana University–Purdue University, Indianapolis, Indiana

---

How to Get Started

If you're new to exercise or have laid off it for quite some time, starting a new program can feel awkward. It's difficult to know how to proceed. The danger is that many men tend to do too much too soon, or fail to overcome initial discouragement—and eventually give up due to soreness or lack of motivation. To gird yourself both mentally and physically, follow these precepts.

Check with Your Physician
A thorough exam will help you anticipate any unforeseen limitations or dangers.

Consult a Trainer
A gym staffer or personal trainer can help you evaluate your goals and program, alerting you to inefficiencies, unrealistic expectations, proper techniques, and safety aspects.

Start Easy
Guys tend to go all-out. Rein yourself in at first, starting out by doing less than you know you can. Then start to increase the intensity, duration, or frequency of your exercise—but by no more than 10 to 15 percent per week.

Invest in Exercise
Funds put toward a gym membership or good piece of gear can increase motivation to see an exercise program succeed. But if you're new to a sport, borrow or rent gear at first, to make sure that this particular activity is where you want to lay your money.

Get Social
The more that friends or family are involved with (or at least support) your exercise program, the more likely you are to stick with it.

greater success with aerobic exercise. If you're stocky and beefy (an endomorph), you have more fast-twitch fiber, and you'll likely do best with anaerobic weight lifting. If you're somewhere in between (a mesomorph), you may enjoy equal degrees of success no matter what you do.

If you've made overall fitness your goal, a well-rounded exercise program should consist of both endurance and strength training. Based on your body type, however, it's likely that one form of exercise will be easier, produce greater gains, and perhaps be more fun.

Home or Gym?

Ideally, you'll exercise at both home and a gym. That's the arrangement that most reliably ensures you'll stick with a program. But it's often a choice between one or the other. Here are the relative merits of each.

Home

- Convenient, open all hours
- No crowds or annoying patrons
- Total control of the radio or TV dial
- After initial outlay, cheaper to maintain
- Less self-consciousness
- Workouts take less time

Gym

- Better equipment, and more of it
- Trained staff to advise you
- Scene provides validation, encouragement, motivation
- Surroundings more appealing
- Social opportunities
- Larger clubs may provide childcare

Recognize Yourself? You and Your Body Type

Do you yearn for a leaner, more muscular look? A flatter belly, more powerful arms, a sculptured chest?

The truth is that each of us has inherited a genetic blueprint for one of three physical types, and this basic frame is going to define us all our lives, setting some natural limits. The good news is that even though we can't change our bone structure, we can learn to make the best of it, modifying and shaping what's on those bones through diet and proper exercise.

Ectomorphs
These are the light, lean types, lacking in muscle but long on speed and agility. They have slender frames and fast metabolic rates. Their muscles are mainly of the slow-twitch variety, making them ideal candidates for aerobic exercise. Even moderately active ectomorphs will always remain essentially lean.

Mesomorphs
Strong and muscular, with broad shoulders, narrow waists, and only a small proportion of body fat, these guys are the natural athletes among us. The model of manhood in our culture, they only have to show up to make most of us feel inferior. Their only drawback is that if they're not careful they can put on weight, even grow a spare tire.

Endomorphs
Blessed by nature with a large build full of muscles containing fast-twitch fiber, endomorphs can easily grow muscles and develop great strength. If they exercise and watch what they eat they can maintain excellent health. But with their slow metabolism, if they're not careful they will almost certainly pack on the pounds.

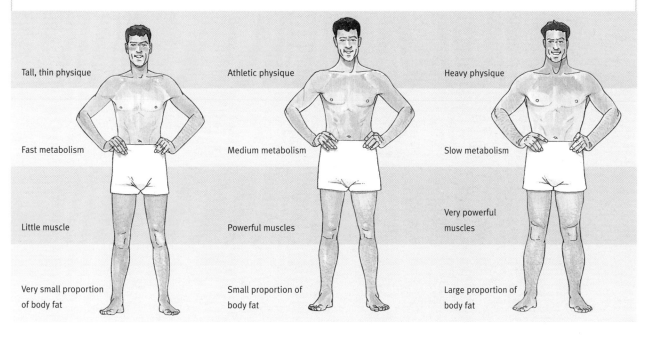

Tall, thin physique

Fast metabolism

Little muscle

Very small proportion of body fat

Athletic physique

Medium metabolism

Powerful muscles

Small proportion of body fat

Heavy physique

Slow metabolism

Very powerful muscles

Large proportion of body fat

Types of Exercise

There are three basic forms of exercise—aerobic and anaerobic exercise, and stretching. Each of these forms corresponds to the three elements—strength, endurance, and flexibility—that go together to make up overall fitness. How exactly do these three differ from each other?

AEROBIC EXERCISE

Aerobic exercise promotes both endurance and cardiovascular fitness. Activities tend to be long in duration and call upon not only the muscles required to sustain movement, but also upon the entire cardiovascular system—the heart, lungs, and blood vessels—whose job it is to oxygenate and circulate energy-bearing blood.

Efficient delivery of oxygen is the end-all of aerobics. With increased aerobic conditioning, the lungs become better at taking oxygen in, and the heart and blood vessels become better at delivering it to muscles. Diet is involved as well, with energy from food (particularly carbohydrates) being stored as glucose in cells awaiting a chance to be unleashed by contact with oxygen. With improved aerobic capacity, individual cells are also better able to accomplish the alchemy of energy transformation.

ANAEROBIC EXERCISE

Short and sharp, anaerobic exercise doesn't involve the aerobic system. Instead, energy is derived for the most part directly from glucose stored in the muscles themselves. Glucose is quickly exhausted with intense effort, so anaerobic effort rapidly fatigues muscles. Weight lifting is anaerobic, and strength, in part, is a function of how much effort muscles can put forth before failing.

In anaerobic exercise, muscles must work against some form of resistance—that's why weight lifting is sometimes referred to as resistance training. Progress is measured by increasing amounts of resistance rather than increases in distance or time. For example, if you are bench pressing 150 pounds in two sets of 8 to 12 repetitions, your goal generally speaking is not to lift the same amount of weight more times as you

What's on the Exercise Menu?

Which exercises you choose to do are as much a matter of preference as necessity. Your body type may determine which exercise is best for you, but other factors include what you like doing, what equipment you have (or are willing to invest in), and what fits best into your social or family schedule.

Golf
Benefits: Mild aerobic benefit, but only if you walk the course. Gets you outdoors. Social aspect valuable for mental health.
Drawbacks: If you ride a cart, it's just not exercise. High potential for back and spine injury. On-going cost of greens fees.

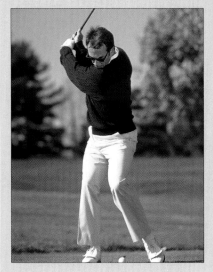

Bicycling
Benefits: Builds aerobic conditioning and tones leg muscles. Excitement comes from speed (for road bikes) and navigating natural obstacles (for mountain bikes). You can bike to work or to the store and count it as exercise. Easy to do indoors with stationary equipment.
Drawbacks: Muscle benefits largely limited to legs. Can be dangerous because of cars (road riding) or logs, rocks, and steep descents (off-road riding).

Swimming
Benefits: Combines aerobic and whole-body muscular conditioning. Low-impact. Water keeps you cool even in most vigorous workouts.
Drawbacks: Need training in basic skills and safety. On-going cost of pool access.

Weight Lifting
Benefits: The most effective way to build total-body strength. Equipment is simple to use. Results come quickly.
Drawbacks: Can be dull. Without proper technique, may be tough on joints. Free weights in particular can be dangerous.

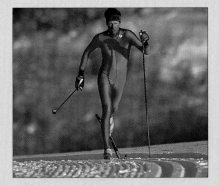

Cross-Country Skiing
Benefits: Super calorie-burner. Works both upper and lower body. Less injury potential than downhilling. Don't need mountains, ski lifts, or snooty powder scene. Machines allow you to take it indoors.
Drawbacks: When outdoors, more dependent on weather than downhilling (no snow machines in nature). Rentals a problem outside of ski resorts, so you may need your own gear. Lacks the excitement of downhilling.

Inline Skating
Benefits: Aerobic training that also conditions the lower body. Fun and fast. Can be done close to home. Gear relatively inexpensive.
Drawbacks: Instruction on skill and technique advisable. High injury potential.

become stronger, but to lift a heavier weight within the same range of sets and repetitions.

STRETCHING

Beyond the benefits of providing greater range of motion, flexibility does little to improve physical conditioning as such. But it's important nonetheless, because limber muscles are less prone to injury and soreness. Loss of flexibility is one of the earliest signs of aging. Attention to this aspect of fitness will help retard the creakiness that can set in as early as the twenties or thirties, and make you less tentative in your movements while performing a wide range of activities, from mowing the lawn to making love.

Five Essential Training Tips

Think of a workout less as a routine than a ritual, characterized by familiar movements and rhythms that evolve into a discipline. Each part of the ritual serves a physical purpose, but also provides a solid mental structure to your efforts. Here are the essential elements.

1 Warm up. For the first 5 to 10 minutes, do a light aerobic activity, such as running on the spot. It'll get your blood moving, loosen up muscles, and prepare the nervous system for vigorous movement.

2 Stretch. Now that muscles are warm and pliable, stretch them gently to open up your range of motion while focusing on what you intend to accomplish in your workout. Stretching should take only about 5 minutes.

3 Push yourself. After the first few weeks, you should work muscles to fatigue if you want to make measurable gains. When muscles nearly can't take it, think, "This is the part that counts."

4 Cool down. Just as you started gradually, end the same way. Do 5 to 10 minutes of light aerobics, walking or stretching. It'll keep your muscles from becoming overly tight and provide a mental transition.

5 Drink water. During vigorous aerobic activity, your body loses sweat at an hourly rate 258 times greater than at rest. Losing just 2 percent of your body weight in water can cut your capacity for prolonged effort by 10 percent. Refresh body and soul often, and don't wait for thirst to hit.

Racket Sports
Benefits: Vigorous aerobic and muscular exercise. Highly competitive nature makes it exciting.
Drawbacks: Exceptionally tough on joints. Need access to courts. Highly competitive aspect may make it intimidating for some.

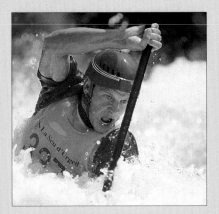

Kayaking
Benefits: Great for upper body conditioning. Satisfies manly attraction to water à la Melville—and seagoers can get as close to whales as Ahab (though experts advise against it).
Drawbacks: Prospect of hanging upside down underwater. Learning to do an Eskimo roll is daunting, but essential.

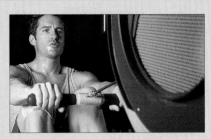

Rowing
Benefits: An aerobic activity that also tones muscles in both the upper and lower body. Low-impact.
Drawbacks: Monotonous after a while if indoors. Mass-market rowing machines are sometimes shoddy.

Running
Benefits: The quintessential aerobic exercise. Good shoes the only equipment needed. Can do anywhere, anytime.
Drawbacks: High-impact; can be hard on lower-body joints. Shoes need to be replaced regularly.

Downhill Skiing/Snowboarding
Benefits: Great exercise for legs. Changing conditions provide endless variety and thrills. Use of reflexes in brisk outdoors invigorating.
Drawbacks: Premium on skill. High injury potential. Need to bankroll gear, clothes, travel, and lift fees.

Stairclimbing
Benefits: Good aerobic workout that's easy on bones and joints. Can do year-round. Movement is one you actually use in real life.
Drawbacks: Steppers work only lower body. Can be boring.

Hiking
Benefits: Good, low-impact aerobic exercise. Natural surroundings a balm for the soul. Only a sturdy pair of shoes needed for daytrips.
Drawbacks: May need to travel to trails. Low on action.

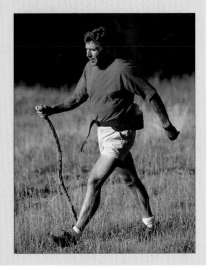

Exercise According to Your Age

The older you are, the more careful you need to be about embarking on an exercise program. But aging is certainly no reason to give up exercise. In fact, although many men taper their activity levels as they get older, remaining active is the surest way to retain youth as the years steadily advance.

Keep Fit through the Years

The basic weight-training exercises described in "Exercises for Improving Strength" on page 92 provide the core routine for any age, but the mix of resistance training, aerobics, and stretching changes slightly from decade to decade. Here are some considerations and suggestions, decade by decade.

YOUR TWENTIES

At this age, you're at your physical peak and exercise may seem unnecessary, if not a waste of time. But now is when you establish habits and priorities that will carry you forward later, when keeping active will matter more.

In your twenties is a particularly good time to begin lifting weights. By starting now, you establish a higher setpoint for the gradual (about 1 percent a year) reduction in muscle mass and bone density that begins in your thirties. Your gains from weight lifting may be greater at this age than in later decades, because your body is still pumping out ample amounts of testosterone, a hormone that plays a key role in muscle development, but which tapers in production as life goes on.

Beyond that, the body of a twenty-something man has more recuperative power. That offers a certain amount of protection from permanent injury that older men lack, and gives younger men more reason to participate in aggressive sports. You're also able to work at a higher intensity, which allows you to cram more effort into a shorter space of time than may be practical or safe for older men.

YOUR THIRTIES

Age-related decline in muscle mass, strength, aerobic capacity, and metabolic rate begin at this age, but is barely noticeable, especially if you're active. Still, activity becomes more of a problem, with increased demands from work and, in all likelihood, family. Perhaps the most noticeable physical decline will be in flexibility.

During the thirties, it makes sense to start backing off from contact and high-impact sports (but not entirely avoiding them). For example, if you run three times a week, run twice instead, substituting biking or swimming on the third day. Likewise, if you're just starting an exercise program, don't assume you can tolerate the kind of punishment you took when you exercised at school. Pay closer attention to distress signals from your body.

As for your workout mix, take longer to do aerobics (since you should be doing them a bit less intensely), and add more stretching. To make up for lost time, subtract one set from your weight routine.

YOUR FORTIES

The effects of age begin to show during this decade, but they needn't

---

When You Shouldn't Exercise

Before undertaking any exercise program, check first with your doctor, to rule out any conditions that vigorous physical activity might aggravate. The final word on when to exercise—or when not to—comes from your physician. In the meantime, you should generally avoid a workout or stop exercising (and even see a doctor) if you:

Feel Pain
Pain is the body's dashboard warning system, and an alarm usually means something is wrong. Don't try to "work through" pain. The old maxim, "no pain, no gain" is thoroughly discredited—by sticking to it, you'll cause yourself more pain and aggravate injuries.

Feel Dizzy
Unexplained dizziness is often trivial, but it's also a symptom of over 350 ailments, the more serious of which include heart attack, stroke, diabetes, and internal bleeding.

Feel Chest Pressure
Not every chest pain means a heart attack, but it's an important enough symptom to warrant attention no matter what. Other signs of blood blockage to watch for include difficulty breathing, clamminess, nausea, and tingling in your neck or left arm.

Exercise Programs Tailor-Made for You

How much aerobics at my age? How much strength training? As the decades pass, your exercise needs change, and a good exercise program takes these changes into account.

The programs below, grouped by decade, should form the basis of your fitness program. Try to work out at least three times a week, with a rest day between each workout.

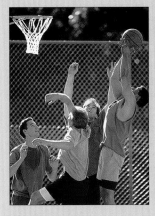

▲ Utilize your body's resilience in aggressive play.

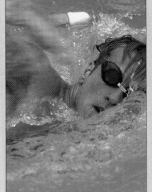

▲ Take longer to do aerobic activities such as swimming.

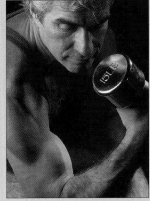

▲ Reduce strength training— but don't abandon it.

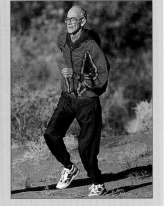

▲ Do weight-bearing exercise to keep bones strong.

Your Twenties

Strength Training
30 minutes Monday, Wednesday, and Friday, doing three sets of each exercise.

Aerobic Training
15 to 20 minutes Monday, Wednesday, and Friday, at 80 to 85 percent of maximum heart rate.

Stretching
5 minutes at each workout.

Special Concerns
Protect knees and shoulders—joints are especially vulnerable to damage during intense exercise and competitive sports, such as football, basketball, and hockey.

Your Thirties

Strength Training
20 minutes Monday, Wednesday, and Friday, doing two sets of each exercise.

Aerobic Training
30 minutes Monday, Wednesday, and Friday, at 70 percent of maximum heart rate.

Stretching
5 to 10 minutes at each workout.

Special Concerns
Don't push your body to the point of complaint. If you're just starting out, take it slow until you're sure you've defined your limits.

Your Forties

Strength Training
20 minutes Monday and Friday, doing two sets of each exercise. Do 45 minutes of circuit training on Wednesday, using lighter weights; do the circuit three times.

Aerobic Training
25 minutes Monday and Friday, at 60 to 70 percent of maximum heart rate. On Tuesday and Thursday, do 30 minutes of light activity.

Stretching
5 to 10 minutes at each workout.

Special Concerns
Add more abdominal exercises to offset midriff padding.

Your Fifties and Beyond

Strength Training
20 minutes Monday and Friday. On Wednesday, do 45 minutes of circuit training.

Aerobic Training
20 minutes Monday and Friday, at 60 to 70 percent of maximum heart rate. On Tuesday and Thursday, do 30 minutes of brisk walking.

Stretching
5 to 10 minutes at each workout.

Special Concerns
Joints and the back are vulnerable to injury—be extra cautious about putting undue stress on these areas.

---

slow you down much if you're already active. If you're not already active, time's a-wasting.

A number of major health problems, ranging from heart disease to cancer, start becoming an issue in your forties. Of course, that doesn't mean they'll inevitably occur, but they are becoming more statistically likely. It's time to get a thorough

exam from a physician no matter what your exercise plans, but especially if you're planning to begin a workout program.

On a less dire note, a reduction in metabolism—the rate at which the body burns fuel—has slowed the removal of excess calories. As a result, you may be witnessing the birth of middle girth, as calories

stored as fat begin accumulating in the belly, the natural repository for flab in men. You'll need to pay more attention to proper diet and fat-burning aerobic activity.

Your workout mix should shift even more firmly toward aerobic activities that are low-impact, to keep stress on the body to a minimum. Don't entirely abandon your weight routine, though; you need muscle because it burns more calories than fat (even at rest), and protects against injury. Try promoting both strength and aerobic fitness with circuit training.

YOUR FIFTIES AND BEYOND

The older you get, the more difficult it becomes to generalize. If you've been active since your twenties, your physical needs and abilities will differ dramatically from a man who's been sedentary all his adult life.

Your overall state of health and the restrictions it places on you may also be vastly unlike another man your age. Increasingly, you and your doctor are the sole arbiters of your exercise options. Still, there are a few aspects of seniority that you should bear in mind.

Loss of bone mass, which kicks in later for men than for women, is now becoming an issue, with your goal being to minimize the likelihood of a hobbling fracture at any point in the future. It's important to do weight-bearing exercises in which you're on your feet, supporting your body. Walking is one example, as is running (within appropriate limits) and even dancing.

What you put into your body becomes more and more important after you turn 50. You may not notice it, but nutritionally, your body's needs change with age—for example, you tend to need fewer calories—and there's a greater premium on choosing good, nutrient-dense foods that are low in fat, sugar, and salt. Any medications you may be swallowing can also affect the absorption of nutrients; this and other drug side effects should be part of the dialog with your doctor regarding exercise and its effects.

QUIZ

Q. Why can people sometimes seem stronger in an emergency?

A. The central nervous system normally holds back untrained muscles in the interests of preventing injury and keeping the body working smoothly, but this safety valve is released during a life-or-death struggle. By one estimate, untrained muscles are actually 40 to 60 percent more powerful than they seem. Initial gains with exercise come largely from neurological changes, not physical ones.

As you age, you also become increasingly vulnerable to injury, but here, too, the risks vary greatly among individuals. Some men run marathons at this age, but that's hardly to be recommended across the board. Again, consult your doctor about what's appropriate for you.

Five Ways to Stay Motivated

Ideally, exercise is fun. Realistically, it often isn't. How do you maintain energy when it's flagging, find time when there's none, keep up interest when you're bored?

1 Set goals. It could be to look better, climb a mountain when you retire, or compete in a sporting event. It's good to have an outcome in mind. But it's just as important to set specific, short-term goals that are action-oriented and measurable. For example, "I will run three miles twice this week" is better than "I will take up running." When one set of goals becomes stale, set different ones.

2 Don't compare. There will always be other men who are more fit, more skilled, more buff than you. Ignore them. Also ignore the athletic accomplishments of your youth. The only measure to focus upon is your own immediate capacities (and limitations) and how they improve.

3 Lighten up. Exercise isn't an all-or-nothing endeavor. If you slack off, fine. Fitness losses, like gains, occur slowly. Maybe you need a break. That's not a failure, and it's not a reason to quit.

4 Have fun. Working out should be a pleasure, not a chore. Cruising down a trail on a bike, snowboarding through powder, or making love is work, but not drudgery. Neither are long hours training on the weights or stationary cycle if you know they'll make those more exciting activities better later.

5 Prioritize life. There are two types of tasks. One type is urgent—it clamors for immediate attention, but has little long-term significance. The other type is vital—it has long-term importance and will ultimately deliver greater satisfaction. Exercise is one of the second type. Write workouts into your calendar to elevate their status. When tempted away from exercise, ask if the alternative is as vital in the long run.

▶ *One way to keep motivated is to find an activity that you enjoy for its own sake. Training with a friend makes exercise that much more pleasurable.*

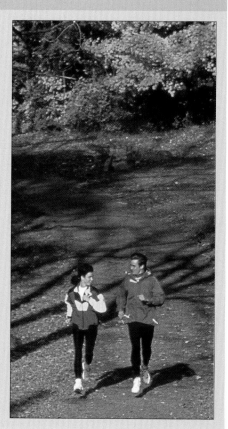

Environment and Equipment

We appreciate all manner of tools that help us go faster, become more efficient, enter hostile environments, and otherwise go beyond our natural limitations. But good exercise gear is not merely a case of toys for the boys, it's one of the essential ingredients to your fitness success.

Get the Right Equipment

You already have enough excuses not to exercise. You don't want shoddy surroundings or inadequate equipment to become another.

An investment in an environment in which you are comfortable and enjoy spending time vastly increases your likelihood of sticking with your program. Likewise, getting gear that meets your needs and doesn't leave you pining for something better, or lamenting the inefficiencies of an item bought too cheaply, will make your workouts more effective and also allow you to take pride in what you do.

Evaluating exercise and sports equipment depends, naturally enough, on what it is you're buying. There are, however, a number of general principles that can be applied to all forms of equipment.

- Consider your needs. Will you be using your equipment a lot or only occasionally? Will you be subjecting it to vigorous use, or going easy on it? Will you be the only person using it, or will you be sharing it? What's your level of ability? Your answers affect the specific models you choose and the price you pay.
- Don't skimp. You're making an investment in gear that should hold up to years of use. If you don't spend enough now, you'll be dissatisfied later. Equipment you don't like tends to end up as a coat rack—far more expensive in the long run than springing for superior goods that you'll actually use.
- Buy from a serious store. Specialty outfitters sell better gear and have more knowledgeable sales people to help guide you than do department stores and discount retailers.

- Test it out. Buy only what you can see, touch, and use. Most reputable stores will allow you to try out equipment either on the sales floor or the nearby outdoors.
- Let the experts assemble. Putting equipment together yourself is time-consuming and fraught with peril—the bike shop gearheads or multi-station gym masters are likely to put your stuff together quicker and more safely than you are. Stores should deliver your gear assembled, installed, and ready to go.

Clothes and Shoes

The good news for your bank balance is that in general you don't need special clothing for a fitness program. Cold conditions, however, do require a few precautions.

Setting Up a Home Gym

It sounds appealing to simply walk into your basement for a good workout, but a successful home gym depends on taking stock of a number of factors.

- Your partner's stuff. If the space you want to develop is already filled with boxes, clothes, and old love letters, you need a plan for removing them.

- The spider factor. A dank, dark room of cobwebs lit by bare bulbs is not much of an enticement to exercise. Brighten things up with paint, lamps, carpet, and even a TV.

- Environmental control. Make sure you've got a source of heat in winter and air conditioning or fans to keep cool in summer.

- Floor space. Bulky exercise machines are space hogs. Measure your floor and the equipment you intend to put on it to make sure everything will fit.

- Ceiling height. It's just as important as floor space, but easier to overlook. And don't just measure the equipment, measure how much up-and-down space you take while using it.

Resistance-Training Equipment

Strength-training gear provides the foundation for any home gym, but there are a number of methods for providing muscles with resistance. What you decide upon depends on what you're comfortable with, how much space you have at home, and how much money you're willing to part with. Here are some of the basic considerations.

Dumbbells

The first major distinction between types of equipment is free weights, such as dumbbells and barbells, versus machines. A free-weight setup ideally should have both dumbbells and barbells. Dumbbells consist of short bars bearing weight plates on each end, with one bar held in each hand so that each arm supports an independent weight. The advantages of free weights are that they are compact and versatile—you can do dozens of different exercises with them—and they require greater balance and control than machines, mimicking real-life motions and thus working more of the body's muscles.

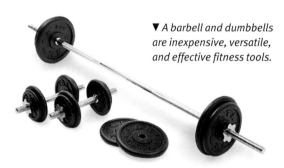

▼ *A barbell and dumbbells are inexpensive, versatile, and effective fitness tools.*

Barbells

A barbell is like a dumbbell, only the bar is much longer, designed to be supported by both hands at once. Because of this, the amount of weight held at the ends of the bars is generally far greater than with dumbbells. With both forms of equipment, it's important to secure the weights with a collar. There are a variety of collar mechanisms. The types that are most easily removed and reliably secured involve a self-locking mechanism, such as expansion springs that let loose when you squeeze the ends of a hand grip. Because of their heaviness, barbells can be dangerous, especially when held above the head, and use of a spotting partner is recommended.

Bench

If you use free weights, you'll need a bench that you can use to sit or lie on, and to hold a barbell on a rack. It's usually worth paying extra for features such as being able to incline the bench at different angles and adjust the height of the barbell rack. Look for sturdy tubing and a stable width at least as long as the distance between your elbow and fingertips, in order to adequately support the shoulders.

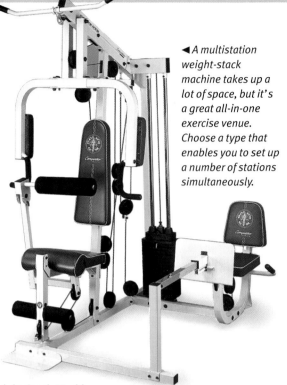

◄ *A multistation weight-stack machine takes up a lot of space, but it's a great all-in-one exercise venue. Choose a type that enables you to set up a number of stations simultaneously.*

Weight-Stack Machines

Machines do a superior job of guiding muscles through a full range of motion with proper form and control, making them easier and safer to use than free weights. (Just keep fingers clear of moving parts—a special consideration if you have children.) Machine motions also tend to isolate muscles, making them ideal for targeting specific areas. Weight-stack machines use a system in which pulling or pushing a bar lifts steel plates via a system of cables and pulleys. Multistation weight-stack machines allow different types of exercises to be done using the same stack of weights. The easiest machines to use allow a number of stations to be set up at the same time; machines that require you to dismantle one setup and reconfigure it to do the next exercise can add significant time to your workout.

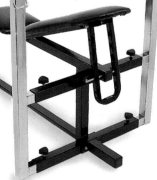

▼ *A bench with a rack for holding barbells comes in handy for exercises such as bench presses.*

Non–Weight-Stack Machines

Instead of weight stacks, some machines employ some other form of resistance, such as flexible cords or bands, hydraulic cylinders, or bent wood or plastic. These machines tend to be lighter, take up less room, and cost less than weight-stack machines. They can deliver a good workout, although they often don't work your muscles as effectively as plate-and-pulley gear; sturdiness may also be a problem. Another drawback is that it's not as easy to accurately monitor increases in resistance (and thus fitness improvements) as it is with weight machines, in which a pin in a slot lets you know exactly what resistance you're working against.

In cold weather, clothing does indeed make the man. The objective, whether running, bicycling, or heading off for a backcountry excursion, is to keep not only warm, but dry, which, in the cold, is often the same thing. Some rules to live by:

• Avoid cotton. It holds moisture against your skin, which makes you clammy and cold. Layers next to skin should be polyester, polypropylene, nylon, or lamb's wool.

• Wear layers that can be stripped off to keep you comfortable, as conditions warrant: Wear two layers of shirts that wick moisture away from skin toward the outer layers; add a third layer of insulation, such as fleece or wool; as cold, wind, or rain threaten, put on a moisture-proof, breathable outer shell or parka.

• Don't forget a hat. You lose something like 50 percent of your body heat through your head.

Outfitting Yourself for Exercise

A general-fitness workout demands very little in the way of special attire, as long as you feel comfortable and safe. There are, however, a few basics—shirts, shorts, socks, and shoes—that it helps to have on hand.

Shirts
A T-shirt is really all you need, but if your upper body looks good enough, a sleeveless shirt with deep arm openings can show off shoulders, chest, and arms to good advantage. Keep in mind that shirts that are cut off at the bottom make you leave more sweat behind on machinery at the gym and fail to cover your gut. For aerobic sports like biking, it makes sense to buy shirts made of a moisture-wicking fabric such as CoolMax, which keeps skin cooler in the heat and warmer in the cold.

Shorts
Go for maximum comfort and minimum embarrassment. It's largely a personal matter: At opposite ends of the spectrum are basic cotton or cotton/polyester athletic shorts that can be used for a variety of purposes (weight lifting, running, biking), versus skin-tight Lycra shorts that provide support and wick moisture away, but cleave to every contour of your body.

Socks
Cotton feels best to a dry foot, but absorbs and holds moisture. Sweating feet will do better in a poly/cotton blend, which is less absorbent, moves moisture away from skin, and dries faster when wet.

Shoes
Whatever activity you're into, you'll need well-fitted, comfortable shoes that give adequate support. Do you need a sport-specific shoe? That depends on how much time you spend doing the one thing: Buy a specialty pair only if you do an activity at least three times a week. The exception is running. No matter how little you do, the high-impact nature of this sport demands a good-quality running shoe.

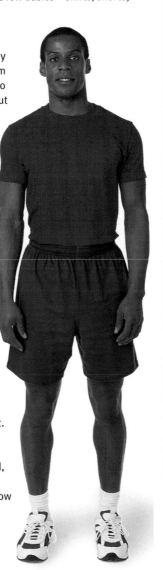

THE SHOE-BUYER'S GUIDE
Shoes—perhaps no single item plays a crucial role in so many different sports. Being improperly shod can make any activity hellish. That's one reason there's such a dizzying array of specialty footwear, with models for running, walking, hiking, playing court sports, bicycling, doing aerobics—virtually every sport has its own design. Do you really need a separate shoe for every activity?

Broadly, no, although some sports demand specialty footwear more than others, and the more you do one thing, the more you could use a special shoe. One rule of thumb is that if you do an activity three or more times a week, a sport-specific shoe is a good idea, to avoid putting excessive stress on your feet and simply to enhance your performance. Running, however, is one sport in which any amount of regular participation demands a good shoe, due to its repetitive, high-impact nature.

Here are some shoe-shopping tips.

• Don't rely on sizes marked on boxes, which in reality can vary from one shoe to the next. Avoid ordering by mail, unless the supplier has a generous return policy.

• Insist on proper fit. Toes should clear the tip of the shoe by about a thumb's width, the ball of the foot should fit comfortably into the shoe's widest point, and the heel should fit snugly without slipping. Don't let sales people convince you that a shoe will be significantly more comfortable when it's "broken in." It should be comfortable now.

• Put on both shoes. Often, one of your feet is slightly smaller than the other. Make sure both shoes in the pair fit well.

• Try to shop late in the day. Feet swell by as much as 5 percent from morning to evening, and buying when you're full size will ensure shoes are not too tight.

Once you've decided what kind of equipment you'd like, the real choices begin. There's always a range to choose from, starting with cheap, entry-level machines with fewer features or less durable components, and ending with expensive, top-of-the-line units that may have features or materials that make little real difference to the average person. Here are some guidelines on buying the most common types of equipment for both the home and outdoors.

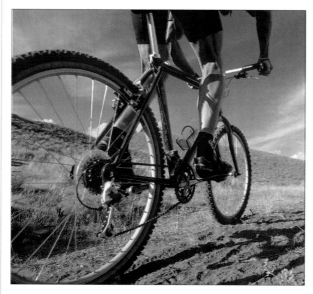

▲ *A mountain bike has a gear to suit just about every terrain.*

Bicycles

Mountain bikes, which now dominate the bike market, have an appealing ability to ride off-road, thanks to their fat and knobby tires, wide range of gear ratios, and suspension systems. The most popular and affordable frame materials are steel alloy (strong and supple, but heavy) and aluminum (brittle and stiff, but light). Suspension in the fork or frame is desirable for rugged terrain, but unnecessary for smooth or level trails. Don't forget the road bike: Sleek and fast, it's a better choice if most of your riding will be on pavement.

Bike Attire: For bicycling (whether on a mountain or road bike), a number of accessories are important.
• A helmet. It's essential: The vast majority of serious biking injuries are to the head.
• Padded shorts. They keep the grind of endurance pedaling from numbing your backside.
• Padded gloves. They prevent the pressure of palms against handlebars from pinching blood vessels or nerves.

Stationary Bikes

Stationary bikes are relatively inexpensive due to their simple mechanics. Pedals make a wheel turn against a weighted flywheel or some other form of resistance. Caliper brakes that hold back the wheel's rim tend to wear out and feel awkward, but wheels that use wind resistance or magnets provide elegant and quiet means of generating a force to work against.

Rowing Machines

Rowing machines fell out of favor after a spurt of enthusiasm in the 1980s, partly because mass-market goods were often shoddy, but good units have survived. The best operate by having the user pull a handle attached to a cable or belt that turns a flywheel. Avoid units that provide resistance by means of a hydraulic or pneumatic cylinder, which may be prone to breakdown, and which also feel less like real rowing.

Cross-Country Skiers

NordicTrack-style indoor skiers (and this high-quality brand has long dominated the market) are one of the best fitness bargains around, since they deliver a good aerobic workout using both the upper and lower body, and don't cost the earth. Still, the movement of a skier machine feels awkward at first and takes some getting used to. You'll need to choose between models that have the feet move independently of each other, and those in which foot movement is interconnected (that is, when one foot platform moves forward, the other automatically moves back, and vice versa). NordicTrack has traditionally kept to independent motion, which is more like real skiing, but tandem motion is easier to master. Extra cash buys you more electronic displays, but you don't need them for a good workout.

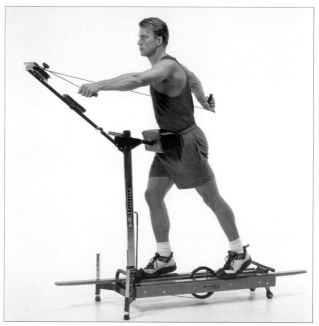

▲ *A cross-country skier is a good-value, all-round fitness machine.*

Treadmills

Go for a unit with a motor that drives the belt on which you walk or run. Aim for at least 1.5 horsepower, labeled for "continuous duty," which won't suffer problems with underpowering over long periods that mar the performance of cheaper units. Make sure the belt is big enough to move around on. Motorized treadmills are among the most expensive pieces of sports equipment. If you can afford it, get a model that can elevate to imitate the effect of a hill.

Stairclimbers

There are two types: Steppers exercise only the legs, while climbers additionally involve the arms in a motion akin to scaling a ladder. You'll also need to choose a foot platform style. With some models, one foot automatically moves up when the opposite foot moves down. With other models, both feet move independently. Both methods work well. The best units forsake hydraulic or pneumatic cylinders to provide resistance, opting instead for cables or chains that move a flywheel. High-end machines also feature better construction on details like hand bars, and superior ergometry.

Inline Skates

Skates are categorized by intended use: street hockey, fitness, recreational, speed. A well-fitting boot (consisting of a foam liner inside a molded plastic shell that bolts to the wheel frame) has obvious importance. Boots that lace often fit better, but boots that buckle are easier to get on and off. One measure of quality is the wheels' bearings. Look for models with an odd-numbered ABEC (Annular Bearing Engineering Council) rating of one or three.

Inline Skating Gear: Like bicycling, inline skating has its own set of requirements.
• A helmet. You can injure yourself a lot of ways on skates, but hitting your head is generally the worst.
• Protective pads. Also extremely vulnerable to injury are elbows, wrists, and knees, and no skating outfit is complete without inexpensive pads to protect them.

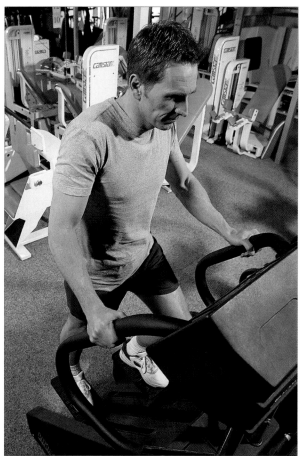

▲ *A stepper gives the lower body an effective workout.*

Skis

There are more options in gear for the slopes than ever before. Traditional categories like slalom (good for snappy turns and moguls) and giant slalom (an all-purpose responsive ski for skilled downhillers) have been supplemented by easily controlled parabolics, powder skis, and all-terrain skis for both powder and hardpack. Aim to get a good grade of P-tex, the slippery material on the bottom of the ski, and pay special attention to getting boots that fit well. Also, consider moving into snowboards, which are relatively easy to get the hang of. Cross-country skiers also have a wide range of equipment from which to choose.

Kayaks

What you get depends on where you want to go. Whitewater or river kayaks have more rounded hulls for greater maneuverability in turbulent, rocky water. Touring or sea kayaks are longer, flatter, and more stable, for superior tracking over lakes, harbors, and oceans. Polyurethane is a durable, inexpensive material suitable for most people, although experienced paddlers often get custom-fitted in fiberglass. Whatever type you decide to invest in, make sure you have enough legroom.

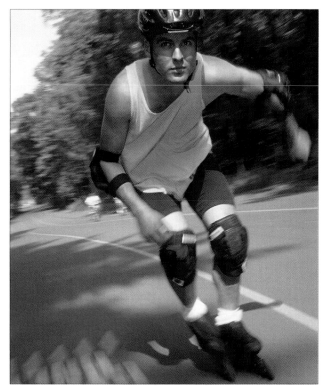

▲ *Well-fitting boots are essentials for inline skating.*

Warming Up

The warmup. Seems like a waste of time, doesn't it? As long as you're exercising, why not proceed directly to the main workout? That's certainly allowable if you're in good physical shape and really pressed for time, but the fact is, your workout will be better if you warm up first.

Why You Should Warm Up

Don't make the mistake of bypassing a warmup and rushing straight into vigorous aerobic activity or a tough weight-training session. "People are impatient. They want to go hard right away so they can get something from their exercise," says Scott Tinley, three-time Ironman World Series champion. "What they usually get is compromised performance or, worse yet, injuries."

Warming up raises body temperature, making muscles, tendons, and ligaments more pliable. That makes them more resistant to injury, including the microscopic tearing that produces soreness.

Engaging in light activity also prepares the body and mind for the more strenuous workout to come. One result is that blood flow is redirected to muscles from organs such as the spleen and stomach.

Your Warmup Routine

Perform any one of the exercises in this section as an entire workout, or for variety, do a couple in combination. Your warmup should take between 5 and 10 minutes.

Stretching

Once you've worked your muscles at moderate intensity for 5 to 10 minutes, don't forget your stretching regimen, which exercise physiologists usually consider to be part of the overall warmup routine.

Stretch for 5 to 10 minutes, holding each stretch for 30 seconds. For a selection of stretches, see "Exercises for Improving Flexibility" on pages 98 to 101. It's important to choose routines that will stretch each part of the body.

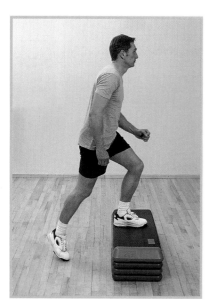

Stair-Stepping

Find a fitness step or an ordinary household stair. Step up with one foot, then the other, then step down with one foot, then the other, continuing this movement at a steady pace. Every minute, alternate the lead-off foot. Don't aim for great speed: 5 to 10 minutes at a moderate pace should be enough to raise body temperature.

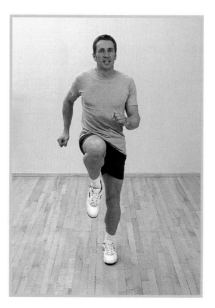

Running in Place

If you don't have a fitness step, running in place on level ground is a good alternative, providing a moderate amount of physical exertion. Try to get your upper body involved. Do this by making exaggerated running movements with your arms, or by swinging your arms in circles gently (not rapidly like a propeller, which can put stress on joints).

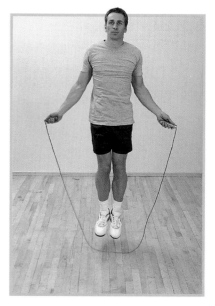

Jumping Rope

A more vigorous alternative to running in place is jumping rope, which is not only aerobic, it works muscles throughout the body. For warmup purposes, jump with both feet simultaneously (jumping with one foot at a time is more strenuous). Keep movements small, keeping jumps close to the floor and spinning the rope with minimal arm and wrist motion.

This gives muscles more nutrients and oxygen, which translates to greater power and endurance.

A warmup is not meant to take a lot of time—only 5 to 10 minutes—or be very strenuous. In fact, you should only work hard enough to break into a light sweat, not to breathe hard, which could take away the energy you'll need for the main part of the workout.

This section details five common warmups. You can, of course, come up with alternatives that make a better fit with your lifestyle and temperament. Take yard work, for example. Seriously. On your way out the door, take 5 or 10 minutes to do a chore like weeding, raking, or sweeping. The American College of Sports Medicine says that such activities contribute significantly to overall fitness, and their moderate intensity makes them well-suited for warmups.

The Art of Cooling Down

If warming up often gets short shrift, cooling down is ignored even more. But it, too, has significant benefits, especially after a vigorous workout in which you've really taxed your muscles.

Cooling down's importance has to do with blood flow. When exercising, the heart beats faster and the blood vessels expand to deliver more oxygen and nutrients to working muscles. If you stop exercising suddenly, your heart begins to slow down, but blood vessels remain temporarily opened. As a result, blood tends to pool in the extremities instead of being efficiently circulated to, for example, the brain. That can cause you to feel light-headed or dizzy. More seriously, if you're very much out of shape or at risk for heart disease, it could put undue stress on your heart. Beyond that,

keeping up blood circulation after exercise helps to remove metabolic wastes such as lactic acid, and to restore energy to muscles.

A cooldown doesn't necessarily demand its own set of exercises. The most sensible approach is to keep doing what you were doing during your main workout, but at only 50 to 60 percent of your previous, more intense effort.

For example, if you were running, slow down to a jog or a brisk walk. Picture yourself doing a victory lap, and you've got the idea. If you're exhausted by a given form of training, you can substitute any of the warmup exercises in this section, which do just as good a job of cooling the body after a strenuous workout as preparing the body for exercise ahead of time.

A cooldown should last from 5 to 10 minutes. Keep in mind that the higher the intensity of your workout, the longer your cooldown should be. Always move gradually from higher intensity to lower. For example, if you've been working out on a stationary cycle for 30 minutes at level 6, notch down to level 5 for a few minutes, then drop to level 4, and so forth.

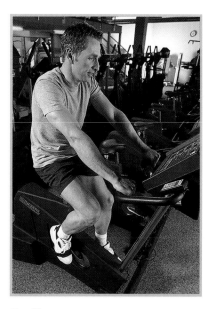

Cycling

If you have a bike, take a short ride. If you have a stationary cycle or trackstand, hop on that. Don't aim for the vigorous pace of aerobic spinning, but program enough resistance or pedal with enough speed to make you draw deeper breaths (the cooling wind on a real bike may make sweat an inaccurate gauge of increased metabolic activity).

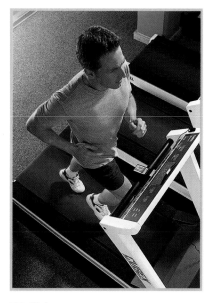

Walking

Start with an amble, then gradually pick up the pace: After 2 minutes or so at a casual pace, increase speed so that your upper body becomes more involved with overall movement. After another couple of minutes, boost yourself to a brisk stride, swinging arms widely and taking longer steps. Maintain this pace for the rest of the warmup.

The Complete Aerobic Workout

Whatever your age, whatever your weight, if you want to be healthy, you should be doing aerobic exercise. Why? Aerobic activity boosts the efficiency of your heart, lungs, muscles, and circulation, burns off excess fat, and protects you against a range of disorders, from heart attacks to brittle bones.

Make Strides toward Fitness

Your heart and lungs work together to deliver oxygen to muscles, which need it to release the energy that powers movement and exertion. Aerobic exercise forces the lungs and heart to work harder. In doing so, it conditions them, which means that your whole body benefits because it gets oxygen and nutrients delivered more efficiently. That translates into a more energized you, a speeded-up metabolism, greater endurance, and protection against heart disease and a host of other ailments.

Being aerobically fit does have a particularly direct effect on the cardiovascular system. If done consistently, aerobic activity can make your risk of a first heart attack 64 percent lower than the risk for sedentary men, according to a study of health patterns among some 17,000 graduates of Harvard University.

The Workout Schedule

The Twenties
15 to 20 minutes Monday, Wednesday and Friday, at 80 to 85 percent of maximal heart rate.

The Thirties
30 minutes Monday, Wednesday, and Friday, at 70 percent of maximal heart rate.

The Forties
25 minutes Monday and Friday, at 60 to 70 percent of maximal heart rate. On Tuesday and Thursday, do 30 minutes of light activity such as brisk walking.

The Fifties and Beyond
20 minutes Monday and Friday, at 60 to 70 percent of maximal heart rate. On Tuesday and Thursday, do 30 minutes of brisk walking.

How Hard Should You Push Yourself?

You've got to work yourself hard to become aerobically fit, but not so hard that you tire quickly. This sustained effort depends on your functioning at a percentage of maximum—high enough to challenge the heart and lungs, but not so high that their ability to provide oxygen and nutrients is exceeded by your muscles' demands.

Knowing your maximum heart rate is a way of determining how intensely you should be functioning during aerobic exercise. The chart shows the "training zone"—70 to 90 percent of maximum. Find your age on the bottom scale and trace upward till you hit the percentage you're aiming for, then go across to the right-hand scale to see how many times per minute your heart should be beating. That figure is what you should aim for over the course of your workout.

Aim to stay around the bottom of the zone, 70 percent. Depending on age and fitness you could aim a little higher or lower—consult a trainer to clarify this. Begin slowly and build up over time.

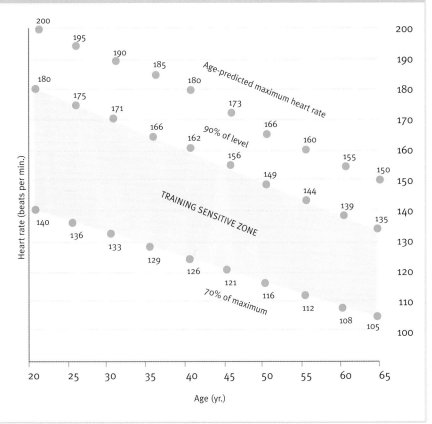

Your ability to improve aerobic fitness has its limiting factors, notably your current level of fitness and your genetic inheritance. Even so, anyone can improve aerobically by following the three fundamentals: intensity, frequency, and duration.

HOW HARD?

To get aerobic benefit you need to exercise so that your heart beats at about 70 percent of its maximum capacity. For details, see "How Hard Should You Push Yourself?"

For your target rate to mean anything in real life, you'll need to take your pulse during your workout, by stopping for a moment and placing two fingers on the throbbing arteries of either your inside wrist or throat. For accuracy, count beats for 10 seconds, then multiply this number by 6. (Counting for 60 seconds underestimates exertion because your heart slows while you've stopped.)

HOW OFTEN?

Experts recommend that you do an aerobic workout three times a week, with a day off between each workout. The day off is important. Not only does it give you time for other interests, it allows your body to repair microscopic damage to the exercised muscles, a process that makes the muscles (and you) stronger.

How Workouts Burn Calories

Start an aerobic exercise program slowly, adding to intensity (how hard you push yourself), frequency (how often you exercise), or time (how long you exercise) as you become fitter.

To illustrate how such adjustments affect exertion, the chart below shows the number of calories burned for several activities, according to how much time is spent doing them.

Activity	15 min.	30 min.	45 min.	60 min.
Bicycling				
12 mph	142	283	425	566
18 mph	213	425	638	850
Rowing	104	208	310	415
Running				
10-min. mile	183	365	548	731
8-min. mile	223	446	670	893
Swimming				
35 yd./min.	124	248	371	497
50 yd./min.	131	261	392	523
Circuit Training	189	378	576	756
Cross-Country Skiing	146	291	437	583

HOW LONG?

Aerobics is a sustained activity. In practical terms, that means each workout should last between 20 and 30 minutes.

What many men don't realize is that you can also get almost the same benefit by doing shorter bouts, for example 10 minutes of aerobic exercise three times in a day.

Testing Your Fitness

Your resting heart rate gives you an indication of the overall state of your aerobic fitness. Because an out-of-shape heart has to work harder to pump blood even while the body is in repose, the resting heart rate goes down as fitness improves; that is, the fitter you are, the more efficiently your heart performs even while you are lying in bed.

The average sedentary man has a resting heart rate of between 80 and 100 beats per minute. A highly conditioned athlete, by contrast, has a resting heart rate of 30 to 40 beats per minute. A moderately active man normally has a resting heart rate of about 60.

To find your resting heart rate, take your pulse at the neck or wrist just after waking up in the morning. That's the time when your body is truly at rest. Simply count the beats for a full 60 seconds.

Two Types of Endurance

It may not seem like it, but there are actually two distinct types of endurance: cardiovascular and muscular.

• Cardiovascular endurance refers to your ability to walk a flight of stairs without gasping for breath or having your heart pound.

• Muscular endurance refers to your ability to sustain movement such as running without your legs turning to noodles.

Aerobic exercise boosts both forms of endurance at the same time, although which muscles benefit and in what proportion depends on the specific activity. For example, running promotes cardiovascular endurance because it works your heart and lungs. It also boosts muscular endurance in your legs, which are doing most of the work. Running doesn't, however, have much effect on muscular endurance in the arms and upper body, which are not used very much.

Choosing an Exercise

Virtually any activity that speeds up your heart and makes you a little breathless qualifies as good aerobic conditioning. So the activities you choose are basically a matter of individual preference. Each will deliver aerobic fitness, but be sure to choose one that you're likely to stick with over the long term.

BICYCLING

Aerobic conditioning on a bicycle requires a consistent pedal cadence—or leg speed—without much coasting (although occasional coasting is fine to control speed or take a breather if you feel overexerted). Elite cyclists aim for a "spinning" cadence of high revolutions per minute (rpm) of between 80 and 100. Casual riders fall more within the 50 range, a minimum for training; 60 to 90 is about average for accomplished riders.

Work out your rpm by counting the number of times your right foot comes up to the top of your pedal stroke. Aim to increase your cadence by about 10 rpm per week. As you reach higher rates of spin, you'll want to shift into higher gears, which takes more effort, making you both stronger and faster.

CROSS-COUNTRY SKIING

This sport provides a great total-body aerobic workout: Make sure to dress in removable layers because you'll get very warm from the sustained movement of both upper and lower body that cross-country demands. While the tactile and contemplative pleasures of outdoor skiing are ideal, there are, nevertheless, practical limitations. The need for snow, skiable land, and the time to get to them may keep this from becoming a frequently practiced activity.

If you move it indoors with a ski machine, start off gradually, especially if you're not familiar with the awkward movement of the equipment. Aim for 10- to 15-minute practice sessions in the first week, then move into real workouts as your conditioning and confidence with the gear improve. Start with 20-minute sessions, then gradually work your way toward a 30-minute workout over the course of three weeks.

ROWING

Rowing provides an excellent aerobic workout, simultaneously working every major muscle group in the body. It's important to get some instruction on proper form before starting—many men use their back muscles more than they should.

The first time you get on a rower, exercise for no more than 5 minutes. Over the course of the next few weeks, as you get accustomed to the motion, gradually work up to 20 to 30 minutes of steady rowing. As that becomes monotonous, mix things up with short intervals of hard rowing to build strength.

RUNNING

It's among the most natural forms of exercise—something you've done all your life. But if you haven't done a lot of running lately, you need to start slow. In fact, don't be ashamed to start out walking. Gauge your effort initially by time, not distance.

Always try to go out for 20 to 30 minutes two to four times a week. In the first week, take a brisk stroll for 20 minutes; expand this to 30

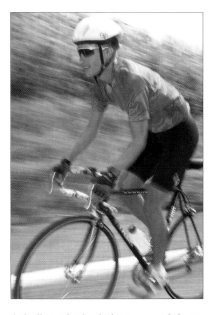

▲ Cycling, whether indoors or out, brings significant aerobic gains. Aim for a cadence of at least 50 rpm.

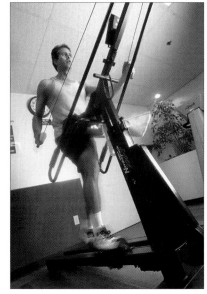

▲ A cross-country skiing machine takes time to get used to, but the effort is soon rewarded: It's a fantastic calorie-burner.

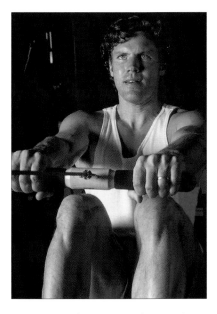

▲ Rowing works every muscle group in the body. Get some instruction on correct technique before starting in earnest.

minutes the second week. Or, if you're up to it, alternate running and walking: Run for 2 minutes, for example, then walk for 4. As you become more conditioned, devote more time to running and less to walking. When you're up to full 30-minute runs, you should start tracking progress by measuring distance, increasing by no more than 10 percent per week—and even then, only if you feel ready for it.

To reduce stress on the body, avoid pavement when possible in favor of soft, even surfaces such as graded paths or smooth fields of grass.

SWIMMING

Here's a sport in which aerobic condition needs to be (or become) extremely good—after all, you're holding your breath for much of it. Start with a warmup, jumping or diving into the water, swimming to the nearest ladder, and walking briskly to the starting point. Repeat this process 6 to 10 times.

Doing laps next is the cornerstone of most swimming workouts. For fitness swimming, you should be able to do 10 laps of an Olympic-size pool nonstop, although most beginners will find this difficult: Make it a goal to work toward gradually.

One way to improve conditioning is through drills in which you concentrate on one part of the body. In stroke drills, for example, you propel yourself freestyle using only one arm, keeping the other outstretched in front of you. In kick drills, you keep both arms motionless, outstretched in front of you, while propelling yourself solely by kicking.

CIRCUIT TRAINING

Circuit training is half aerobic exercise, half strength training. It involves lifting weights, but unlike most weight-lifting routines, you don't do multiple sets of a single exercise in a given sitting. Instead, you move quickly to the next exercise. A "circuit" might be made up of 6 to 12 exercises. After doing one, you may repeat the entire circuit.

Do at minimum the same basic lifts described in the next section, "Exercises for Improving Strength" (on page 92). Do 8 to 12 repetitions of

How Much Is Enough?

For overall health, the rule was once that you should exercise aerobically 20 to 30 minutes a day, three days a week. Now, studies have revealed that many of the health benefits of exercise can be realized in shorter bouts, and that exercise benefits accumulate. Thus, doing 10 minutes of moderate aerobics three times a day is about as good as doing 30 minutes once. And the definition of "moderate exercise" has been broadened to include a wide range of ordinary activities such as painting the house, carrying a bag of golf clubs, or fly fishing.

each exercise, taking about 6 seconds for each lift. (Although you're moving through the circuit fast, the lifts themselves should be performed slowly.) Rest between stations for only about 15 seconds (30 at most), to keep your heart rate up.

On a three-day-a-week schedule, do just one circuit per workout for the first month. Add a second circuit during the second and third months, and a third circuit during the fourth month.

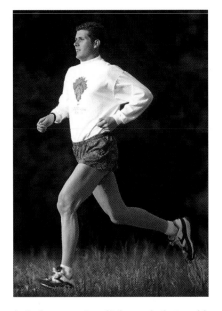

▲ Go for a run: Four little words that could change your life. Beginners should start out slowly, mixing running with walking.

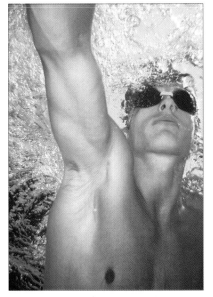

▲ Cutting swiftly through the water is one of the attractions of swimming—no need to be an Olympian to make gains, though.

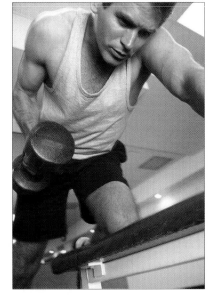

▲ Circuit training is a sequence of aerobic and anaerobic exercises that together work every part of the body.

Exercises for Improving Strength

Training with weights has a muscle-bound image attached to it, but pumping iron is not just for Schwarzenegger wannabes. Strong, powerful muscles will not only make you look good, they'll protect against injuries and back pain, as well as helping with everyday activities from shopping to sex.

Successful Weight Training

Working out with weights will make you stronger, and boost your appearance as muscles grow and become better defined. You'll have a flatter abdomen, a bigger chest, stronger-looking arms, and better-looking legs. And strong muscles mean you'll be better able to do all those ordinary, everyday things around the house much more easily.

New muscle also has a specific fitness payoff: It helps the body burn fat. That's because muscle requires greater amounts of energy to sustain than fat does. The more muscle you have, the easier it is to keep it on.

To get the most from a weight-training program, follow these four basic principles.

Take It Slow and Steady

How fast should you lift weights? Actually, it's more a question of how slow. Rapid movements should be avoided because they place stress on muscles and tendons. Slow and steady is good not only to avoid injury, but because it ensures that momentum is not doing any work for you. The best advice is to take six seconds to execute a complete lift: two seconds up and four seconds down. Spending more time on the "down" part (known as eccentric or negative movement) is an advantage because it actually builds muscle as much as 20 percent faster than the "up" part, known as concentric or positive movement.

• Load up. The weight on any given exercise should be heavy enough to bring targeted muscles to fatigue within 8 to 12 repetitions.
• Progress gradually. If you're just beginning a program, start the first two to three weeks lifting weight that feels light to you—enough that doing 12 reps is fairly easy. This allows muscles to adapt to the new activity. After two to three weeks, load up so that doing 8 is easy (but 12 is hard). As you get stronger, do more reps. When you can finish 12 reps without feeling completely fatigued, add more weight (but no more than 5 percent of what you're currently lifting).
• Rest. If you do multiple sets, take a breather for about 90 seconds in between, to allow muscles to recover and perform sufficiently on the next set. Rest periods can vary according to your goals.
• Target the big muscles. The body has hundreds of muscles, but they are organized in several major muscle groups. Performing exercises that work groups of muscles together allows you to do a full-body workout with only the seven basic exercises that follow.

The Workout

All of the exercises in this section are performed with free weights, which are most likely to be found at both home and the gym. It's a good idea to consult a trainer to help monitor your technique, as well as to obtain machine alternatives. Note that the core routine consists of seven exercises: lunges, bench press, one-arm dumbbell rows, alternating dumbbell press, concentration curls, seated triceps press, and squats (on pages 93 to 96). The others (heel raises, dumbbell flies, and side dumbbell raises) can be added.

In addition to the core weight-training exercises, do at least one of the abdominal exercises from "The Total Abdominal Workout" on pages 110 to 116.

The Workout Schedule

Your Twenties
30 minutes Monday, Wednesday, and Friday, doing 3 sets of each exercise.

Your Thirties
20 minutes Monday, Wednesday, and Friday, doing 2 sets of each exercise.

Your Forties
20 minutes Monday and Friday, doing 2 sets of each exercise. Do 45 minutes of circuit training on Wednesday, using lighter weights and moving quickly from one station to the next; complete the circuit 3 times.

Your Fifties and Beyond
20 minutes Monday and Friday; 45 minutes of circuit training on Wednesday.

> "Muscle cells are pretty stupid. They have a short memory and need to be shocked on a regular basis to keep on improving."
>
> Tom Baechle, Ed.D., chair, exercise science department, Creighton University, Omaha, Nebraska

Program Principles

Weight training can boost muscle strength, size, and endurance, but it helps to know which of these is most important to you. That's because slight changes in the elements of your routine—amount of resistance, number of reps, number of sets, and amount of rest between sets—can make your gains faster for one goal, but slower for another. Here are the principles for most effectively getting what you want.

Goal	Resistance	Reps	Sets	Rest
Strength	Heavy	3–8	3–5	2–5 min.
Size	Moderate	8–12	3–5	30–90 sec.
Endurance	Light	12–20	2–3	15–30 sec.

Lunges

Works the legs and hips.

1 Stand with feet shoulder-width apart. Hold a dumbbell in each hand with palms facing your legs and each arm fully extended. This is your starting position.

2 Take a large step forward with your left foot. The left leg should be bent at a 90-degree angle, but your knee should not be positioned beyond the point of your toes. Your right foot should be bent at the knee, and should remain in its starting position, although the heel may come off the floor. Push off with your left foot to return to the starting position. Lunge with the right foot. Do 20 reps (10 on each leg).

(!) *If starting a program, do this exercise without the dumbbells at first, making sure you can perform the range of motions without soreness before using weights.*

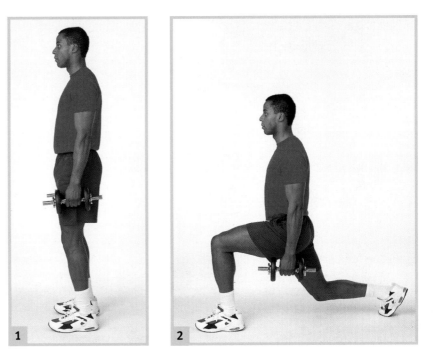

Bench Press

Works the chest.

1 Lie on a bench, with a barbell above your chest (a bench equipped with a bar rack makes this safer and easier). Grasp the bar shoulder-width apart or slightly wider, with palms facing legs, feet flat on the floor and back straight against the bench.

2 Slowly lower the barbell to your chest, so that elbows are pointed to the side, with the rest of your body held in position (don't arch your back). Pause slightly at the bottom of the lift, lightly touching the weight to your chest, keeping the bar under complete control (never bounce the bar off your chest). Raise the bar back to the starting position and repeat.

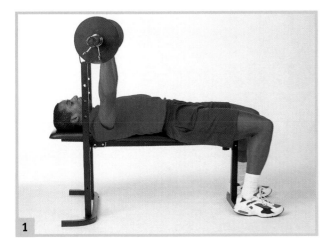
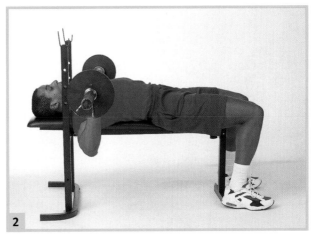

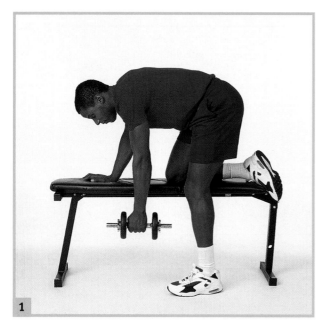

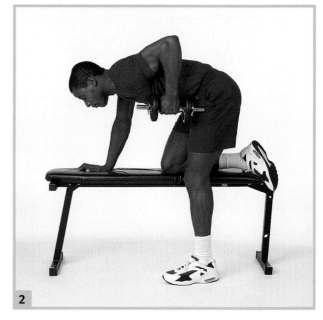

One-Arm Dumbbell Rows

Works the back.

1 Put your right knee and right hand on the surface of a bench, with your left foot flat on the floor. Grasp a dumbbell with your left hand, keeping your back straight and your eyes looking toward the floor. Extend your left hand toward the floor, keeping the elbow unlocked. This is your starting position.

2 Pull the dumbbell up toward your torso, bringing it into your lower chest muscles so that your left elbow is pointing toward the ceiling. Lower to the starting position and repeat. Perform the same exercise with your right hand.

(!) *Always keep your back straight. If you start to feel tired, make sure you don't arch your back.*

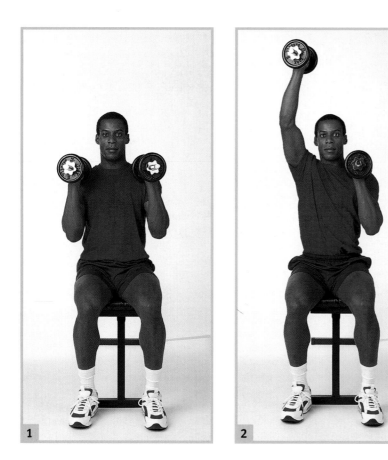

Alternating Dumbbell Press

Works the shoulders.

1 Sit on a bench with legs apart and feet flat on the floor. Grasp a dumbbell in each hand, holding them at shoulder level, palms facing each other. This is your starting position.

2 Keeping your back straight and leaning slightly forward, raise the left dumbbell until your arm is straight — but make sure to keep elbows unlocked. Lower to the starting position, then raise the right dumbbell in similar fashion. Repeat.

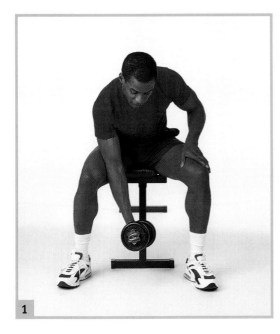

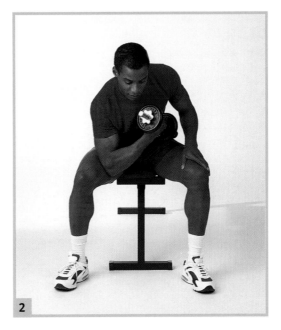

Concentration Curls

Works the biceps.

1 Sit on a bench, feet flat on the floor and shoulder-width apart. Extend your right arm between your knees, grasping a dumbbell in your right hand with palm facing out. Rest your right elbow and upper arm on your right thigh, and place your left hand on your left knee.

2 Slowly raise the dumbbell to your shoulder, bringing it through an arc so that the palm now faces in. Keep your movements slow and controlled. Your bracing stance of right elbow against right knee and left hand on left knee will provide support. Lower to the starting position and repeat. Perform the same exercise with your left hand.

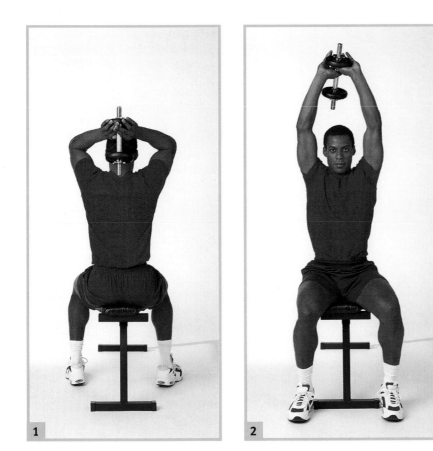

Seated Triceps Press

Works the back of the upper arm.

1 Sit on a bench holding one dumbbell vertically behind your head, grasping it by the uppermost weight using both hands, with fingers interlacing or overlapping for support. Your elbows should be pointing up, with arms held near your head.

2 Slowly extend both arms, pushing the dumbbell toward the ceiling, keeping your back straight. Stop when arms are straight, but do not lock your elbows. Bend your elbows to lower the weight back to the starting position. Repeat.

(!) *Take care that you have a secure grip on the dumbbell at all times.*

Squats

Works thighs and hamstrings.

1 Place a barbell across your shoulders behind your neck, holding the bar with palms forward. Start by standing straight with feet shoulder-width apart.

2 Keeping your knees unlocked, lean slightly forward, then bend your knees, lowering your body as if preparing to sit in a chair. Stop when your thighs are about parallel to the floor, then slowly raise back to the starting position, keeping feet flat on the floor. Repeat.

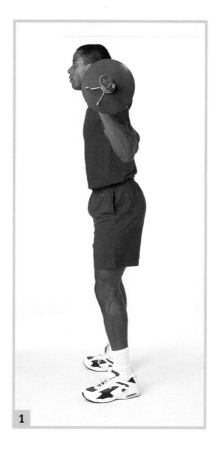

1

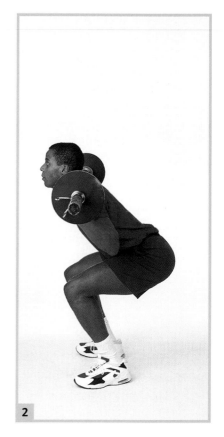

2

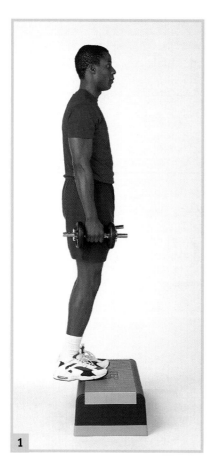

1

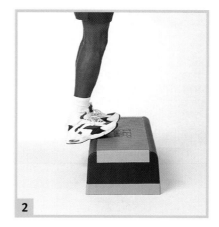

2

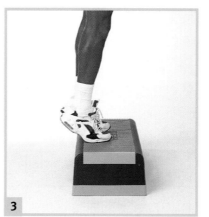

3

Heel Raises

Works the calves.

1 Stand with both feet on an elevated surface such as an exercise step, stair, or even a thick weight plate or wooden block (height should be at least 2 or 3 inches), holding a dumbbell in each hand, palms facing legs. Position feet so that your heels protrude off the edge of the platform, with your weight on the balls of your feet.

2 Slowly lower your heels to a point slightly below the level of the platform.

3 Raise yourself all the way up on your toes, pausing briefly at the top. Repeat.

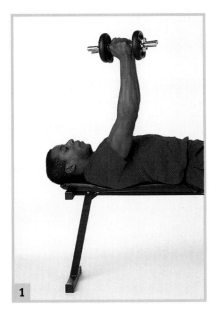

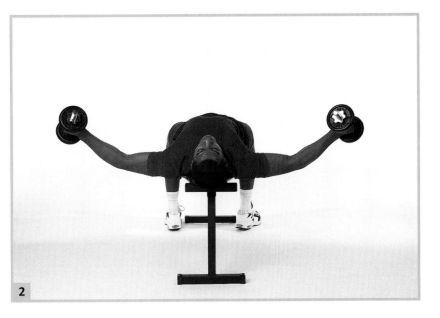

Dumbbell Flies

Works the chest.

1 Lie on your back on a bench, with feet flat on the floor. Hold two dumbbells in the air over your chest, one in each hand, palms facing each other. Your back should be straight and pressed against the bench, and your elbows should be slightly bent, not locked. This is your starting position.

2 Keeping elbows bent and wrists firm, slowly lower the dumbbells away from each other to the sides until they are at chest level. Elbows should be bent at about a 45-degree angle. Raise the dumbbells back to the starting position and repeat.

(!) *Focus on making your chest muscles do all the work: Don't let your shoulders get involved, or you may injure them.*

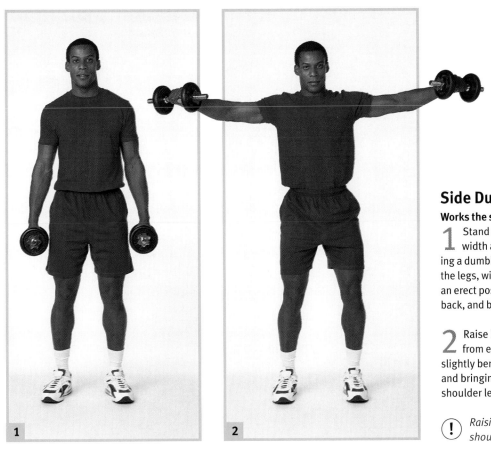

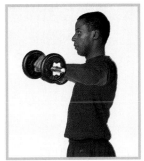

Side Dumbbell Raises

Works the sides of the shoulders.

1 Stand upright with feet shoulder-width apart, arms at your sides, holding a dumbbell in each hand, palms facing the legs, with elbows slightly bent. Keep an erect posture: chest out, shoulders back, and back straight.

2 Raise both dumbbells straight out from each side, keeping elbows slightly bent (see side-angle view, above), and bringing the weights no higher than shoulder level. Lower and repeat.

(!) *Raising dumbbells higher than shoulder level may cause injury.*

Exercises for Improving Flexibility

Watch an Olympic gymnast at work and you'll be mesmerized and maybe astonished at the flexibility of the trained human body. But you don't have to be a gymnast to be flexible. A range of simple stretches can easily be incorporated into your fitness program to bring you all the benefits of increased flexibility.

Flexibility Fundamentals

Flexibility is the ability to stretch, bend, twist, and turn though a full range of movement. The body can make these movements because of well-stretched muscles.

Compared to stiff muscles, flexible ones can exert force through a fuller range of motion, and are able to contract more rapidly. This translates into a more powerful golf or tennis swing, better coordination, and a faster stride while running. Flexible muscles also ensure a safe aerobic or strength-training workout—which is why you should always stretch before vigorous activity.

KEYS TO SAFE STRETCHING

Although there are several different methods of stretching, most are intended for use by top-class athletes; only one form, known as static stretching, is safe and effective for people of all fitness levels.

With static stretches, you move slowly and easily, using gravity and body weight to apply only a small amount of force that pushes targeted muscles slightly past their usual range of motion. To stretch

Are You Flexible?

Try these simple moves to assess how limber you are in several crucial areas.

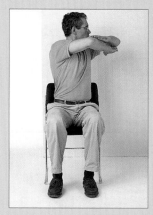
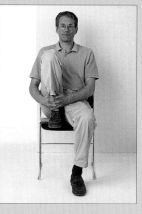
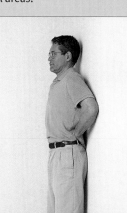
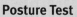

Chair Twist

Sitting upright in a chair, twist your torso to one side. You should be able to rotate so that a line connecting one shoulder to the other would cross a line connecting one side of your hips to the other at a 90-degree angle, forming a T-shape. If you can't, you're tight in your torso and back.

Toenail Touch

Sit upright in a chair. Bring up one foot from the floor and try putting it on the seat so that the heel touches your buttocks (you can guide your foot with your hands if you have to, but don't force it). If you can't, your hips, gluteals, lower back, and upper hamstrings are likely tight and need help.

Posture Test

Stand against a wall, then reach behind and place your palm flat against the wall. Try to slide your hand between the small of your back and the wall. If you can push your hand in up to the wrist, your lower back muscles are tight. If you can only fit your fingertips into the space, you likely have tight hamstrings.

Ceiling Reach

Interlock your fingers with both palms facing away from you, then reach over your head with both hands, extending your arms upward as straight as you can. If you find that you can't easily go beyond a bent-elbow position, you could use more flexibility in shoulders, chest, and upper back.

safely and effectively, always stick to the following guidelines:

• Warm up. A few minutes of activity that makes you break into a light sweat makes muscles warmer and more pliable, allowing them to stretch further without injury.

• Be gentle. You should stretch only until you feel a slight tug on the targeted muscle, using slow and controlled movements. That way, you won't force muscles to go further than they should.

• Hold. During the initial part of a stretch, muscles reflexively contract to automatically guard against being overextended. Holding the stretch for 30 seconds allows muscles to relax and stretch further.

• Don't bounce. Pushing stretched muscles "just a bit further" in short and quick bursts increases the risk of tearing muscle fibers like overextended rubber bands.

• Breathe normally. Some people seem to think that holding a stretch requires holding their breath, too. But taking slow, rhythmic breaths contributes to the stretch by helping you to relax.

HOW LONG IS A GOOD STRETCH?

In studies of hamstring stretches, researchers have found that 30 seconds is ideal for providing significant, measurable weekly improvements in flexibility.

In contrast, holding for less than 15 seconds was not much better than not stretching at all, and holding longer than 60 seconds provided no greater benefit than holding for 30 seconds.

The Workout

As with weight lifting, targeting several major muscles, or groups of muscles, provides an excellent basic routine. This entire stretching program can be completed in 5 to 10 minutes. The exercises can be done in any order you wish.

Advanced Techniques

Apart from static stretching, there are a number of more specialized methods. These should be tried only with the advice of a trainer.

• Dynamic stretching. This is a "bouncing" move, in which you power the targeted muscle into an expanded range of motion. One example is swinging your foot to stretch the hamstrings before running. It's best for muscles that are already in good condition, in preparation for sports that involve sudden, forceful movement.

• Ballistic stretching. Similar to dynamic stretching, but movement is quicker and more violent.

• PNF (proprioceptive neuromuscular facilitation) stretching. A partner holds your stretch position for you while you isometrically contract muscles. In the hamstring stretch, a partner holds your leg while you contract either the hamstrings or the quadriceps.

Shoulders

1 Lie on your back on the floor, legs extended, with toes pointed. Extend your arms above your head, with fingers interlocked and palms pointing toward the ceiling.

2 Keeping your arms straight, slowly lower your hands until they rest on the floor behind the crown of your head. Hold.

(!) *Take care not to arch your back. If you feel your back starting to arch, push your lower back into the floor.*

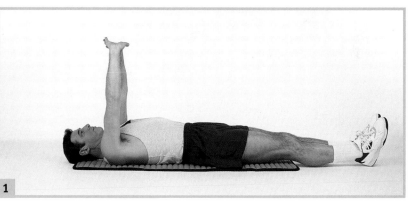

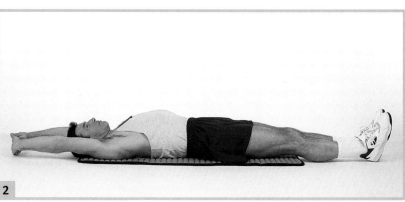

Hips

Mobilizes pelvic joints and improves the flexibility of muscles around the pelvis.

1 Lie on your back, legs extended. Lock your fingers together at the back of your right upper leg.

2 Slowly pull your right knee toward your chest. Hold. Return to starting position and repeat with your left leg.

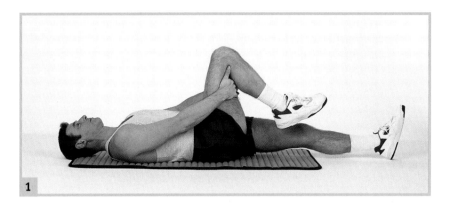

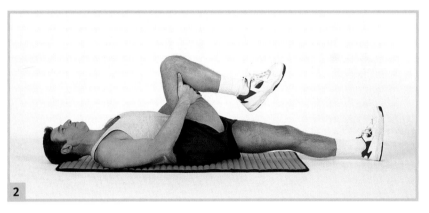

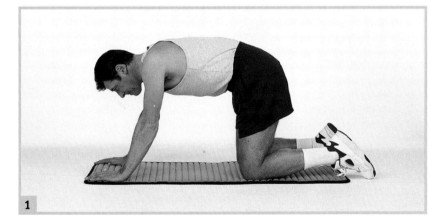

Lower Back

1 Get onto your hands and knees, with hands under your shoulders.

2 Keeping your hands in one place, sit back onto your heels so that your arms are outstretched.

 Don't let your back sag. If you do, you'll put stress on the spine.

✱ **Alternative:** Without sitting back on your heels, arch your back so that it's rounded toward the ceiling like a cat's.

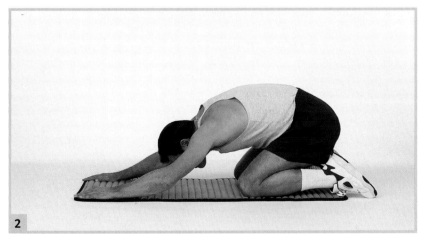

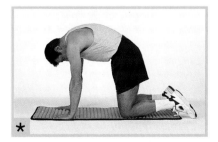

Hamstrings

1 Sit on the floor with your left leg straight out in front of you, right foot tucked against your left thigh so that your legs make a figure-4.

2 Reach your left arm as far as you can toward your toes. Hold, and repeat with the right leg.

★ **Alternative:** For a similar exercise that puts less stress on the lower back, sit on the edge of a bench (or bed) with your left leg extended on the bench and your right foot flat on the floor. Resting your right hand on your right knee, extend your left hand toward your left toes. Hold and repeat with the right leg.

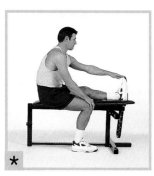
★

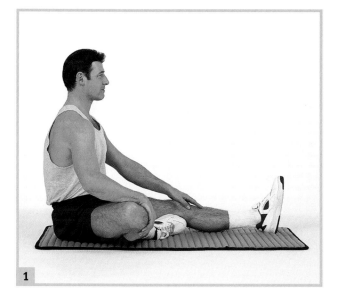
1

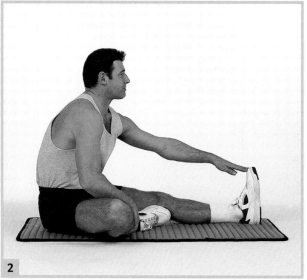
2

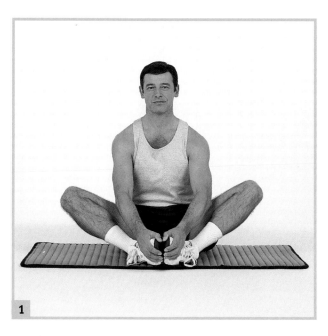
1

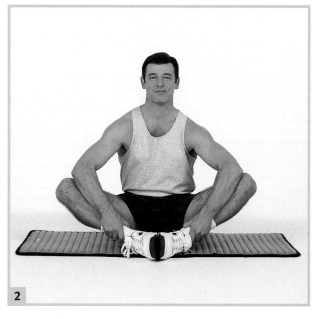
2

Groin

1 Sit up on the floor and bend your legs like a frog's, touching the soles of your feet together.

2 Keeping your soles in contact, gently press your knees toward the floor with your hands or elbows. Hold.

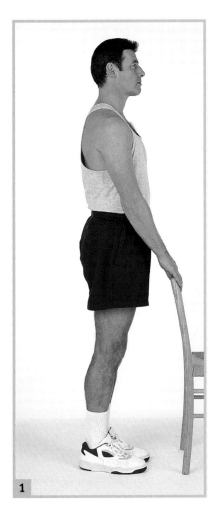

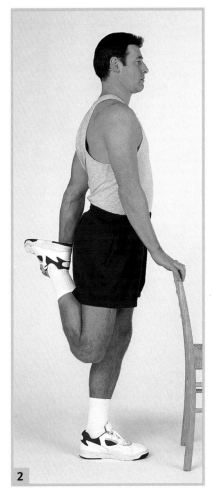

Thighs

Targets the much-used thigh muscles.

1 Stand up, with feet about shoulder-width apart. Have a chair ready as a support, or use the wall.

2 Bend your right knee and grasp your right foot or ankle with your left hand, using your right hand to support yourself against a chair or wall. (Note that the hand and foot making contact are from opposite sides.) Pull your right foot up so that the heel presses against your buttocks. Hold and repeat with the left leg.

(!) *To reduce stress on the knee, keep the leg you're standing on slightly bent.*

Lower Back and Buttocks

1 Lie on your back with your arms straight out at your sides, palms facing the floor. Bend your left leg, leaving the right leg extended, placing your left foot on the floor beside your right knee.

2 Twisting your hips at the waist while keeping your upper body in position, drop your bent left knee toward the floor on your right side, lowering it as far as feels comfortable. By keeping your left shoulder from lifting off the floor, you'll get an added benefit to your upper back and shoulder. Hold. Return to starting position and repeat on the other side.

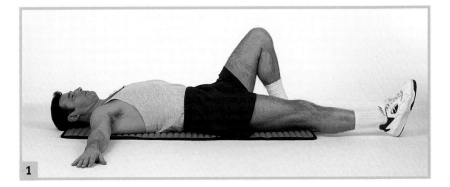

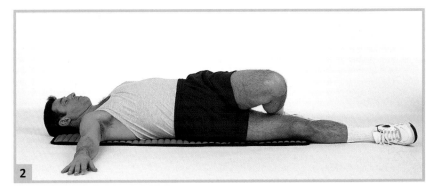

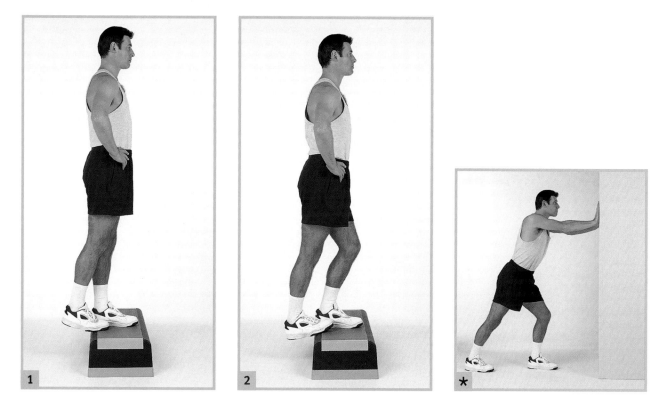

Calves

1 Stand on a step with the heel of your right foot sticking over the edge of the step.

2 Drop your heel below the level of the step until you feel a tug at the back of your lower leg. Hold and repeat with the left foot.

★ **Alternative:** Stand 3 to 4 feet in front of a wall with feet shoulder-width apart and toes pointing forward. Step forward with your left foot, allowing the left knee to bend, placing your hands against the wall for support, while keeping the right foot in place, heel flat on the floor. Lean forward as far as is comfortable. Stand further from the wall with increasing flexibility.

Side and Lower Back

1 Stand upright with feet shoulder-width apart and knees slightly bent. Put your right hand on your hip and extend your left arm above your head, palm facing away from the body.

2 Bending at the waist toward your right hand-on-hip, reach your left hand over your head and as far to the right as feels comfortable. Hold. Repeat on opposite side.

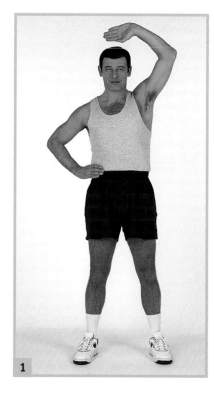

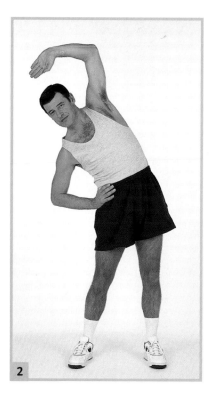

Hip and Thighs

1 Place the ball of your left foot on a bench, the third step of a flight of stairs, or a firm platform of similar height, with your right foot flat on the floor slightly behind you, with the knee slightly bent.

2 With your hands on your hips, lean forward into your left leg, pushing your hips forward and keeping your torso straight. (Don't let your left knee extend past the point of the toes on your left foot.) Hold. Repeat on the right side.

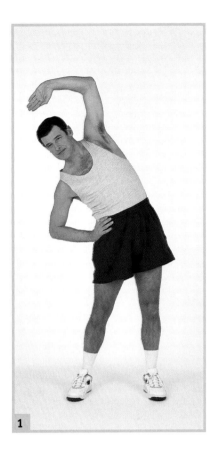

1

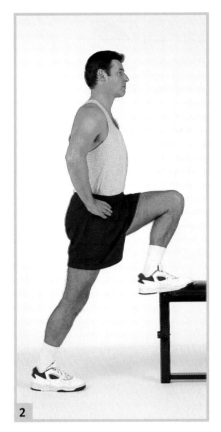

2

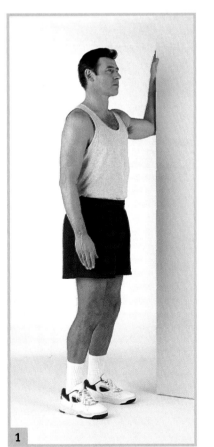

1

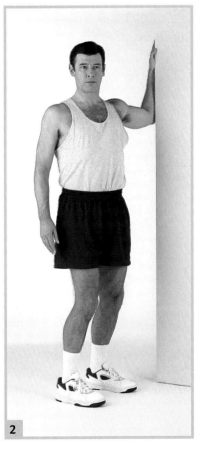

2

Chest

1 Stand in a doorway or at the edge of a wall with your feet shoulder-width apart. With your left arm bent at a 90-degree angle, place your hand and forearm against the wall, so that your upper arm is parallel with the floor and your forearm is vertical on the wall.

2 Slowly rotate your body toward your right shoulder so that your elevated left arm is drawn slightly behind your torso. Hold. Repeat on the right arm.

Triceps

Stretches the muscles in the backs of the arms.
Stand with your feet shoulder-width apart and knees slightly bent. Raise both hands over your head, elbows bent. Grasp your right elbow with your left hand, and gently pull the right elbow toward your left arm until you feel a tug at the outside of the upper right arm and shoulder. Hold. Repeat on the left arm.

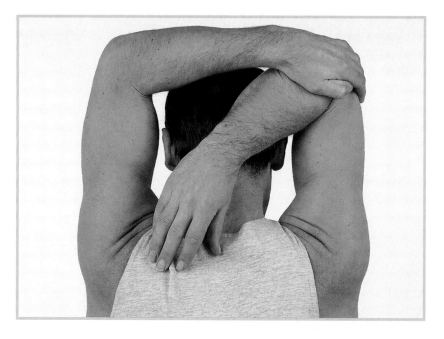

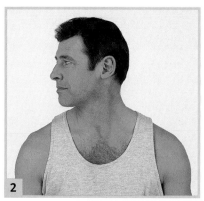

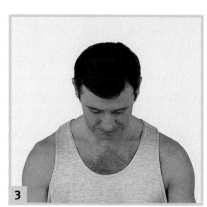

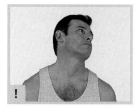

(!) *Don't roll your head in a continuous motion—this puts pressure on the upper spine, especially as the head moves back so that eyes face the ceiling.*

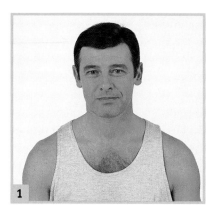

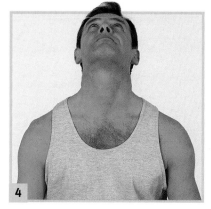

Neck

1 Stand with feet about shoulder-width apart, back and neck straight, and shoulders relaxed and eyes straight ahead. This is the starting position.

2 Slowly turn your head to the right as far as feels comfortable. Hold. Repeat to the left.

3 From the starting position, slowly lower your chin to your chest (without rounding your shoulders) so that you feel a mild pull on the muscles at the back of your neck. Hold.

4 Slowly tilt your head upward until you are looking straight up. Hold.

Training for an Endurance Event

There'll always be guys who want to prove to themselves and perhaps to the world that they've got what it takes to pull off an endurance event. Whether it's an above-average personal best or a triathlon, high-aiming goals take dedication and time, but those who succeed say it's worth the effort.

The Training Regimen

So you want to achieve more than the longer life, better health, and sharper looks that general fitness provides? Well, you're about to move onto another fitness plane. That's because training for an endurance event is fundamentally different from mere exercise: You're moving toward a specific goal within a specific amount of time.

Training requires a more serious approach because there is not much room for slacking. While the occasional unscheduled day off won't necessarily ruin your program, a consistent pattern of missing workouts will fail to put you in peak condition at the time of your event. That will make the event more difficult

and, in all likelihood, leave you disappointed in your results.

Here's what you'll have to do to get started in the three basic triathlon sports of bicycling, running, and swimming.

BICYCLING

The endurance target for amateur bicyclists is the century, a 100-mile ride in one day, the preparation for which takes weeks of training.

This is certainly a worthy objective if your body can deal with it, but most experts advise beginners to aim for a less-grueling but still-impressive feat, the metric century, which is 100 kilometers (62 miles) in one day. Even if you train for a mile century, you'll need to reach the

metric century mark during your training. So aim for the lower goal, then continue your training if you still want to strive for more.

The key to the program (see box, below) is to ride six days a week. One day (try to make it Saturday) is a long-distance day, and one day (preferably Thursday) you have off. Each week, you gradually increase the weekly distance total—especially on your long-distance day—by about 10 to 12 percent.

The distance you ride each day varies, with long rides followed by shorter ones. Speed varies as well, according to three measures: pace, brisk, and easy.

• Pace. This is the speed at which you'll ride on the day you complete the century. Plan for a metric century to take you between three and four hours to complete, depending on how hilly the terrain is. Most of your training rides will be at this moderate speed.

• Brisk. About two or three miles per hour faster than century pace.

• Easy. A leisurely ride.

The combination of different distances and speeds provides a balance of exertion and recovery that will propel you to your goal.

Bicycling: The Metric Century Schedule

The metric century (100 kilometers or 62 miles) is a challenging goal for novice endurance riders. The program below gives a mix of distances and speeds to build endurance over a five-week period. Distances are given in miles.

Week	Monday	Tuesday	Wednesday	Thursday	Friday	Saturday	Sunday	Total Miles
1	6	10	12	Off	10	30	9	77
2	7	11	13	Off	11	34	10	86
3	8	13	15	Off	13	38	11	98
4	8	14	17	Off	14	42	13	108
5	8	14	17	Off	10	5	62	116

- ☐ Easy
- ☐ Brisk
- ☐ Pace
- ☐ Century Day (pace)

Swimming: The 100-Meter Buildup

Mondays and Wednesdays
Cover 1,500 to 2,000 meters in segments of your choosing, such as 100 meters or 500 meters, resting for 30 seconds after each set. For example, you could swim 1,500 meters in 15 sets of 100 meters, or three sets of 500 meters. Change the distance of your segments as you achieve greater endurance and power. For example, if you start with segments of 100 meters, you might later favor 500-meter segments. Swim at a pace that's about 70 percent of an all-out effort.

Tuesdays and Thursdays
Build endurance and speed. Swim the same distances as on Mondays and Wednesdays, but work at about 80 percent of maximum effort, and cut the rest period after each segment to 15 seconds.

Fridays
Pour on the intensity: Swim four segments of 100 meters at 90 percent of maximum effort. Don't rest between segments—instead, keep swimming for 50 meters at 60 percent of maximum.

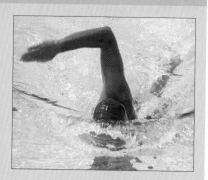

▲ To do well at the 100-meter freestyle, you will need to perfect your form, build strength, and boost speed.

RUNNING

If you want a challenge that's vigorous, yet not so overwhelming as a full marathon of 26.2 miles, aim instead to run a half-marathon—an objective you can reasonably expect to accomplish with eight weeks of training. That's assuming you're already fairly fit, and running three miles three times a week.

The plan (see box, below) involves running more often (four days a week instead of three), gradually increasing your weekly distance. Don't worry about your pace, since your goal—even if you're aiming to compete in a race—is simply to cover the distance comfortably, not get a place in the competition.

SWIMMING

Unless you have the option of swimming in open water, this is one form of training where the scenery can get more than a bit tedious. If you're already swimming a half-hour three times a week in a pool, you'll probably want to swim stronger, faster, better, rather than more often.

What you want to aim for is a competition benchmark, the 100-meter freestyle. And don't just aim to cover the distance at a personal best, aim to win. This will take a different mental approach to training, in which relaxed, meditative strokes aren't going to cut it anymore. Instead, you need to concentrate on perfecting form, building strength, and increasing speed.

To perfect your form, you'll need the assistance of a coach or trainer. The rest you can do on your own. The program (see box, top of page) is based on alternating difficult days with easy days, to the tune of five workouts per week. On Mondays and Wednesdays, concentrate on aerobic and cardiovascular endurance. On Tuesdays and Thursdays, work on muscular endurance and strength. On Fridays, put everything together in an all-out effort.

Follow the program during the eight weeks before the competition. Stick to the same simple directions each week. One exception: During the eighth week, take off the two days before the race.

Running: The Half-Marathon Plan

Week 1	Add another 3-mile run on a fourth day. From here on in, you will be running four days every week, usually covering a longer distance on one of the four days. Schedule a rest day before and after your longest-distance day.
Week 2	Run 4 miles on one of your days.
Week 3	Add a second run of 4 miles, alternating the 4- with the 3-milers, so that your distance schedule is 4–3–4–3. Take rest days when you need them.
Week 4	Time to start really challenging yourself. Run 4 miles on three days, and 5 miles on a fourth day. Take a day off before and after the 5-mile run.
Week 5	Continue boosting your mileage, adding another 5-mile run, and making your longest-distance day a 6-miler, so that your distance schedule is 6–4–5–5.
Week 6	You're still running a 4-miler and two 5-milers, but on the long-distance day, expand your miles to 8. Your distance schedule: 8–4–5–5.
Week 7	Begin by boosting your 8-mile run to 10 miles—a distance that's two-thirds of your goal. If you can do this now, you'll be in good shape next week when you run the half-marathon. Your distance schedule: 10–4–5–5.
Week 8	Taper off as you approach half-marathon day at the end of the week. Go back to the distance you ran in Week 3, 4–3–4–3. Take a day off on Saturday. Run the half-marathon on Sunday.

The Benefits of Cross-Training

Cross-training involves combining two or more different forms of exercise into one workout plan. It sounds like a specialty, but it's a form of exercise you've been doing for years. If you've moved furniture one day, biked to the store the next, and done some heavy yard work on another, you've been cross-training.

The Essence of Cross-Training

Cross-training mixes different forms of exercise. The man who's interested in general fitness almost by necessity engages in cross-training because different forms of exercise are required to achieve basic levels of strength and endurance.

For years, trainers and coaches thought that working on endurance and strength simultaneously was in some ways counterproductive. What they meant was that by trying to do both at the same time, you'd do neither well, and one form of exercise would rob the body of the benefits attained through the other.

There's a basis for this thinking in a fundamental tenet of physiology called the specificity principle. It states that muscles are best able to improve at a specific activity—weight lifting, say, or bicycle riding—when they are trained in just that way. By this reasoning, you don't become a better cyclist by lifting weights, or vice versa.

The specificity principle is still very much alive as a training precept, but even serious athletes now realize that a little variety can break the monotony of stale, repetitive routines, provide balance, and prevent injury. Research indicates that cross-training actually doesn't interfere very much with sport-specific training. One study even suggests that strength training lowers resting heart rate, which helps the heart (although becoming stronger won't necessarily improve aerobic fitness). At the very least, trainers nowadays realize, cross-training does no harm. And for overall fitness, it's a preferred method.

One of the greatest advantages of cross-training is the rate at which it

No-Time Exercises

Cross-training embraces any form of physical activity that fits into your schedule—whether or not you get to the gym or even change into exercise clothes. Here are a few possibilities.

- Walk to work or run for the train.
- Take the dog for a walk.
- Stroll with a baby carriage.
- Take the stairs between floors in the building where you live or work.
- Rough-house with your kids or play sports with them in the backyard.
- Do some yard work with your own hands or nonmotorized hand tools—cutting the grass, trimming hedges, pulling weeds, raking leaves.

How to Be an Ironman

Cross-training has the most meaning to those preparing for a serious event such as the triathlon, a long-distance race that includes segments of running, swimming, and bicycling. If you're a would-be ironman, get a taste of what a triathlete's training program would be like by trying this beginner's routine.

In addition to varying the distances as listed, vary the pace as well. On longer outings, for example, slow the pace to conserve energy. On other days, cover your distance by doing short intervals at a high-intensity pace, followed by longer, less intense intervals in which you maintain a more modest pace.

	Swim	Run	Bike
Mon.	1,200 yd.	4 mi.	—
Tues.	—	—	15 mi.
Wed.	1,800 yd.	6 mi.	—
Thurs.	—	6 mi.	15 mi.
Fri.	1,500 yd.	4 mi.	—
Sat.	—	—	25 mi.
Sun.	—	8 mi.	15 mi.

► *A triathlete runs the last few yards to the finish line. The training program above gives you a taste of an ironman's life.*

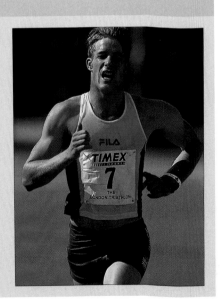

The Challenge of the Triathlon

In the mid-1970s, a group of runners in Southern California, inspired by local lifeguard training, decided to combine running, swimming, and biking into a single exercise program. The triathlon was conceived. One of those pioneers exported the idea to Hawaii, where the granddaddy of triathlons, the Ironman, was born by simply fusing three already-grueling races into a single 140-mile-long exercise in masochism. Incredibly, the idea caught fire and there are now some 2,000 triathlons held in the United States alone, and many others held the world over.

Distances of each segment vary and as yet there is no firm definition of how long a triathlon should be, although the most popular format is the International Standard, consisting of a 1500-meter swim, a 40-kilometer bike race, and a 10-kilometer run. Although more extreme (if not insane) challenges have since been developed, doing a triathlon (especially the Ironman) remains a pinnacle of athletic achievement.

▶ *The start of a triathlon at Parana, Brazil. From modest beginnings, the sport has grown to become hugely popular.*

burns blubber. Doing strength and aerobic training together burns fat better than either form of exercise does by itself.

Cross-training also gives you an opportunity to incorporate exercises or activities into your exercise regimen that make a good match with your schedule and lifestyle. These can be very simple. Taking the stairs at work, rather than the elevator, and pulling weeds in the backyard are two activities that can count as part of a cross-training program.

Mixing and Matching

When you come to mix and match exercises, what should govern your choice? Elite athletes tend to go for activities that exercise the same muscle groups used in their primary sport. So, for example, a top runner might take up bicycling. But for mere mortals like us—who simply want to inject variety into a general-fitness program—it's best to mix dissimilar activities.

The trick is to match exercises that balance one another, each providing an advantage that your other activities don't. It's all a matter of how you interpret the meaning of "balance." Here are three mixing principles to help guide you in your choice.

• Match skill with repetition. Certain forms of exercise, such as running and swimming, involve repetitive, familiar movements in which the mind is free to wander. Mix these with other sports in which high levels of skill are required, so that body and mind are taken in entirely different directions. High-skill activities include snowboarding, soccer, mountain biking, racquet sports, and golf.

• Combine hard and soft. High-impact sports, such as running and tennis, can jar the joints. Mix in some sports that are less abusive to the body. Good examples are bicycling, swimming, and rowing.

• Combine upper and lower. The big problem with running and bicycling is that both target the lower body, but leave the upper body largely unimproved. Aim for a whole-body workout. Possible combinations are listed below. Combine any sport in the left-hand column with any sport in the right-hand one.

- • Walking
- • Running
- • Biking
- • Skiing

- • Swimming
- • Rowing
- • Canoeing/kayaking
- • Tennis

Three Ways to Make Training Easier

Despite good intentions, it's sometimes hard to keep a fitness program going. Having a workout plan is part of the battle, but it won't win the campaign. Here are some tips for adding power to your program.

1 Write it down. Keep track of your progress in a training log. This not only records how well you're sticking to your plan, it provides a sense of accomplishment. Don't just write down times and distances—note things like your frame of mind or how tired you felt as well. These can help give you a sense of what works for you and what doesn't, so you can fine-tune your program.

2 Enlist friends. Training alone can become dull and discouraging. Training with one or more friends or colleagues, however, can provide support, camaraderie, inspiration, and a dash of competitiveness. It also helps motivate you because you're less likely to miss a workout if your buddies are counting on you to be there.

3 Keep it convenient. Make sure the bulk of your training can take place somewhere that's easy to get to, close to your home or workplace. The more you have to travel or otherwise burden yourself with logistical complications, the harder it will be.

The Total Abdominal Workout

Let's get one thing straight: Exercising only your abs won't rid you of midriff flab. You'll need a combined aerobic–strength–abs routine to do that. Beyond firming your belly, strength in the abdominals is essential because the abs' central location in the torso makes them a linchpin of bodily movement.

What the Abdominals Do

The abs consist of four muscle groups layered at the front and sides of the torso. All of them are crucial for keeping your trunk firm, allowing you to bend and twist at the waist while providing the leverage you need to exert force with other parts of the body.

The abdominals support the spine as well, and strengthening your abs shores up the back and protects you against lower back pain. Strong abs also promote a good, erect posture.

Washboard Abs: The Truth

Exercising the abdominal muscles will take inches off your waist, right? Wrong. The spot-reducing theory of exercise is well and truly discredited. Doing a lot of abdominal exercises won't burn off fat around the belly, although you'll probably end up with nicely toned abdominal muscles underneath the flab.

The belly is the first place fat is stored in men, and the last place the body turns to for energy. Not only are men genetically predisposed to having pot bellies, they're also programmed to put on more fat with advancing years, due to a slower metabolism and lower calorie requirements combined with a diet that typically stays the same.

To get rid of the gut, you'll need a healthy diet, fat-burning aerobic exercise, and whole-body muscular fitness. Oh, and keep up the abdominal exercises if you want to see those washboards in the end.

The Workout

You don't have to do all of the exercises described in this section, but you should give some attention to the obliques as well as the two abdominis muscles. It's a good idea to identify the muscles being described by consulting the illustration in "Where the Abs Are."

Exercises should be performed on a mat to prevent harm to the back.

Where the Abs Are

When performing your abdominal exercises, these are the muscles you're targeting.

Internal obliques
These lie beneath the external obliques, connecting the last four ribs with the pelvis. They also help you bend and twist, but pull in opposite directions from the external obliques.

Traversus abdominis
These lies underneath the rectus abdominis, forming a complementary sheet of muscle that runs across the gut instead of up and down it, to provide a supportive girdle for internal organs.

Rectus abdominis
This flat sheet of muscle runs from below the chest to the pelvis. It's the muscle most often associated with the term "abdominals," because when exceptionally toned, it provides a washboard look.

External obliques
These run down the sides of your torso between the chest and pelvis. Working in opposition to each other (one side of your body relaxes while the other contracts), the external obliques power bending and twisting motion.

The Workout Schedule

The abdominals are among the few muscles in the body that can stand up to being worked every day, although it's best to concentrate on different areas on alternating days.

Abdominal muscles can also stand up to high numbers of repetitions, making progress a highly individual matter that rides on both your strength and endurance. Keep track of how many you do each day, and try to boost the number of reps by about 10 percent a week, exercising to exhaustion.

When choosing exercises, strive to hit the major muscle groups from at least two angles on the days you work them. You should create your own workout schedule, but here's one way to do it.

Monday	Crunches and vacuums
Tuesday	Obliques
Wednesday	Crunches and vacuums
Thursday	Obliques
Friday	Crunches and vacuums
Saturday	Obliques
Sunday	Your day off

Target Your Abs

It's a misconception that there are upper and lower abdominal muscles. The rectus abdominis is actually one large muscle. You can, however, choose exercises that mostly train the upper or lower area of the one muscle. For example, crunches work upper ab muscles at 90 to 100 percent of their capacity, while pelvic lifts work them at only about 30 percent. If targeting the lower abdominals, however, those figures are roughly reversed.

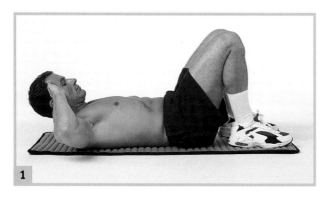

1

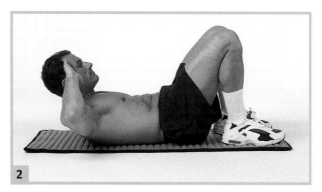

2

Basic Crunches

1 Lie on your back with elbows out to the sides, hands at your temples or cupped behind your ears (not grabbing the back of the neck), or cross arms over your chest. Your head should be a few inches off the mat, chin tucked slightly forward. Feet should be flat on the floor, placed next to each other about 6 inches from your buttocks, with knees bent at 45 degrees. (Keep legs slightly apart.)

2 Pushing the small of your back into the floor, slowly curl your upper torso up toward your knees, raising your shoulder blades (but not your lower back) off the ground. Hold for a second. Lower to the starting position, but do not relax between repetitions. Do as many as you can, or do multiple sets of 10 repetitions.

(!) *Don't hold your breath. Exhale as you crunch forward, inhale as you lower yourself to the starting position.*

Vacuums

The reflexive sucking in of your gut at the beach can actually condition your abs if done systematically.

1 Sit in a kneeling position, feet crossed behind you and hands held at the hips or thighs. Keeping the upper body erect, let the air out of your lungs.

2 Immediately suck your gut in and up as far as it can go. Hold for 5 seconds, then release. Take a normal breath, and repeat. Do 2 to 3 sets of 10 repetitions.

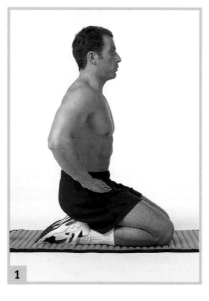

1

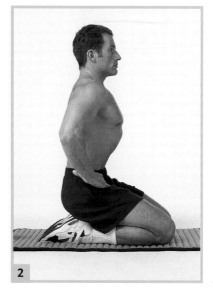

2

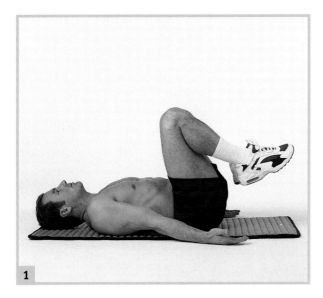

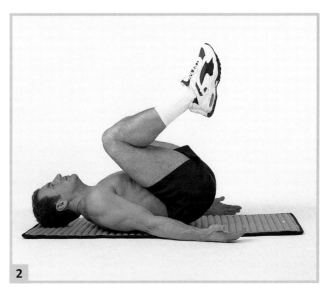

Reverse Curls

Works the lower abdominals.

1 Lie flat on your back with your head resting on the mat and hands by your side, palms up. Bring up your legs so that your thighs are at a 90-degree angle to the mat. Your knees should be touching each other. This is your starting position.

2 Pull your knees toward your chest, then slowly shift them back to the starting position. Keep the movements slow and controlled. The muscles in the lower abdomen should be doing the work, so try not to use momentum to help you. Remember to breathe out as you curl the knees toward you and breathe in as you lower them.

Oblique Twists

1 Stand with feet shoulder-width apart, hips facing forward and knees loose. Hold a broomstick across your shoulders behind your neck, hands grasping the outer ends of the broomstick.

2 Keeping your hips motionless and facing forward, slowly twist to the left as far as you can. Return to the starting position and pause. Twist to the right, then return to the starting position. Continue alternating, keeping a slow and steady pace.

⚠ *This exercise can strain the lower back, so make sure you move slowly, keeping control at all times.*

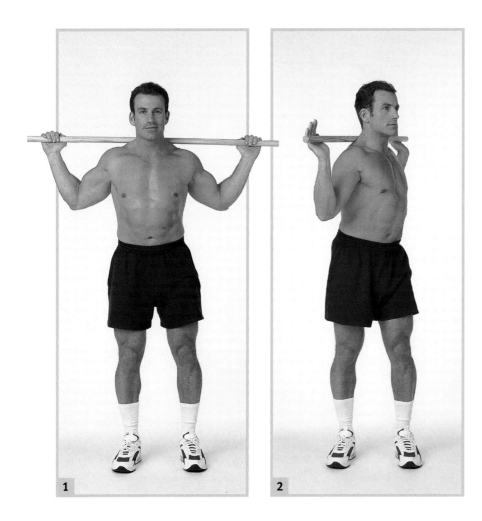

Crossover Crunches

1 Take up the same starting position as for basic crunches: Lying on the floor, feet flat and together, knees bent at 45 degrees. If you crossed your arms over your chest on crunches, make sure you have your hands at your temples or cupped behind your ears for these, elbows to the side of your head. Raise shoulders off the floor, curling your torso up toward your knee.

2 Slightly twist your trunk so that your left elbow points toward your right knee. Hold for a second, return to the starting position (without relaxing your abdominal muscles), then repeat, raising your right elbow toward your left knee. Continue alternating, doing as many as you can, or doing multiple sets of 10 repetitions.

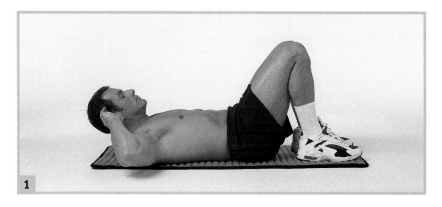

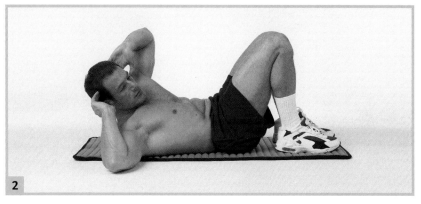

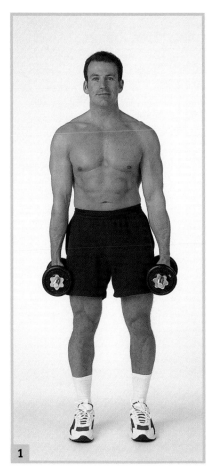

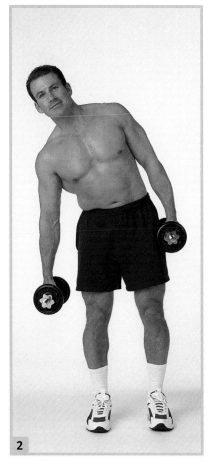

Dumbbell Side Bends

Adding weights makes this move harder on your muscles than other oblique exercises—a good booster for advanced training, but not one that's necessary for the majority of men.

1 Stand with feet shoulder-width apart, holding a dumbbell in each hand, arms at your side with palms facing in. As a rule, light weights and high repetitions (12 to 20) are better than heavy weights and low repetitions.

2 Keeping your torso facing straight ahead at all times, slowly bend to the right side, letting the dumbbell drop down your leg until you feel the obliques on your left side working. Don't allow your torso to twist in the direction of the bend. Slowly bring yourself to the starting position, then repeat on the same side without resting between reps. After as many reps as you are comfortable doing, repeat on the left side.

Oblique Crunches

These provide an extra dose of exertion to the obliques.

1 Lie flat on your back, hands at your temples or cupped behind your ears. Let your legs fall to the right side, so that your upper body remains flat on the floor while your lower body lies on its side.

2 Keeping the shoulders as parallel to the floor as possible, lift your shoulder blades off the floor. (Do not aim an elbow at one knee.) Hold for a second, then lower to the starting position. Do 10 to 20, then drop knees to the opposite side and repeat. If you can, do multiple sets.

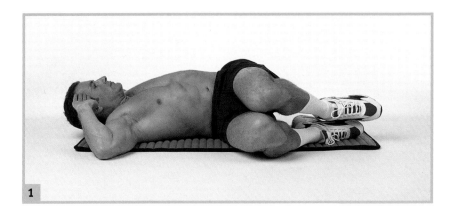

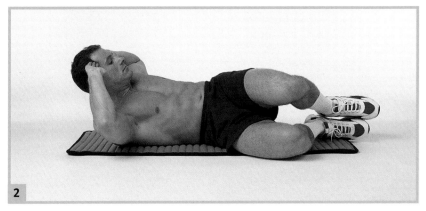

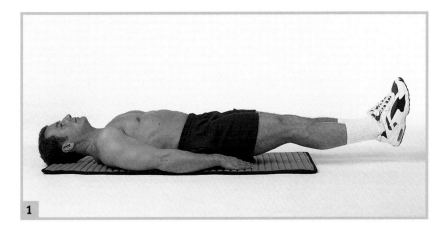

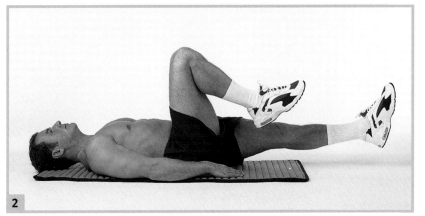

Lying Knee Raises

1 Lie on your back on the floor with legs straight and arms close by your side, hands palm-down and tucked slightly under your buttocks. Press the small of your back against the floor and lift your heels about 3 inches.

2 Lift your right knee toward your chest, keeping your left leg elevated and straight. Hold for a second, then straighten your right knee to the starting position and repeat with the left knee. Do as many as you can, or do multiple sets of 5 to 10 repetitions with each knee.

 It's best not to do this exercise if you have a weak back.

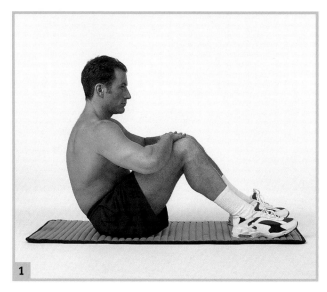

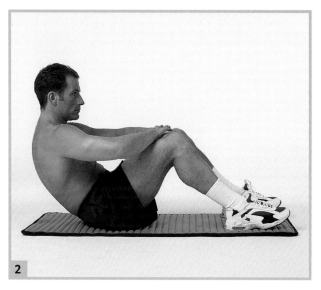

Sit-Backs

A twist on the situp, this move works the same muscles in a different way.

1 Sit on the floor, knees bent and feet flat on the floor about shoulder-width apart. Rest hands lightly on your knees, fingers interlocked with palms facing your knees. Your torso should be tilted back slightly from a 90-degree angle to the floor.

2 Lower your torso back toward the floor, curling your upper body forward, rounding your lower back. When your torso reaches a 45-degree angle to the floor, return to the starting position. Do 2 sets of 10.

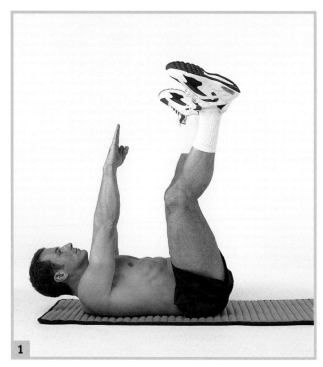

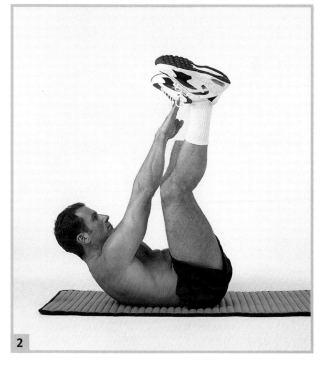

Lying Toe Reaches

1 Lie flat on your back, with legs extended toward the ceiling in a "V" shape. Keep your knees loose and unlocked. Point your arms toward the ceiling, placing the palm of one hand over the back of the other.

2 Curl your shoulder blades up, reaching toward the right foot with your outstretched hands. Hold for a second, then lower to the starting position, keeping your abs contracted. Raise your hands toward your left foot. Repeat 5 to 10 times to each foot, then do 1 or 2 more sets.

Raised Leg Crunches

Lie flat on your back with your knees bent and lower legs supported by a bench or chair. Your thighs should be at 90 degrees to the mat. Tilt the head forward to 45 degrees and hold your hands at your temples or cupped behind the ears. This is the starting position. Slowly crunch forward, breathing out as you do so, then slowly move back to the starting position while breathing in. Repeat, but don't relax between reps.

ⓘ *Never pull on your neck during a crunch. Doing so may injure your neck or upper back.*

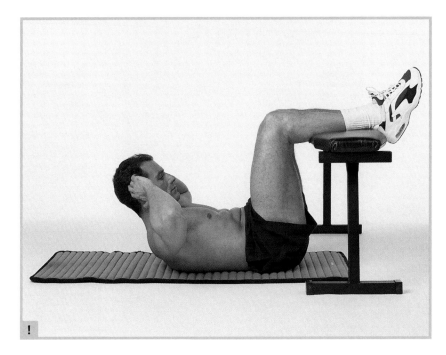

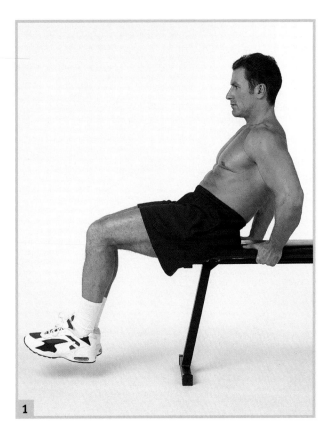

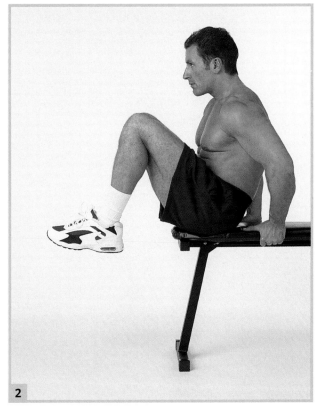

Bench Crunches
Works upper, lower, and oblique abs.

1 Sit on the narrow end of a bench with feet flat on the floor, hands grasping the sides of the bench. Lean your torso back about 45 degrees and raise your feet a few inches off the floor, keeping knees slightly bent.

2 Bring your upper body to an upright position while pulling your knees into your chest. Hold for a second, then return both the upper and the lower body to the starting position. Do 2 sets of 10.

Rest and Recovery

It's a little-known fact that becoming fitter depends to a large extent on *not* exercising. That's right: Sitting on the sofa, lying in bed, or doing only light activity is at least as important as working out. This is called rest and recovery, and without it, exercised muscles can't become more powerful.

Why Rest Is Important

Most of us harbor a misconception that muscles become stronger or more efficient while we're doing a strenuous activity such as running, cycling, swimming, or weight lifting. Likewise, we feel that muscles break down and become weaker when we sit doing nothing.

The reality is very different, however. Exercise is what breaks muscles down and makes them weaker. Rest and recovery after exercise is what builds muscles up and makes them stronger, thanks to the body's ability to repair damaged tissue so that it's better than before.

Most concern about rest focuses on top-class athletes. They have such vigorous schedules that coaches and doctors worry about overtraining, a syndrome in which muscles are repeatedly taxed beyond their abilities, adversely affecting performance for weeks, even months in some cases. But getting adequate rest is also important to the rest of us, who are in danger of "overreaching"—a kind of short-term overtraining from which muscles can usually recover in a matter of days.

Overreaching often takes place when you begin a new program by overly exerting yourself, or if you suddenly push yourself harder in an activity you're already doing. In all your efforts, you should aim for a balance between challenging muscles enough, but not too much. The penalty if you overdo it is pain, fatigue, loss of motivation, and the risk of a permanent layoff.

TOO MUCH REST?

Some may say that there's more danger in resting too much and losing what you've gained than in exercising too much.

The truth is that declines in conditioning don't occur quickly, and more is not always better. For example, swimmers who train for 3 or 4 hours a day have been shown to improve no more than peers who swim 1 to 1½ hours. In other research, swimmers and runners who cut back their training by 60 percent showed no loss of endurance even after three weeks. Weight trainers who stop their programs don't begin a noticeable decline in what they've gained for as long as a month.

Four Ways to Balance Workouts with Rest

Finding a proper mix of exercise (but not too much) with recovery (but not too much) is as much art as science. It largely depends on how much exertion you feel you're putting out. Here are some guidelines.

1 Hold back when beginning. Even if muscles are capable of it, strenuous activity will make them sore if they're not used to it. When beginning an exercise program or resuming one after six months or more, at first do less than you think you can. Increase intensity by no more than 10 percent per week, whether in terms of pace, distance, sets, resistance, or repetitions.

2 Take time out to rest during the workout. Allowing muscles momentary relief can help them to continue sustained effort and ultimately deliver superior results from your workout. This is especially true of resting between sets while weight lifting. Remember that you may want to vary your rest periods according to your goals.

3 Give your muscles a day off. Between intense workouts, allow exercised muscles 48 hours to recover before exercising them again, especially if you're doing the same activity. You don't have to be completely inactive, however. Weight lifters often do what are called split routines, in which they work on the upper body one day and the lower body the next. That's a strategy which allows daily workouts while at the same time providing ample recovery time for every muscle group.

4 Do active recovery. Another way to stay moving is to do some sort of light activity on your off day, especially if it's different from the previous day's workout—walking, for example, after a hard bike ride the day before. Such "active rest" may even have the positive side effect of reducing any soreness by helping to flush waste products out of the muscles.

Protecting against Injury

Most injuries sustained during exercise are preventable if you follow basic safety practices, use good form, and anticipate common problems before they occur. Even small traumas can provoke lingering complaints years or perhaps decades later. Here's how to avoid some of the most likely problems.

How to Keep Out of Trouble

A quick review of the most important exercise practices is in order. Following these will go a long way toward keeping your body in action and your program on track.

• Progress gradually. Men who have the least amount of training have the most injuries.

• Warm up. Warming up not only makes muscles more pliable, and less likely to tear, it lubricates joints and improves muscle cells' ability to convert oxygen to energy.

• Stretch. Increasing flexibility further reduces risk of injury.

• Use safety gear. Believe it or not, it was invented for a reason.

> "We often say that you shouldn't play your sport to be in shape; you should be in shape to play your sport. Training for the demands of the sport prevents injury."
>
> Edward R. Laskowski, M.D., co-director of the Mayo Clinic's Sports Medicine Center, Rochester, Minnesota

• Get some expert instruction. You can pick up a lot by doing, but always try to learn proper form from a coach, trainer, or publication before attempting something new.

• Pay attention to pain. It's a sign that something is wrong.

When to See a Doctor, When to Do It Yourself

There are times in most sportsmen's lives when something goes very wrong indeed. The illustration shows some of the signs of serious injury in a selection of the body's more injury-prone parts. If ever in doubt about sport-related pain or discomfort, see the doctor—take his or her advice, not ours.

If your injury is minor, however, you don't have to take it lying down. Muscles ache because minor internal blood and fluid spillage is causing pressure. To staunch the flow, use the RICE method of rest, ice, compression, and elevation.

• Rest the injured area, to reduce circulation and allow damaged tissue to mend.

• Ice the ache to constrict blood vessels and numb the pain. Don't apply ice directly to the skin, however, and avoid leaving the ice pack in place for more than about 20 minutes, to reduce the risk of frostbite.

• Compress the area with a snug bandage, to squeeze blood vessels and reduce swelling.

• Elevate the damaged area, for 20 minutes or so, to a level above the heart, to increase the flowing-out of accumulated fluid while decreasing the flowing-in of more blood.

Head
A blow to the head followed by disorientation or loss of consciousness, even for a moment, are signs of concussion. Also be alert to dizziness, confusion, headache, nausea, weakness, or fatigue.

Shoulders
Your shoulder feels like it's come out of its socket; you can't move the shoulder or raise your arms above your head. It could be dislocated.

Elbows
A persistent numbness or tingling "funny-bone" feeling might indicate nerve damage. If you develop Popeye-like small bumps that protrude from the elbows, you could have bursitis.

Back
Pain radiating down below the knee, or accompanied by any numbness or loss of coordination or body control could indicate a nerve or disk problem.

Knees
Not being able to fully extend or flex your knee might signal a loose piece of bone or cartilage.

The Benefits of Massage

Many athletes swear that massage helps them both avoid and recover from injury, by relaxing muscles and flushing wastes out of them. The scientific proof is largely lacking for these claims—that's true of any therapy whose results are not measurable beyond the fact that beneficiaries say it makes them feel better. But who can argue with that? Here are a number of simple self-massage techniques for several areas especially prone to soreness or stiffness.

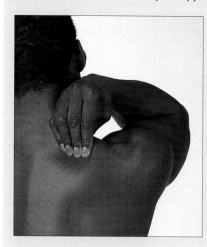

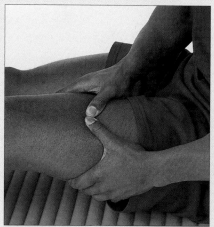

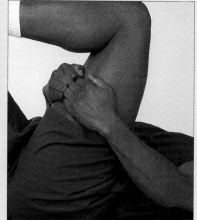

Neck and Shoulders

Reach your right hand onto your right shoulder. Dig into the thick muscle at the base of your neck, tilting your head away from your hand while dragging your fingers toward the right shoulder. To also massage the shoulder, press and squeeze the muscle at the top of the shoulder, rocking fingers back and forth. Repeat on the other side.

Thighs

Sitting on the floor or on a mat, use both hands to knead, squeeze, and shake the muscles at the top of one of your legs so as to loosen them up. Then place one hand on either side of your thigh so that your thumbs meet at the top of the leg. Press down firmly with both thumbs, pushing them along your thigh toward your knee. Repeat with the other leg.

Hamstrings

Sit against a wall with one leg propped up. Loosen the back of the propped leg by kneading and squeezing, then lie flat, right knee bent and right foot flat on the floor. Rest your left ankle on your right knee, grab the back of the left leg with both hands. Press with fingers bent so that the backs of the fingers of your hands make contact with each other. Slide your fingers to your butt.

Keep Your Cool

Maintaining a safe body temperature while working out is often well down the list of the average man's fitness concerns. It's time to think again. A breakdown of the body's ability to regulate its internal temperature is itself a form of injury, with possibly life-threatening consequences. Here's how to keep your thermostat set properly in extreme conditions.

OUT IN THE COLD

Low temperatures can threaten the body's regulation of vital functions such as heartbeat and metabolism. Hypothermia is particularly likely if you get wet, which accelerates heat loss from the body.

For protection, wear clothes that wick moisture away from the body rather than holding it close to the skin. If you tire, find shelter because your body heat will start to drop as soon as you become less active.

THE TORRID ZONE

When it's hot, the muscles and skin become undersupplied with the fluids necessary for temperature regulation and the production of sweat. Avoiding heat exhaustion is largely a matter of staying out of heat when you're most active. Do strenuous activity on hot days before 8:00 A.M. or after 6:00 P.M., wear loose-fitting clothes and drink lots of fluid. Be alert to warning signs such as goose bumps, light-headedness, and cramps.

The Best Pain Relievers

Prevention is far better than cure, of course, but when all else fails, you need effective pain relief.

For sportsmen, ibuprofen (Advil, Nuprin, Motrin) is the analgesic of choice. Its anti-inflammatory properties mean that it reduces swelling and with it, pain. The drug acetaminophen (Tylenol) works a different way. It kills pain by acting on signals to the brain, but does little to reduce inflammation.

Second-best choice is aspirin. It's weaker than ibuprofen, but does have anti-inflammatory properties. Be careful, though. It can irritate the stomach, and it interferes with the clotting of the blood, which makes it inadvisable for use in contact sports.

Exercises involving speed, balance, high-impact movement, heavy lifting, or some combination of these factors, produce the highest rates of injury, but with proper mechanics, the most likely pains and problems can be avoided. Here's what you should be aware of if you're running, cycling, inline skating, weight lifting, stairclimbing, or rowing.

Running

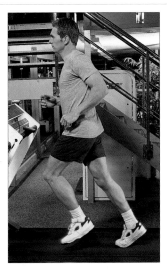

▶ *Beat cramped muscles by adopting a looser running style.*

Problem

High impact, from landing on one foot with full body weight, can stress muscles, tendons, and joints.

Solutions

• Walk a bit. Alternating walking with running, especially in the early weeks of a program, allows the body to get accustomed to the strains of running.

• Wear shoes made for running. Running is one of the few sports that absolutely demands sport-specific footwear, to cushion impact and promote smooth stride.

• Use soft, even surfaces. A path that's hard-packed, pitched, or full of holes invites twists, sprains, and fractures.

• Take short steps. A stride that's too long overextends muscles and tendons, and may actually slow you down, due to a braking effect when your leading foot hits the ground.

• Relax. A tense, closed, clenched-fist running style can cramp your muscles. A looser style is easier to sustain, and can be faster as well.

Bicycling

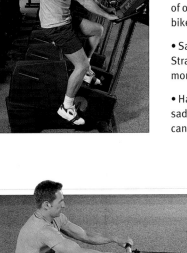

▶ *The bike seat is correctly adjusted when your knee is only slightly bent at the bottom of the stroke.*

Problems

Outdoor cycling risks accidents, and crashes involving head injuries can kill. Both outdoor and indoor biking can be hard on the back and knees.

Solutions

• Always wear a brain bucket. A helmet is cheap and necessary insurance. To avoid crashes, secure shoestrings, outerwear, and cargo away from spokes and chain, beware of opening car doors and other obstacles, and keep the bike's speed within your abilities.

• Save high gears for when you have sufficient speed. Straining against them at slower speed makes knees more susceptible to overuse injuries.

• Have a bicycle mechanic check your position on the saddle, handlebars, and pedals. Improper positioning can cause knee and back pain.

Rowing

Problem

Driving rearward with too much effort from the torso can strain back muscles.

▶ *Push back with your legs before pulling the rower's handle toward you.*

Solution

• Move fluidly. To row properly, you need to move smoothly and steadily through a precise sequence of movements. With upper body pitched forward slightly, push back with the legs first. Lean slightly back and pull the handle toward your torso with your arms. As you return to the starting position, extend your arms, bend your legs, and lean slightly forward again.

Weight Lifting

Problems

Improper form can not only damage joints and strain muscles, it can cut the effectiveness of your workout.

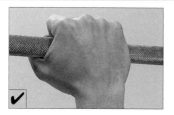

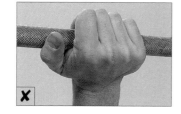

▶ *When you grip the bar, fingers should be on one side, thumb on the other (top). A bad grip (bottom) has the thumb on the same side as the fingers.*

Solutions

• Keep joints loose. Locking joints such as the elbows or knees takes pressure off muscles (that's cheating), and puts it on bones, which can irritate or injure complex joints. Keep movements slow and controlled.

• Breathe. Avoid the tendency to hold your breath while lifting: Lack of oxygen during exertion can cause dangerous blackouts. As a rule, breathe out when lifting a weight and breathe in when returning to your starting position.

• Use a proper grip. For stability and control, grab bars by wrapping your thumb on one side and your fingers on the other. Avoid placing all fingers on one side, which allows the bar to fall if it slips. Place your hands evenly on the bar to keep weights balanced.

Stairclimbing

Problems

Poor stance can cause tingling in the feet and pressure on the neck and back.

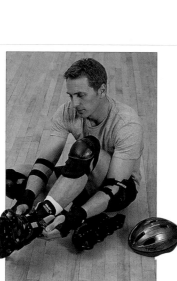

▶ *Always keep an upright stance—don't be tempted to lean forward.*

Solutions

• Be flat-footed. Stepping with the toes puts pressure on nerves in the balls of the feet. Keeping feet flat, covering the entire platform area with the soles of shock-absorbent shoes, spreads out the pressure. Loosen laces to help improve circulation. Use short, shallow steps to reduce pressure, which also burns more energy.

• Stand straight. Bending over seems more relaxed, but it puts pressure on the neck and lower back, especially if you're craning to view the TV or aerobics class.

Inline Skating

Problems

Falling is easy, and injuries to head, wrists, elbows, and knees are common.

▶ *Inline skating demands proper protective gear—a helmet, as well as pads for the elbows, knees, and wrists.*

Solutions

• Don a helmet. Injuries to the head are less common than to joints, but are disastrous when they occur.

• Wear pads. The wrists are by far the most common injury sites; guarding them with protective gear cuts their risk of injury by something like six times. But don't forget the elbow and knee pads.

• Take lessons. Learning how to properly brake, stride, and fall can help eliminate injuries in beginners, and also advance your skills beyond self-taught levels.

• Remember to look up. Watching your feet, as many beginners do, tends to throw you off balance. Keeping your eyes on the horizon helps put your center of gravity over your feet, where it belongs.

The Office Workout

You're wearing your best clothes. There's little room and even less equipment. And there are certain positions you just don't want your boss to see you in. But the office is where exercise is most necessary, thanks to a combination of inactivity, poor posture, and mental and physical strains.

The Toll of Work

Our bodies are designed to be in motion, but instead we spend all day sitting in meetings or slouched down in front of computers performing repetitive tasks. Beyond our being sedentary, the positions we take at work tend to strain and fatigue certain muscles, while the mental stress we feel makes us tense.

The purpose of the office workout is not only to offset our lack of normal physical activity, but to take out the cricks and kinks we feel from poor posture, as well as relieve overall tension.

In addition to the exercises shown in this section, take the following simple physical steps to keep tension and strain at bay.

• Shift positions often. Holding the same position too long is the primary cause of stiff and tense muscles. Even if your work is engrossing, take a small break every 10 to 15 minutes to stretch your legs, move your arms, flex your fingers.

• Hobnob on the hoof. Wherever possible, try to speak with your colleagues while walking, especially if you know the topic is going to be a stressful one. It may seem strange, but talking while walking invites a casual, open attitude.

• Go for a walk at your lunch break. Even if you can't schedule a workout, at least get out of doors for a brisk stroll, to let your mind expand and give your legs a chance to do what they're designed for.

• Stand up whenever you answer the phone: It gives muscles and circulation a change of pace, and makes you sound more dynamic as well.

Wall Sits

This is a good all-round leg exercise.

Stand with your back against a wall, feet about shoulder-width apart. Slowly slide your back down the wall as you walk your feet forward, until you reach a bent-knee position that looks as if you're seated in a chair. (To avoid stress on the knee, keep your thighs positioned above the level of the knee.) Hold for 5 to 10 seconds, then slide back up to the starting position. Do 5 repetitions.

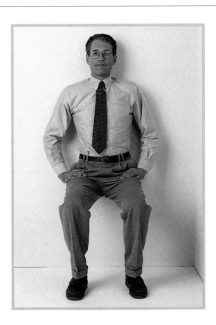

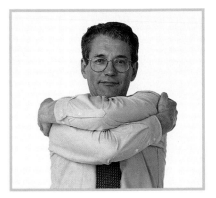

Shoulder Hugs

To relieve shoulder and upper-back tension, cross both arms over your chest, reaching around your right shoulder blade with your left hand and your left shoulder blade with your right hand.

Chair Dips

Chair dips will give you an excellent upper-body workout.

1 Sit on the edge of a chair with your heels flat on the floor. Place your hands on the chair's forward edge and carefully inch your buttocks off and away from the chair while supported by your hands. Keep your back straight.

2 Slowly lower yourself until your upper arms are more or less parallel with the floor, then lift back up. Do 8 to 12.

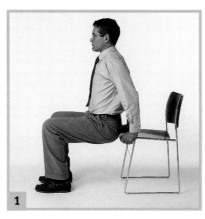

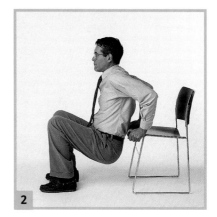

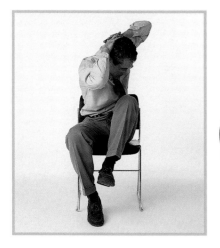

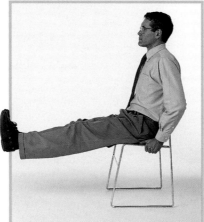

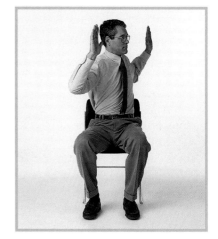

Knee-to-Elbow Touches

Works the abdominals.

Sit upright in your chair, feet flat on the floor and link fingers behind your head. Lift your left knee, and bend your right elbow down toward the knee. Return your left foot to the floor, then lift your right knee, touching it with your left elbow. Repeat at least 5 times.

Seated Leg Lifts

Works the thighs.

Sit up straight in a chair with both your legs extended and with feet flat on the floor. Lift both feet off the floor together, keeping the legs straight, so that your legs and torso make an "L" shape. Hold for 5 seconds and lower your legs back down. Repeat.

Twists

Works the chest and abs.

Sit up straight on the edge of your chair, holding arms in an "I surrender" position. Keeping your hips steady, turn your torso and head to the left as far as possible. Hold for about 2 seconds, then return to the starting position. Repeat 3 times on the left, then do 3 twists to the right.

Let Go of the Tension with Mind Games

Pressing deadlines, ringing phones, angry bosses—they're here to stay. But you can still escape occasionally with these microreleases throughout the day.

• Take your mind on vacation by visualizing a faraway place. You're high on a peak, above it all. You can see for miles around and there's no one in sight. The wind is hissing through pines below. Concentrate: Part of your mind is really there, and it is relaxed.

• Gaze out the window, and fix your eyes on something—a bird, a bug, a distant tree, a taxicab. Let your senses momentarily take over: If you do more looking and listening, you'll do less thinking and worrying.

• Having a sense of control is perhaps the most potent of all stress-busters. When the phone rings, think, "They will just have to wait a moment." Take a deep breath first, then let yourself pick up the receiver.

• Every hour or so, stop what you are doing and do a mental rundown of how stressed every part of your body feels. Pay particular attention to your hands, shoulders, neck, and jaw. Then take a moment to mentally relax the tense areas.

• Have a toy handy. It could be a physics gizmo (a floating magnet, a top), an action figure, a squirt gun. Just looking at it lying in your drawer puts you in carefree-kid mode.

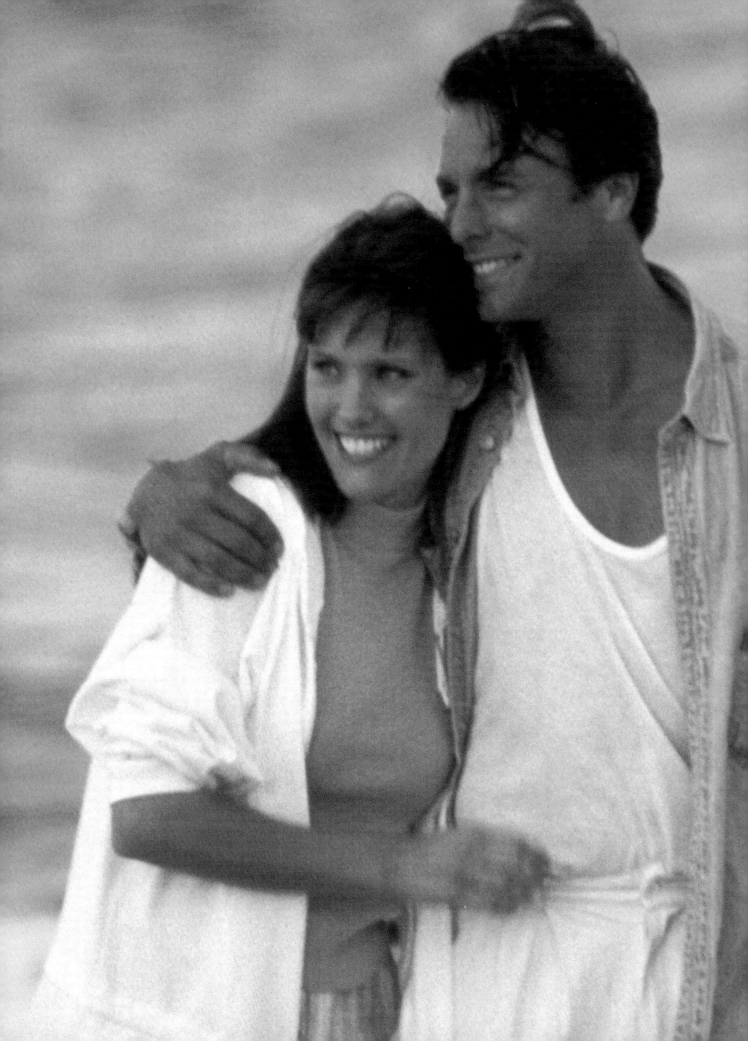

Improving Relationships

Effective Communication

Communication comes easily to some people, but—as the women in your life may have hinted once or twice—most of us could use a little help. This is something men need to master. The old cliché contains more than a grain of truth: Good communication is the heart of every successful relationship.

Talk, Talk, Talk

Through talking together, sharing hopes and dreams, making plans, you build a partnership and learn about each other. And because sharing your thoughts and feelings creates intimacy and trust, it's also the key to great sex.

Good communication is also the key to resolving love's inevitable little conflicts, as well as to avoiding the big ones that could destroy your relationship. "It's important to be able to talk about what's going on in your relationship, even the unpleasant things," says Louanne Cole Weston, Ph.D., a sex therapist in Sacramento, California, who writes the "Sex Matters" column for the *San Francisco Examiner*. "If not, you may have a relationship that seems smooth on the outside, but you really don't know each other very deeply. That leads to trouble."

There's another reason why talk is essential. Scrapping traditional ideas about gender differences had its liberating side, but we may have gone too far. As John Gray, Ph.D., put it in his best-selling book *Men Are from Mars, Women Are from Venus*, "Not only do men and women communicate differently, but they think, feel, perceive, react, respond, love, need, and appreciate differently."

For example, have you noticed how, in relationships, women seem to crave intimacy and fear separation, while men want independence and fear getting trapped? It seems that the more you want your own space, the harder she tries to hold you close. If we're going to get along, we obviously have to talk about this.

"It's very common in our culture for couples to avoid the tough talk because they don't want to rock the boat. But if you don't rock the boat by talking about the important things in your relationship, one day she may suddenly say 'I'm outta here.' And it will hit you like a brickbat because you didn't see it coming."

Louanne Cole Weston, Ph.D., Sacramento, California, sex therapist and sex advice columnist

So talk to her. Tell her how you feel, what you need. Even more important, listen. Listen closely to what's important to her, what upsets her, or what makes her happy. Really make an effort to hear what she's saying instead of projecting what you're thinking. For example, Dr. Weston says, "Try not to predict where she's going with her conversation. If you think you know what she's going to say, you tend to hear that instead of what she's really saying."

In other words, give her a chance to talk about whatever she wants to talk about. This may not seem terribly important to you, but for her it is the lifeblood of the relationship.

NONVERBAL COMMUNICATION

It's not only the spoken word that's important in communicating—there are many ways to "talk" without words. For example, fixing the sink or planning a vacation may be your way of communicating your feelings about her.

Those are nice thoughts, but they don't tell her what she needs to hear. What works better? Try using your

Reading Body Language

Does she take your arm when you're crossing the street? When you're talking, does she sit facing you, looking you in the eyes, nodding, listening, smiling? Or does she gaze off into the distance, her body slightly turned aside, arms folded protectively across her chest, legs crossed? You say you've never noticed? Well, you'd better; she's talking to you.

And, even when it doesn't seem like it, you're talking to her—constantly. Before you speak a single word, she may have already made up her mind about you from such things as the way you stand or walk, whether you hold yourself with confidence or slouch like a loser, whether your glance is gentle and kind or aggressive and predatory.

Experts say that as much as two-thirds of the information we convey is through body language. Some signals, like the defensive stance of crossed arms and legs, are pretty obvious and universal. But there are highly individual "dialects," too. Each of us—whether we're aware of it or not—puts out his or her communiqués all the time.

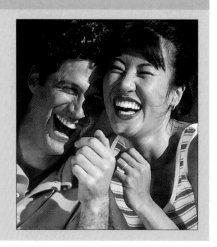
hands, suggests Timothy Perper, Ph.D., a biologist who wrote *Sex Signals: The Biology of Love*. "A caress here, a hug there are very useful ways to express affection," Dr. Perper says. "Use touch as communication, not just as an overture to sex."

Talk Your Way to Great Sex

"A healthy sex life means different things for men and women," says Aaron Vinik, M.D., Ph.D., director of research at the Diabetes Institute in Norfolk, Virginia. For him, "Men tolerate closeness to have intercourse, while women tolerate intercourse to have closeness."

A man's life outside the bedroom typically has little room for tenderness or passion. But to have a life *inside* the bedroom, he usually finds his heart is capable of opening up.

For the majority of women, the process is reversed. Intimacy—closeness, warmth, trust—has to come first. When a woman feels secure in love, she is ready to move toward sex.

So if you want great sex, these two approaches are going to have to be accommodated. Again, the solution is talking—and not just about sex. Listen to her. Connect with her. And confide in her. Tell her how you're feeling about your life, and about the relationship. If you're worried or

hurting, don't hide it from her. Compared to you, she's an expert on feelings, and she's not afraid of them, either in herself or in you.

Sharing feelings with you is a turn-on for her. So take it slowly. Cuddle her, talk openly together. When you're both relaxed and comfortable, deep physical intimacy will

be almost inevitable. Nobody's saying this is easy. "It takes courage to talk about the things that are important in your relationship," Dr. Weston says. "And it takes courage on a daily basis."

But if you do find that courage, you'll find her heart. And if you have her heart, you have all of her.

Understanding Your Partner's Needs

For a relationship to work, each partner's needs have to be met, and each of us tends to believe that the other's needs are just like our own. But that attitude doesn't take account of the very real differences between men and women. Your partner's needs are her own and nobody else's.

> **"Though a man loves a girl ever so much, he never succeeds in winning her without a great deal of talking."**
> *Kama Sutra, Indian love manual*

You Need to Know Her Needs

Men tend to offer women the same kind of support *we'd* like to receive; women treat us as *they'd* like to be treated. But in reality this approach may not always work.

For example, if you see that your buddy is upset over something, you'd normally either back off and leave him alone until he cools down, or offer some words of encouragement: "Don't worry, you can handle it." A woman doesn't want to be left alone with her troubles; she wants your active support. She needs to talk and be listened to; she needs a hug and your undivided attention. One of the most important ways you can build a successful love relationship is to learn everything you can about your partner.

So how do you do that? It's pretty simple, really. Tune in to what she likes, then listen, watch, and learn.

TUNING IN

Part of your job description in a relationship is to fulfill your partner's needs and, as much as you can, to make her happy. And you can't do that if you have no idea what she likes and needs.

So how do you know? Louanne Cole Weston, Ph.D., a sex therapist in Sacramento, California, who writes the "Sex Matters" column for the *San Francisco Examiner*, offers this truly revolutionary approach: Ask her. "That's the best way to find out for sure what she'd really like," Dr. Weston says.

Problem is, sometimes it may not be as simple as it sounds, especially if the subject is sex. "If she's been feeling deprived, she may vent her frustrations and shoot for the moon when you finally ask her what she'd like from you," Dr. Weston says. "That's when it helps for you to calmly ask what she'd be reasonably happy with. The idea is to ask clarifying questions so you can get a workable answer."

Naturally, it's better to know your partner's desires before things get to this point. So make her your full-time project. Listen, watch, and learn. Is she a reader? What kind of books does she like? On vacation, does she prefer a day in the mountains to a day at the beach? What are her favorite foods and restaurants? Does she like sports, or would she rather go to the opera or a concert?

How to Be a Better Listener

Relationship gurus say the best gift a man can give his female partner is to listen to her. John Gray, Ph.D., author of *Men Are from Mars, Women Are from Venus*, notes that 90 percent of the people in therapy are women. "And why is that? Because women will pay to have somebody listen to what they're feeling."

The following suggestions will help your listening skills. But, warns sex therapist Louanne Cole Weston, Ph.D., who writes the "Sex Matters" column for the *San Francisco Examiner*, it's not enough to just go through the motions. "You've got to mean it when you follow these guidelines," Dr. Weston says. "Just saying 'uh-huh' when you're not really hearing her is patronizing and self-defeating."

• Pay attention. Don't drift off, or start preparing an answer before you fully hear what she has to say.

• Listen with your heart as well as your head. Listen to the words, but also to the feeling being conveyed.

• Listen with your head as well as your heart. If you tend to react emotionally, use your head to keep from getting upset.

• Try to grasp the essence of what she's getting at.

• Maintain eye contact. It shows her you're paying attention.

• Give her encouragement and feedback with smiles, nods, and an occasional "uh-huh."

• Paraphrase back what she has said. Like this: "So, when I said, 'that's the dumbest idea I ever heard,' you felt invalidated, right?"

• Ask questions. If you're not sure what she's saying, ask her to clarify. Asking questions also shows her you're paying attention.

• Most of the time, keep quiet and don't interrupt.

• Always follow the golden rule. Be the kind of listener you would like her to be for you.

Tune in to what turns her on. And this, of course, means in bed as well as everywhere else.

Little Things Count

You don't need 40-yard touchdown passes to make a woman happy. A few yards at a time is better. For example, suggests Gena Ogden, Ph.D., a certified sex therapist in Massachusetts and author of *Women Who Love Sex*, "Make eye contact with her during the day." That's the kind of little expression of love and intimacy that's most meaningful to her. So is asking her how her day went—and listening while she tells you. Or bringing her flowers when it's not a special occasion. Or when it is. Or telling her she's beautiful.

"Sexual response begins long before you get into the bedroom and it lasts long afterwards," says Dr. Ogden. "One woman told me the sexiest thing her husband could say is 'Let me wash the dishes.'"

Loving words and actions—expressions of love—not only build trust between you, they also add up to what some experts call "all-day foreplay." A woman needs them in order to fully open to you sexually. That's because for her, sex is not just a Saturday night's recreation, something apart from life, like going to a movie; ideally, she wants it to take place in the context of a secure, loving relationship.

Be Her Best Friend

Most women want their partners to be their intimate friends. They want us to cherish them, to listen to their feelings without judgment or impatience, and to care for their well-being. They need to feel that we respect them and consider their preferences and needs. And they need us to repeatedly let them know all this. And if a woman does things with us and for us—takes an interest

What Does a Woman Want?

Toward the end of his career, Sigmund Freud confessed a deep frustration: "The great question, which I have not been able to answer despite my 30 years of research into the feminine soul, is, what does a woman want?" Here's a thought-provoking answer.

In a major study conducted by David M. Buss, Ph.D., professor of psychology at the University of Texas, Austin, and reported in his book, *The Evolution of Desire*, 10,000 people in 37 cultures were asked what they wanted in a mate. Across all cultures (including our own), women universally desire in a man the following things:

• Money and wealth

• Social status and power

• Someone older (average 3 ¹/₂ years older than she is)

• Ambition

• Dependability and intelligence

• Love and commitment

The first five provide a woman with the security she needs in order to fulfill her biological imperative of raising a family. (Even if she doesn't have children, these deep-lying desires still guide her choices, suggests Dr. Buss.) Older, more intelligent, and ambitious men of higher social standing can offer her offspring all the evolutionary advantages: better food, better housing, better education, better health care. Love and commitment make it all enjoyable and deeply rewarding.

▼ *What does she want in a mate? Knowing a woman's deepest agenda helps us understand why she craves security in a long-term relationship.*

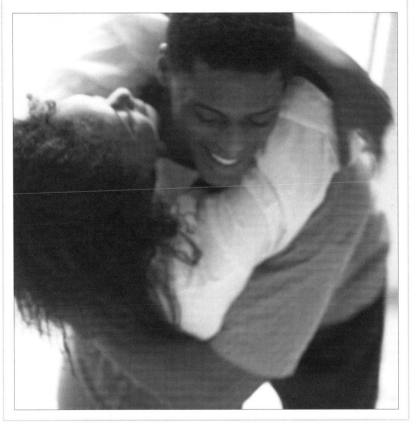

in our lives, cooks, shares sex and recreational activities, creates a beautiful living environment, shares the economic burden of a household—we feel secure that she loves us.

"The steps of the relationship dance are nurturing, equality, mutuality," Dr. Ogden says. "Each partner's desires are equally important. So listen to your partner—and to yourself."

Rekindling Passion and Romance

The two lovers started out blazing like a meteor in a dark summer sky, but the passion began to subside, sex became routine or even boring, and now they wonder where all the love went. So how do you ensure long-term passion and romance in a long-term relationship? Here's how.

> **"Twelve years doesn't mean you're a *happy* couple. It just means you're a *long* couple."**
>
> Neil Simon, American playwright

Is the Honeymoon Over?

Do all relationships inevitably wind up a pallid reflection of the first months of passion? Looking around, you might think so. But experts disagree. And studies conducted at the University of Chicago show that the people having the most emotionally fulfilling, physically satisfying sex are married or in long-term, monogamous relationships.

A decline in passion is entirely normal. The energy of being in love, with its romantic intensity and insatiable sexual desire, can't be sustained indefinitely. Work, children, and other responsibilities all rightfully claim some of your attention. The problem comes when they take *all* your attention, and you stop feeding energy into the relationship.

The key insight here is that over the long haul, you get out of something what you put into it. As San Francisco therapists Lonnie Barbach, Ph.D., and David L. Geisinger, Ph.D., point out in their book, *Going the Distance: Secrets to Lifelong Love*, you wouldn't open the doors of a new business for six months and then just go in once a week; it requires time and attention every day. It's the same thing with nurturing a relationship. "Keeping love alive," they explain, "requires ongoing thoughtful attention to the things that nourish a relationship: laughter, sex, social activities, vacations, tenderness, good conversation, adventure, dreams, romance."

A Return to Romance

Women want romance. But you knew that, didn't you? In the courtship stage of a relationship, men are all too willing to be romantic. Flowers, nice clothes, best behavior, candlelit dinners, fine wine—to

Start Dating Again

We're all so busy these days there's hardly a chance to be alone and romantic with our partner. But without some special quality time, romance, passion, and deep, fiery sex are almost certain to remain a memory of times gone by.

So seize the initiative. Tell her you want to take her on a date next Saturday night. Here are some ideas that various relationship experts have suggested.

• Get tickets to something you know she'll love, like the ballet, a concert, or a play.

• Call for reservations at a restaurant she always wanted to try. Make sure it has lots of atmosphere. Dress up for the occasion, and don't forget to buy her a corsage.

• Take her dancing.

• Reserve a room at a hotel, or a country inn in a beautiful location. All week, let her know you're planning to rival those sweaty all-night love feasts of your early days.

• Don't take your beeper or your cell phone, and if possible, don't call the babysitter.

• If you can't spend a lot of money, use your imagination. Borrow a friend's apartment or go camping. The idea is just to be away from your usual environment, free of responsibilities, able to focus on each other.

• Most of all, don't make this a one-time thing. Plan on regular intimate dates together at least once a month.

▶ *Here's looking at you: Refresh the relationship by starting to date again. The honeymoon may never end.*

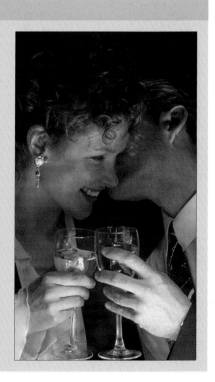

get the girl, nothing is too good or too expensive. But once we've got the girl, our attitude seems to be: It's time to get real. Who's got time for romance? Once the hunter's caught his quarry, he can relax.

For women, however, the need for romance never goes away. Romance makes a woman feel feminine, cherished, and protected. She needs this attention, especially if she is working all day in a man's world and also taking care of children and a home. Romance sheds a magical glow that helps her transcend the dull details of day-to-day living.

When those fancy threads of yours turn into sweaty T-shirts, and candlelit dinners and expensive wines become an order-in pepperoni pizza and a six-pack, your Cinderella may start to feel like a pumpkin. Just as she was turned on by your ardent attention to her and the relationship, she'll be equally turned off when you're too busy to listen to her, too busy to shave, dress nicely, or take her out to special places.

PUTTING BACK THE ZING

It often doesn't take much to put the zing back into a relationship. "Sometimes just the details are enough to change things for the better," says Louanne Cole Weston, Ph.D., a sex therapist in Sacramento, California, and columnist for the *San Francisco Examiner*. "Little details can trigger spontaneity." Here, then, are some details that sex and relationship experts often suggest.

• Buy her flowers. There may be a woman who doesn't respond with delight to a bouquet of fresh-cut flowers, but we haven't met her yet.

• Tell her in plain English that you love her. If you like to write, offer her a love poem or love letter. If Shakespeare is not in your family tree, buy a card. Call from work, "just to say I love you."

Fun in Bed

Sex that's getting routine and predictable may signal stormy seas ahead. Stoking the sexual fires may reduce the temptation for either of you to look elsewhere for excitement. "You have to try different things," says sex therapist Louanne Cole Weston, Ph.D., who writes the "Sex Matters" column for the *San Francisco Examiner*. "And then you have to keep on trying different things." Try these:

• Do it somewhere else. If you've been restricting your sexual encounters to the bedroom, expand your horizons. Try the couch, the floor, the kitchen table, the bath tub, the backyard, the back seat of the car . . .

• Spice up your language. Women tend to be more verbal than men. She may enjoy some sexy talk either in bed or to get her there.

• Act out a fantasy. Pretend you're meeting for the first time. Go separately to a singles spot dressed for the kill, and pick her up—or vice versa—and take her to a motel for the night. Or make up your own story.

• Take a look at the sexual positions on pages 150 to 157 and try something new.

You don't have to stop here. Sex toys, phone sex, bondage . . . the options for adventure and experiment are endless. Just be sure to try only what feels acceptable to you both; some things may seem a little too exotic. Don't forget that for her, sex is not just sex. Her sexual openness depends on feeling secure, respected, and loved.

A final word: Have you gotten too busy and too serious to just play? Drop your goal-oriented, fear-of-failure attitude and have a good time!

• Take her on a date.
• Remember special days. Birthdays, Valentine's day, anniversaries are important to her.
• Buy her little gifts, such as chocolates, earrings, perfume, or fragrant bath oil. Expensive is not necessarily better. But be sure it's something she really likes, not something you're attracted to.
• Find a good cookbook and make a special dinner. Be sure to serve it by candlelight.
• Get up early and prepare breakfast in bed on a weekend morning.
• When you go on a trip, bring back something for her so she'll know you've been thinking of her.
• Prepare a picnic basket with a bottle of wine and other treats, and take her for an afternoon in the country—or at least in the park.
• Of course, one of the most powerful ways to keep your romance alive and well is to have great sex. To reignite the fires of sex, be adventurous; try new ways of lovemaking and new places to be together.

Cultivating Passion

For a lot of couples, according to Dr. Weston, it's not a question of rekindling the flame. It's a question of lighting it in the first place. "Some couples never really learned to develop passion," she says. "They enjoyed the novelty of the thing on the front end and then just drifted."

If that's you, don't despair. All it means is that the best part of your marital bliss may lie ahead. "Some people think the best sex is later in life anyway," Dr. Weston says. "Sometimes when we're young we have some rather unrealistic expectations of what sex is supposed to do for us, rather than what we should do for ourselves."

The point is that fanning the flames of passion is an ongoing project in a relationship. For great sex and rich romance on a long-term basis, you need to learn about your partner, explore her wishes, and fulfill them. That provides her with the security she needs to be able to open up to you and give you all she's got.

How to Enjoy a Happy Love Life

Most of us jump into an intimate love relationship thinking—if we think at all—that it will somehow just take care of itself. The truth is that you have to make an effort to maintain a happy relationship. It's tough work sometimes, but the rewards can prove incalculable.

> **"Those who have not known the deep intimacy and the intense companionship of happy mutual love have missed the best thing that life has to offer."**
> Bertrand Russell, British philosopher

Why Bother with Love?

What makes us think we can carry off a marriage with no skill, knowledge, or preparation? Would you take the mound at Yankee Stadium without expert coaching and years of practice? The sad fact is, most of us haven't a clue about how to conduct a long-term relationship that's happy, harmonious, mutually supportive, and fulfilling.

So why is a happy relationship important? Why is it worth pursuing? To find an answer, let's be selfish. What's in it for the guy?

Men need a good relationship as much as women do. It's part of the male self-image to feel we'd be just as well off being single and independent, but for most of us, a loving relationship is just what the doctor ordered. Studies show that happily married men live longer and are healthier than their single (or unhappily married) brethren.

"When you're 80 years old, it's a real comfort to have known somebody deeply, and to have had that person know you," says Louanne Cole Weston, Ph.D., a sex therapist in Sacramento, California, and columnist for the *San Francisco Examiner.* "Sex in a relationship is a really powerful pathway to sharing a part of yourself with another person, and that has a healthy effect on a man."

The Seasons of Love

Feelings of love ebb and flow. Problems and conflicts arise even in the best relationship. One day we realize that the honeymoon is over; things aren't as perfect as they seemed, and if the relationship is going to succeed, we'll have to work on it.

This is *not* the time to bail out. "Looking for relief with a new person is the cheap way out," Dr. Weston says. "Besides, the novelty that it might offer doesn't last anyway." The more rewarding approach involves the dreaded "C" word—commitment. In the long haul, you get out of something only what you put into it. Whether it's a business, an exercise program, a garden, or a relationship, if you don't put much in, you don't get much out.

Commitment means that when conflicts come up, the relationship means enough to you that you'll work together to find a solution. It means being there for the other person, no matter what.

Keys to a Happy Love Life

If you want the relationship to get better, start with a good look at yourself. Don't blame your partner for the problems, or expect her to change. No list can possibly be complete, but here are some factors that relationship experts often cite as key ingredients in making any relationship work. Examine each of the points and see how you stack up, and where you can make improvements.

COMMUNICATION

Experts say that a good relationship requires face-to-face communication every day, to keep things going smoothly, repair hurt feelings, and defuse tension.

INDIVIDUALITY

You're distinct entities. Your partner is who she is and who she's going to

Marriage Is Good for Your Health

"It is a woman's business to get married as soon as possible, and a man's to keep unmarried as long as he can," wrote George Bernard Shaw, and many of us feel that way. Yet research has consistently shown tremendous benefits for married men, in physical and mental health as well as longevity. As sociologist Jessie Bernard wrote in *The Future of Marriage*, there is a "sometimes spectacular and always impressive superiority on almost every index...of married over never-married men." For example, death rates for divorced, single, and widowed men are significantly higher than for married men. Married men have also been found to have fewer illnesses than unmarried men. Why? No one knows for sure. But having a steady, loving companion—with better food, more regular sex, and more comfortable surroundings thrown into the bargain—certainly couldn't hurt.

be; you are who you are and who you're always going to be.

HONESTY

Issues of truth and how to tell it without hurting feelings come up often in a relationship.

SEX

A good, warm (and sometimes hot) sexual connection is good for a happy love life. Sexual compatibility is essential.

FRIENDSHIP

Doing things together, talking freely to each other, relying on each other in difficult times—having someone like that in your life is one of life's greatest gifts.

COMPATIBILITY

In a love relationship, compatibility means more than sharing similar interests, values, political views, and dietary habits. It also means the ability to accept life together lovingly despite your differences.

COMPROMISE

The need for compromise comes up each and every day, and how fairly and graciously it's handled helps define a relationship.

FORGIVENESS

As John Gray, Ph.D., points out in his book, *Mars and Venus in Love*, forgiveness "is the action of love...it exercises our love and makes it stronger."

STRESS

It's inevitable. How much explodes does much to decide the tone of a relationship.

Giving and Caring

Care for your partner, cherish her, and give as much as you possibly can to her. Any successful relationship revolves around mutual giving.

Smoothing It Over

Conflicts are inevitable, and sometimes, despite your best efforts and intentions, you'll have a fight. According to Wendy Fader, Ph.D., a psychologist and sex therapist, the following strategies should help you resolve those conflicts with your relationship in one piece.

• Remember that your goal is not to win or to be right, but to restore harmony and love to the relationship.

• Treat your conflict as a common enemy, and work together to solve it. If you can do this, you're halfway home.

• Practice listening skills. Be the kind of listener you'd like her to be for you.

• One of you (probably you, since this is a typical male pattern) will want to deal with conflict by avoiding confrontation and working it out on your own. You may run, take a long walk, get absorbed in a project—eventually your feelings will settle down. She'll probably need to express her feelings and talk it out, though she can learn to give you some time and space first.

• Make love. Some people say it's inappropriate to use sex to smooth over problems, and it certainly shouldn't be used every time. One or both of you may still be harboring resentments and she, especially, may not be ready to open up to tender feelings. But if you generally have a good sexual rapport, lovemaking can be a very effective means of dissolving tensions and restoring harmony. It's especially effective to take you the rest of the way once you begin to resolve the problem.

▼ *Sex can be an appropriate—and very pleasurable—way to resolve conflicts and restore peace and harmony.*

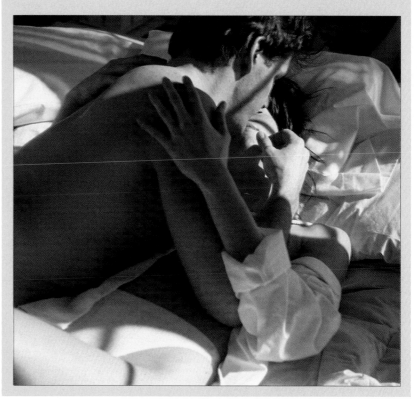

If you're both in it only for what *you* can get, neither gives, so no one receives. If you care about each other, support each other, listen to each other with respect, learn to give each other what each one really needs and desires, you've got yourself a win-win situation that can carry you forward through life, year after year in happiness and love.

Re-Entering the Singles Scene

So you broke up with her and now you feel bad. Very bad. That's only natural, especially if the two of you had been together for a long time. Thing is, though, there's a world out there, and there are a lot of single women in it. Eventually, the time will come to start meeting some of them.

> **"She gave me a smile I could feel in my hip pocket."**
>
> Raymond Chandler,
> *Farewell, My Lovely*

Take It Slowly

If you've been married or in a steady, long-term relationship, being single again can be tough. You may still be hurting, unwilling to open up to a new relationship, yet too lonely not to try. It's a vulnerable time.

Don't be in a rush to settle down again with one person. Stretch your horizons. Get involved in activities that fit your interests, and meet women there. Dating a number of women can help crystallize what you're looking for. "True, there are lots of potential pitfalls along the way," says sex therapist and columnist Louanne Cole Weston, Ph.D. "But you can have lots of fun creating the sexual aspect of a new relationship. You may need to take a deep breath a couple of times to get through unfamiliar things, but it's do-able."

This may sound cold-blooded, but it's important to spend time checking out a potential life-mate. Define what you're looking for. Do you want a long-term relationship or someone to be with tonight? Do you want to get married or get laid? Your criteria for a casual sexual experience will be different from what you're looking for in a partner for life. "What you're looking for is simply the right fit," Dr. Weston says. "There are so many different women out there, you should be able to find a good fit."

The New You

Maybe you got into bad habits in your previous relationship, and became complacent about how you looked. Now's the time to check out your physical appearance. You may not care much about how you look, but women do. Even if you're just going hiking or to the ballgame, wear something nice.

Watch your posture, too; slouching conveys a lack of self-confidence. Is it time for a haircut? And what about starting to work out again? Maybe you could stand to drop a few pounds, or firm up your muscles. A little attention here will increase your self-confidence and your attractiveness to the opposite sex.

And while we're talking appearances, be sure to get your living quarters in shape. Eventually—maybe tonight—you're going to bring somebody home, and you don't want to turn her off with dirt and disarray.

LEARN THE NEW WAYS

You may find that rules and roles of dating have changed since you were last single. With AIDS being a deadly addition to the list of sexually transmitted diseases, the need for safer sex is far greater than in your days as a stud. And dating etiquette—who picks up the check; who asks for dates; who initiates sex—is no longer written in stone.

Your best roadmap through this changing landscape, according to Dr. Weston, is openness and direct communication. "Candor does not destroy sexiness," she says.

Besides, most of the changes are to your advantage. "Twenty years ago, you'd never see so many personal ads and dating services," Dr. Weston

---

Think Positive to Get Back in the Race

Your relationship broke down, you've worked through your sense of loss, and begun to put the past behind you. It's time to get off your duff and start meeting women—but suddenly you feel scared, unsure of yourself. "What'll I say?" "What if I get into another disastrous relationship?" "What if I'm too old?" Too fat? Too anything?

This kind of negative thinking will get you nowhere, and you've got to nip it in the bud, says sex therapist and newspaper columnist Louanne Cole Weston, Ph.D. When you've been down, it takes a positive attitude to get out the

door and willing to take a risk. Accept that you'll get some rejections; you might even make a mistake or two. But think about how great it is when a good relationship is working.

Women are attracted to men who are upbeat, active, and enthusiastic about life. When you meet a woman who interests you, stick to the bright side. Talk to her about what's good in your life, things you enjoy, books or movies you like, things you're looking forward to doing, places you want to go. And, Dr. Weston says, don't forget to remind *yourself* about those good things, too.

says. "That means a lot of the stigma about being single and looking for a mate has gone away."

The Great Seduction Scene

Put away that copy of *101 Guaranteed Pick-up Lines*; using these devices is tacky and guaranteed to turn most women off. Every woman you meet is a person with unique interests, perceptions, and qualities.

Whenever possible, approach her with a remark geared directly to her, such as "That's a beautiful scarf," or "What brings you to a lecture on quantum physics?" In almost any situation, friendly words of greeting are easy to create. They can be as simple as "How's the pizza in this place?" or "That's a great dog."

WHERE TO GO ON A DATE

So now that you've got her attention, where are you going to take her? If your repertoire of dating gambits ends at dinner and the movies, here are some suggestions to stimulate your imagination.

• Outdoor activities, such as hiking, a visit to the zoo, a walk by the river or seashore, a bike ride
• A lecture, class, or workshop on mutual interests
• A drive in the country
• Dancing: ballroom, rock, square, folk, clogging, and so on
• A concert or play
• An art gallery or museum
• Watch a video together
• Wine tasting
• Sports, such as swimming, skiing, canoeing, jogging, inline skating

WHEN TO HAVE SEX

Let's be honest. Even if you're interested in a long-term relationship, you're also interested in a short-term roll in the hay. But you don't want to blow it by being too sexually aggressive or waiting too long to make a move. You have to "read" her carefully, tune in to how she's feeling and responding. If you're not sure, talk about it.

"A woman needs a reason to have sex; a man just needs a place," says Joseph R. Jablonski in *Dating: A Practical Guide for Men*. She may be as eager as you are to unleash her passion, but for her, sex implies emotional involvement. She needs to feel it is okay to move on to this new level of the relationship. "Okay" means that she trusts you, and believes that you care about her and are not just interested in getting her into bed.

A word of caution: Sex creates emotional bonding for both partners, so easy does it. It's always much harder to extricate yourself from a relationship once sex complicates the picture.

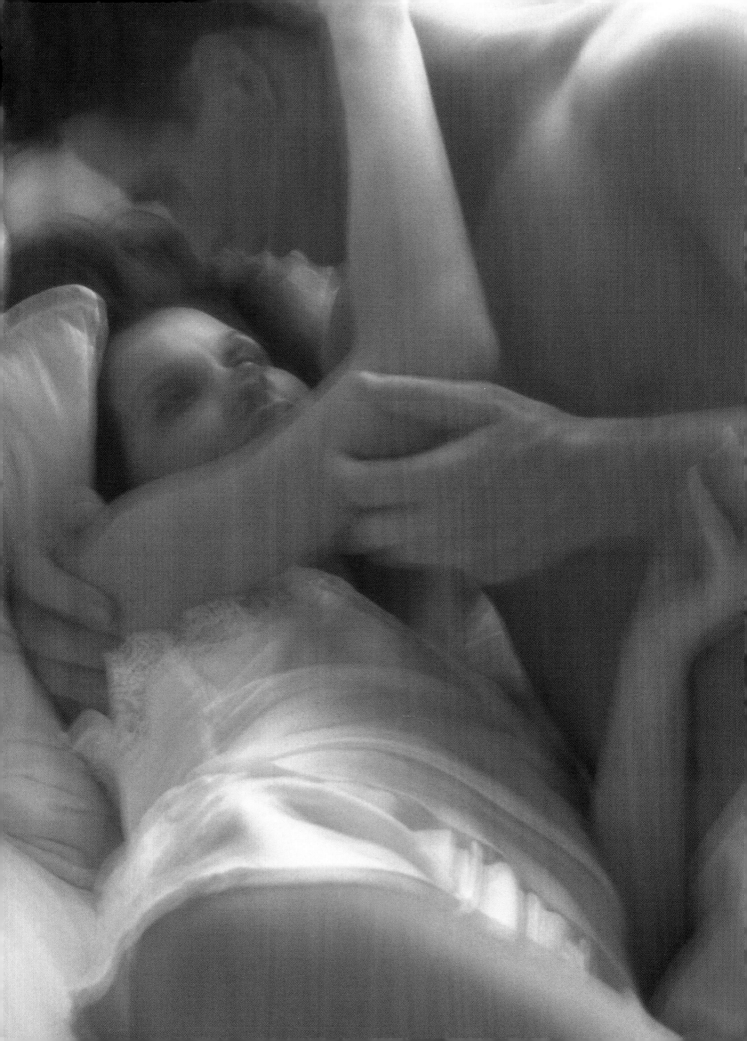

Better Sex

Keeping Up Your Potency

Let's begin this discussion of male potency with two fundamental assumptions: Sex is a great and wondrous thing, and each and every one of us ought to be able to enjoy it throughout the course of our adult lives. The difficult part is how to make sure this happens.

It's Up to You To Keep It Up

One simple way to ensure that you continue to have sex is to continue to have sex. Making love regularly stimulates the production of testosterone, which in turn stimulates the desire to have more sex. It really is a case of use it or lose it.

Another key fact to remember is that while your penis might seem, at times, to have a mind of its own, in truth it is intimately connected to the rest of your body. Therefore the key to maintaining a good sex life is maintaining good overall health. Everything from our cholesterol levels to our muscle flexibility and our waistlines has an impact on our sexual appetites and capabilities, not to mention our attractiveness.

Overcoming Impotence

Most men who struggle with impotence are over the age of 40. As we age, erections occur less frequently and wilt more quickly. Some of that is inevitable, but a lot results from circulatory problems. A penis won't rise if it can't become engorged with blood, so keeping your heart and arteries in good shape is the best gift you can give your sex life.

For those already experiencing difficulties due to purely physiological causes, several types of prescription drugs—such as Viagra—can virtually guarantee an erection. As a last resort, penile implants are also available.

Of course, our minds can short-circuit sex just as effectively as our circulatory systems. In particular, anxiety about getting an erection often leads to erection difficulties. Performance anxiety, as it's known, affects millions of men.

Sex therapists say the first step toward addressing impotence is to communicate your fears to your partner. If that's difficult for you, a sex therapist can help: Building communication between couples, and helping them understand that their struggles are both common and solvable, are chief among the services that therapists provide.

A popular technique for dealing with impotence involves relearning the art of enjoying sex by not having it for a while. See "Cultivate the Caress" on page 140 for details about sensate-focus techniques.

The Sex Organ in Your Head

One particularly important body part that's plugged directly into the penis is the brain. Our emotional health and the health of our relationships is fundamental to maintaining our sexual potency, especially in this time of rampant stress, shifting sex roles, and AIDS.

Sex therapists report that legions of walking wounded are coming to their offices, complaining that they've lost interest in their partners, or that their partners have lost interest in them. Much of the time, therapists report, what these patients need is either more sleep, less pressure from work and family lives, or—perhaps most important—the ability to better communicate with their mates.

Testosterone and Your Sex Drive

Testosterone is a hormone that spurs everything from the development of male sex organs in the womb to the growth of the beard at puberty.

The maintenance of your sex drive throughout your life depends on your testosterone staying within normal levels. In the vast majority of men—roughly 80 percent, according to some estimates—it does stay within normal levels, even though the amount of testosterone in our blood gradually begins to decline after the age of 50.

If you're worried about loss of desire, a doctor can check your testosterone level (before 10:00 A.M.), and give you testosterone replacement therapy, which must continue for life. Chances are good, though, that your problem is in your head, and not in your hormones.

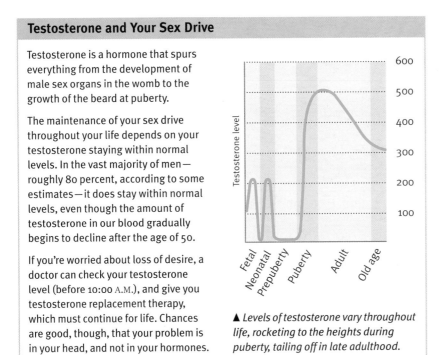

▲ Levels of testosterone vary throughout life, rocketing to the heights during puberty, tailing off in late adulthood.

Mastering Foreplay

There's probably no modern man who hasn't heard the lecture a hundred times: Women require extended foreplay in order to enjoy sex. If you are to be a successful lover, a considerate partner, and a decent human being, you will—you must—supply the requisite amount of foreplay.

> **"Sex is one of the nine reasons for reincarnation—the other eight are unimportant."**
>
> Henry Miller, *Big Sur and the Oranges of Hieronymous Bosch*

Foreplay for Better Sex

The question we want answered is a selfish one: What's in this foreplay stuff for the guy?

The answer, we're delighted to tell you, is: plenty. The difference between hurried sex and leisurely sex is like the difference between a fast-food take-out meal and a full-course banquet at a top restaurant. Sometimes a quick sex session is convenient, fun, and satisfying, but the most luxurious sex takes time.

Part of the reason for that is simply that in the modern world we unconsciously get into a way of thinking that leads to rushing by many of life's greatest pleasures. If it feels good, why be in such a hurry to get it over with?

More important, prolonged sex is also better sex because it is often more intense sex. "For many men, the longer the sex, the stronger the orgasm," says Marilyn Volker, Ed.D., a sex therapist in Miami, Florida.

Of course, getting the most out of relationships involves giving as well as receiving. Dr. Volker says that if your significant other wants time to enjoy extended foreplay and you want to get right to the nitty gritty, you simply need to take turns. "Longer foreplay can help establish a stronger relationship with your partner," Dr. Volker says. "When the man does more to satisfy the woman, she'll be ready the next time to do more to satisfy him."

Be a More Sensuous Lover

Men and women have learned a million techniques over the centuries to drive each other crazy in bed, but a common theme to the vast majority of them comes down to this: Learn how to feel. As the famous American sex therapists William Masters, M.D., and Virginia Johnson once put it, "If words are the currency of poetry, and color is the currency of art, touch is the currency of sex."

Masters and Johnson helped popularize a technique for enhancing the sensuality of sex known as sensate focus. (It's also an important way to treat impotence.) Basically it involves a series of lovemaking sessions in which couples take turns touching each other's body all over without having intercourse. The idea is to shift the sexual focus from reaching orgasm to experiencing the broadest possible range of sensation. If you truly pay attention to your skin's capacity to feel, the whole body can become an erogenous zone.

One reason the sensate-focus technique is so effective at heightening arousal is that it teaches couples to relax during sex, and virtually any sex therapist will tell you that the more at ease we are in the bedroom, the better our sexual experiences are likely to be. "I often tell my clients to drop the 'e' in foreplay," says Robert Birch, Ph.D., a sex therapist in Columbus, Ohio, and author of *Male Sexual Endurance*. "Make it 'for play'. Men need to get out of the mad dash toward intercourse and into the playfulness of sex."

How the Other Half Turns On

What turns a woman on? And how do her turn-ons differ from a man's? Here's what the sex therapists have to say.

• Women almost always like plenty of foreplay while men want to get on to what they consider to be the main event, intercourse.

• Men are more interested in a variety of sexual partners than women are. This doesn't mean, though, that women are any less interested in a variety of types of lovemaking than men are.

• Men tend to be more focused on their genitals, while women's sexual feelings are more generalized.

• Women as a rule are more concerned with the entire relationship; men are more able to focus on sex alone.

• A woman likes a man who isn't afraid to let her take the lead in sex, while many men say they find women who initiate sex a turn-on.

• Men respond to visual stimulation more than women do. Women are more responsive to sound—they love to hear their lovers moan with pleasure.

• Negative emotions kill passion. Feeling angry, hostile, or resentful toward their partner is a turnoff for both men and women.

Do Aphrodisiacs Work?

For centuries men have searched for some magic substance which could arouse women sexually, saving them the bother of doing it themselves. Alas, despite dozens of claims to the contrary—including the legendary capabilities of Spanish fly (made from dried beetles), oysters, royal jelly, ground rhinoceros horn—the search has been unsuccessful.

According to Michael Castleman, author of *Nature's Cures* and *The Healing Herbs*, some natural substances may make us think we're getting horny, but they don't truly produce desire. One example is a tree-bark extract called yohimbine, which in prescription-level doses increases blood flow to the penis. And ginseng and caffeine have stimulant qualities which can help keep you awake for sex, which is a start.

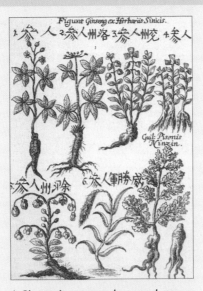

▲ *Ginseng's supposed powers have been valued for millennia, as seen here in this seventeenth-century engraving.*

CULTIVATE THE CARESS

Experienced lovers have a wide variety of erotic caresses in their repertoire, ranging from the "spider's legs" tickle (lightly brushing the fingertips in a dancing motion over the skin) to the gentle love slap. Consider it your mission to explore them all.

A series of sensate-focus exercises devoted to caressing is highly recommended by Barbara Keesling, Ph.D., a sex therapist in Orange, California, and author of *How to Make Love All Night (and Drive a Woman Wild)*. This approach is also good for men battling impotence because it reduces performance anxiety by putting a temporary ban on intercourse.

Dr. Keesling recommends that couples practice touching one another, devoting separate sessions to the face, the back, the front, and finally the genitals. The point of these sessions isn't to massage each other's muscles, or even to give each other pleasure, but to learn to experience how it feels to feel your lover's body. Each session should last 20 minutes, Dr. Keesling says, and each should specifically avoid intercourse.

Again, the point is to train yourself not to rush to the finish line before you've learned to fully savor what might be called full-body (rather than genital) eroticism.

The last stage of sexual caressing is mutual masturbation: Knowing how to pleasure your lover is a skill that can come in handy for every modern man and woman.

TRY A LITTLE TENDERNESS

Many men simply come on too strong, too quick, and too rough. "Women want the three Ts: more time, more touch, and more talk,"

Fantasyland

Virtually everyone has sexual fantasies. They can be an important part of your sex life, juicing you up at the right moment. Fantasies become a problem only if they seem to be more important than the real-life relationship.

Fantasizing about sex while having sex can heighten sexual pleasure by cueing the body to respond more passionately than it otherwise would. Some men have just a few X-rated thoughts, while others construct full-blown blue movies. Lesbian love scenes and picturing a wife or girlfriend having sex with another man (or men) are among the most common types of male fantasy. Fantasies often focus on taboo behaviors, such as having sex in public or with a person of the same sex.

Some people feel guilty about having fantasies; they feel they're being disloyal to their partner. But fantasizing isn't the same as putting it into practice. If it's fun and arousing, well, that's good enough.

It's not always a good idea, though, to share fantasies with your partner. Imagine how she might feel if you told her you've always dreamed about having sex with her closest female friend. Try to sense your partner's feelings about sex and about fantasies in general. Don't force the pace; if you both find it comfortable to talk about sexual topics in general, then the subject of fantasies will probably come to the fore sooner or later.

▶ *Does she feature in your fantasies?* Baywatch's *Yasmine Bleeth.*

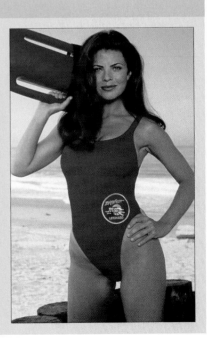

says Marilyn Volker, Ed.D., a certified sex therapist in Miami, Florida. "Those add up to a fourth T: more tenderness." That's not to say that women can't get to a more boisterous place sexually, she adds. They just take some time getting there, and need a little skilful masculine encouragement.

BE A 12-HOUR MAN
Try to turn foreplay into an all-day proposition. For example, call your partner from work. Tell her you're fantasizing about her; ask her what she's wearing underneath her dress, and describe what you want to do with her when you get home. When you actually get there, you'll both be ready to tear each other's clothes off.

CREATE A MOOD
Set the stage for sex by paying some attention to your surroundings. Soft lighting—candles especially—is very important; gentle music helps, too. Make sure the room temperature is comfortable for being naked together, take the phone off the hook, and if you have kids, make sure there'll be no unexpected visitors.

Certain accessories can enhance the pursuit of sensual foreplay, chief among them a lightly scented massage oil. Candles, feathers, and mirrors are also useful to have around.

LEARN TO KISS
Kissing is an art form in and of itself and an essential element of sex. Susan Wright, author of *Driving Your Woman Wild in Bed*, suggests using your lips as if they were fingers to caress your partner's lips and skin. Don't keep your mouth tightly puckered, says Wright—the attraction of lips is their soft, sensual nature.

Also remember that kissing isn't only something for two mouths: Your lover's body is a continent for your lips and your tongue to explore.

The Beauty of Massage
The anthropologist Ashley Montagu once noted that fingertips are erogenous zones, and nowhere is the truth of that statement more evident than in the art of massage.

The skin is our largest organ, and each square inch of it contains anywhere from 14,000 to 18,000 nerve receptors. Stimulating those receptors sets neural impulses racing toward your spinal cord and up to your brain, which fires reflex impulses back down the line. You are literally turned on.

Just as massage can wake up your skin, it can also relax your muscles. When it comes to enjoyable sex, both are important. Stress, anxiety, and tension are all enemies of sensuality; by relieving the tight muscles that modern life creates, massage puts you in the mood for love.

Another sexual dividend massage provides is the breakdown of the subconscious barriers between you

---

Different Strokes

There are three basic types of stroke used in a good massage. Jennifer Barefoot, a certified massage therapist in Emmaus, Pennsylvania, describes them as stroking (also called "effleurage"), pressing ("petrissage"), and percussion.

Stroking
These are long, smooth, gliding movements using a flat hand. Pressure can be either light or firm. "Use stroking at the beginning of your massage, as the warmup stroke," Barefoot says. "It's a good way to prepare your partner's muscles for the other strokes."

Pressing
This type includes kneading and thumb presses. Use pressing strokes when you're ready to work on the specific spots where your partner's muscles and joints are tense, especially the shoulders and larger muscles in the back. When kneading, keep the palm flat on the body and "knead" your partner's skin like bread dough, gently, with your fingers or your thumbs. Thumb presses are the more concentrated pressing and rotating of the thumb directly onto a knot of tight muscle.

Percussion
The sides of the hands are used in a hacking motion to strike the skin, either rapidly or slowly, with varying degrees of intensity. For a slightly softer version, keep your hands loosely closed. Percussion works best on the padded, fleshy parts of the body, like the thighs and buttocks, where there's a little give.

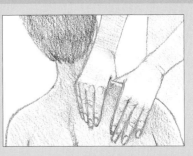

▲ *Applied with either the palm or fingers of the hand, strokes can be either short or long, light or firm.*

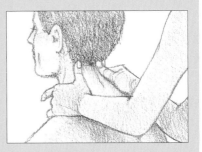

▲ *Pressing includes thumb presses and kneading, and is usually targeted at specific muscles or joints.*

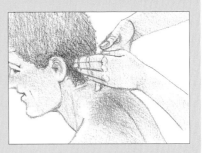

▲ *Percussion uses the sides of the hands to strike the skin with varying degrees of intensity, rapidly or slowly.*

and your lover. Men in particular tend to be encased in a suit of psychic armor, which is a barrier to intimacy. Massage is an effective way to lower those defenses.

Learning how to give a good massage does take a little practice, although we wouldn't exactly call it hard work. Using lubrication is an important first step; warm a teaspoon of scented oil by rubbing it between your palms before you apply it to your partner's body. Try to keep your movements smooth rather than abrupt, gliding gracefully along the body's contours.

THE LOVING TOUCH

Unlikely as it may sound, creating a good massage is much like building a pyramid, according to Jennifer Barefoot, a certified massage therapist in Emmaus, Pennsylvania. You start with broad, easy strokes and gradually focus your attention down to a point, or points: the places where the stresses of life have caused your partner's muscles to become knotted with tension. "Work" the points for a bit, then, as the massage ends, broaden out again.

A good massage doesn't have to last for a long time—15 minutes is usually plenty, Barefoot says—but that does not mean it should be hurried either. Slow, rhythmic, sensual movements are key to setting and maintaining a relaxing mood. And relaxing tense muscles—and minds— is what massage is all about.

Below you'll find Barefoot's "road map" for a successful massage. (See also "Different Strokes" on page 141 for a description of each of the strokes.) She stresses that although this is a good route, it's not the only one. A routine backrub can become as boring as routine sex: Don't be afraid to be creative.

The Sensual Massage

A whole-body massage gives a sense of relaxed intimacy, and makes a great prelude to sex. Start with your partner's neck and shoulders. "This is where everybody is most tense," says Barefoot.

The Shoulders and Neck

After some warmup strokes—don't forget the hand-warmed oil—knead the shoulders, starting from the outside and working in toward the neck. Rub with your thumbs on either side of the neck, then work your way back out toward the shoulders. Repeat several times.

The Back

Use long, smooth strokes all the way from the shoulders down over the buttocks, as if you were finger painting her back. Start with three to four gentle strokes to spread the oil and three to five strokes to work the oil into the skin a little. Then you can start concentrating on specific points of tension with kneading strokes and finger presses.

Hands and Arms

This is a good place to try a variation of kneading called "wringing." Gently grip one of your partner's upper arms with both hands and then move them gently in opposite directions, as if you were wringing out a dishtowel. For the hands, use your fingers, rubbing thoroughly along each of your partner's fingers and on her palms. Don't forget that for us mammals, the hands are among the most sensitive parts of our bodies. It's worth spending a little extra time and attention there.

The Feet

This is finger-work territory, and it's probably as sensitive an area as any on our bodies, along with the hands and the face. In fact, there's a whole branch of physical therapy called reflexology which employs hand and foot massage to provide deep relaxation and relieve the body of stress.

The Face

This sensitive—and sensual—area needs a slow-and-gentle approach. Use some light thumb presses beginning at the bridge of the nose and moving out along the eyebrows to the temples. Stop there and rub gently, in a circular motion, for five seconds or so. Move up a half an inch on the forehead and repeat the movement from the center to the side of the forehead. Gradually work your way up to your partner's hairline.

The Legs

Kneel down beside your partner to work on the legs, which are especially well suited to both kneading and soft percussion strokes. Work your way up the thighs to the buttocks and then down again. Kneading and percussion are also good for the calves. Many people have sore calves, Barefoot points out. It won't hurt to spend just a little extra time and attention here as well.

Oral Sex

Oral sex is hot, ranking as one of the more intense sexual experiences possible for both men and women. Cunnilingus should be part of every modern man's sexual arsenal. But do you have the gift of tongues? Or are you tongue-tied? Read on for a primer in the noble art of oral sex.

Overcoming Oral Anxiety

Polls and sex therapists agree that oral sex is now a standard part of most couple's lovemaking repertoire, especially in more educated and affluent households. This is not to say that there aren't many people who feel ambivalent about oral sex. Many men love to receive it, but don't like to give it, a situation that can understandably cause some resentment on the part of the woman.

A surprising number of women are uncomfortable receiving oral sex. According to sex therapists, women tend to be more fearful than men that their genitals or genital juices will smell or taste bad. There may also be lingering messages from childhood that there's something wrong with letting a man see them down there. Oral sex, after all, is about as intimate as you can get. When contemplating cunnilingus (a combination of the Latin words for "vulva" and "to lick") men should keep these special sensitivities in mind.

Tips for Oral Engagement

Good cunnilingus depends on skill and responsiveness. Here are a few things to keep in mind.

• This is a tough one for many men, but the best way to find out if she's uncomfortable with cunnilingus is simply to ask her.

• Don't go straight for her crotch, as many men do, in the mistaken belief

Passing the Oral Exam

• Gently flick your tongue back and forth across her clitoris. Try increasing and decreasing the intensity of the flick.

• Thrust your rolled-up tongue in and out of her vagina.

• Lick the inner and outer lips of her vagina from bottom to top.

• Gently suck her clitoris.

• Slowly and rhythmically lap at her vulva and genitals as if they were an ice-cream cone.

• Use the tip of your tongue for a while, then switch to a broader, flatter stroke.

• Insert your finger or a dildo into her vagina as you lick her clitoris.

• Hum or purr while you lick. The vibration adds to the sensation.

that their partners want them to jump at their genitals. Instead, work your way slowly south, pausing to nibble, kiss, and stroke at each point along the way. Start kissing and licking her lower belly and thighs, for instance, then gradually move to the labia minora and, taking your time, to the clitoris.

• Different women prefer different things in oral sex, just as they do in intercourse. Try a variety of different techniques (for some suggestions, see "Passing the Oral Exam") and pay attention to her reactions to each one.

• If a woman is insecure, a little verbal reassurance can work wonders. Tell her how beautiful she is down there, and how much you love to taste and smell her.

• She's not going to climax right away, no matter how good you are. Be patient and take your time.

Finding Your Way Around Down There

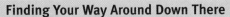

All the external portions of the female genitalia are called the vulva. The outer lips of the vagina are called the labia majora; the inner lips are called the labia minora. If you want your woman to have an orgasm, become familiar with her clitoris; that's her pleasure center. Sometimes it's tucked between folds of skin, but it will often emerge when aroused. The vagina is also more sensitive near the opening than it is further up, so big penises don't make that much of an impression. Like a collapsed balloon, it expands to accommodate the penis.

▶ *The vulva consists of the outer and inner labia, the clitoris, and the entrances to the vagina and urethra.*

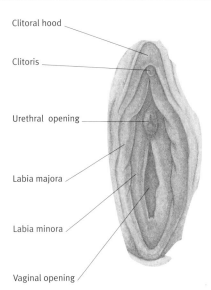

Clitoral hood

Clitoris

Urethral opening

Labia majora

Labia minora

Vaginal opening

The Phases of Intercourse

What exactly happens when you get it on? When things start to heat up, that's probably not the sort of question in the forefront of your mind, and yet knowledge is power—in the bedroom as well as the boardroom. Knowing how your body works—and that of your partner—is part of being a better lover.

Carnal Knowledge

It's a strange image to contemplate: cold-eyed scientists in white coats holding clipboards, watching hundreds of couples having sex, taking detailed measurements and notations on everything from the size, color, and hardness of the men's erections to the convulsions of the women's vaginas during orgasm. It's hard work, but somebody had to do it.

The ones who did were William Masters, M.D., and Virginia Johnson, the U.S. sex researchers who in the late 1950s and early 1960s observed 382 women and 312 men engaging in more than 10,000 sexual "episodes" of various types. Their landmark book, *Human Sexual Response,* was published in 1966, and in it they spelled out in the most graphic possible detail what happens when men and women are getting it on.

Since then other researchers have found reason to quarrel with some of Masters and Johnson's findings, the main objection being that any model of human sexuality implies there is greater uniformity to individual sexual responses than there actually is (a point Masters and Johnson repeatedly acknowledged). In the main, though, Masters and Johnson's text remains the standard point of reference.

The two researchers divided the sex act into four phases: Excitement, Plateau, Orgasmic, and Resolution.

Later they added a fifth, preliminary phase, called Desire, which included all the components of attraction, from overall good health to a sexy dress, which get a man and woman in the sack together in the first place. Here's an overview of what occurs during the opening two stages of intercourse.

THE EXCITEMENT BEGINS

At the start of the Excitement phase, the man's first response is usually an erection, which may or may not fade and then rekindle during subsequent lovemaking activity. The skin of his scrotum thickens and the muscles holding his testicles begin to tighten, lifting them up toward his body.

The woman first begins to lubricate. Her clitoris becomes engorged with blood and expands, and the outer lips of her vulva swell and part. Her vagina extends and darkens in color; her uterus and cervix elevate. Her nipples become erect. In both male and female, the heart rate and blood pressure increase.

THE PASSIONATE PLATEAU

The Plateau is an intermediate phase in which both partners are poised at a high level of sexual arousal. Masters and Johnson stress that it can fly by quickly, heading straight to orgasm, especially if the couple is

What's on Your Mind?

You might think your penis is doing all the thinking during sex, but in truth your brain is still in charge. On a purely physiological level, it's busy coordinating the complex sexual mechanisms firing away throughout the body, from the flush on your cheeks to the tingle in your testicles. But the brain is in overdrive on an emotional and psychological level as well.

The brain can enhance sex when we're thinking passionate thoughts about our partner, or even when we're fantasizing that we're having sex with somebody else. It's when our thoughts keep us from enjoying the sensations of sex that they can cause trouble, says sex therapist Shirley Zussman, Ed.D.

Negative mental messages during sex can range from the "sex is dirty" lectures we heard in grade school to the latest statistics on AIDS. The brain can also distract us with the concerns of the day—"Penises tend to go up or down with the stock market," Dr. Zussman says—or it can simply get bored. Among the most pernicious thoughts a man can have during sex are those which tell him he isn't performing adequately as a lover.

These sorts of worries become so preoccupying for some men that their erections wilt. The remedy for that is learning how to disregard the brain and listen to the body. See "Overcoming Impotence" on page 138 for details.

highly aroused before intercourse commences. On the other hand, couples who indulge in prolonged lovemaking can pass back and forth from the Excitement phase to the Plateau phase several times.

In the Plateau phase the heart rates of both the man and the woman rise higher yet. Their breathing becomes more rapid and shallow; overall muscle tension increases. The head of the penis grows wider and darkens in color. The testicles enlarge as they become engorged with blood. Meanwhile, the testicles continue to elevate, rotating slightly so that they are pressed against the perineum (the point between the anus and the scrotum). A few drops of fluid emerge from the penis. They're not semen, but they can contain some sperm.

The tissues surrounding the lower part of the vagina swell markedly during the Plateau phase. This serves to make the vaginal opening narrower, creating a tighter grip for the penis. Masters and Johnson note that this is one reason why the size of a man's penis is fairly unimportant. The other reason is that most of the vagina's sensory nerve endings are at its lower end. Thus, plunging your penis way, way down inside only reaches a relatively insensitive part of a woman's anatomy.

The clitoris continues to enlarge, but at the same time it pulls back against the woman's pubic bone. Because the vaginal lips are swollen, this retraction can cause the clitoris to seemingly disappear. This can be disconcerting to any male trying at that point to find the clitoris, especially visually.

Also during this phase, between 50 and 60 percent of women develop a deep "sex flush," which can cover most of their torsos, thighs, and buttocks. About a quarter of all men develop a similar flush. From this point, the next stop is the Big O.

His and Hers Sexual Response

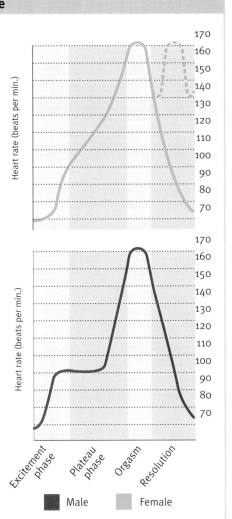

Excitement Phase
Blood flows into the pelvic region. The penis and the clitoris become erect. The vagina lubricates and extends. The labia swell and become erect. The woman's nipples become erect; erection of nipples in some men. Heartbeat, blood pressure, muscle tension increase.

Plateau Phase
The penis and the clitoris become even more erect; the clitoris withdraws as the labia swell. The head of the penis increases in size, and a small amount of fluid is emitted (not semen, but containing sperm). Heavy breathing; heart rate, blood pressure, and overall muscle tension increase.

Orgasm
Rapid involuntary spasms of the pelvic region, including contractions of the womb. The prostate gland contracts, releasing fluids that mix with sperm. Ejaculation occurs as rapid muscle contractions force semen out of the penis.

Resolution
The body's responses gradually return to normal. Multiple orgasms may be possible for women.

Make It Last Longer

So you're enjoying yourself in the Plateau phase. You want to hold off your orgasm. How? Thinking about baseball scores doesn't work. Here are four techniques that will.

• Sex therapist Barbara Keesling, Ph.D., says the way to prolong sex is to relax and focus on the experience, not distract yourself from it. Anxiety contributes to early ejaculation.

• Certain sexual positions, most notably ones in which the woman is on top, help the man last longer.

• The best way to delay orgasm is simply to stop having sex temporarily, according to sex therapist Robert Birch, Ph.D. When you feel yourself moving toward the point of no return, withdraw from the vagina, switch positions, give your partner some manual stimulation, walk around the room. . .whatever it takes to pull back from the brink. Eventually, longer periods of intercourse will become a habit.

• Another way to gain better orgasm control is to exercise the muscles at the base of the scrotum called the pubococcygeal (PC) muscles. They're the same ones you use to cut off your flow of urine. Training these muscles can help you literally squeeze off orgasms and give you stronger erections to boot. They also play an essential role in having multiple orgasms. For more details, see "Train Those Muscles" on page 148.

How to Heighten Your Orgasm

A volcanic eruption, fireworks, climax, reaching the heights: We've got all sorts of expressions to communicate the sheer pleasure of the Big O. The search for orgasm is among our most powerful drives, and it's one that science has dissected in detail. The magic and allure, of course, still remain.

The Big O in Close-Up

Defining the male orgasm as "a series of second-stage expulsive urethral contractions," as U.S. sex researchers Masters and Johnson once did, is like defining a Bruce Springsteen concert as a "lengthy exposition of popular song forms in a public setting." Purely technical descriptions can miss the essence of the experience.

The classic *artistic* description of orgasm was the one used by Ernest Hemingway in the novel *For Whom the Bell Tolls*, later picked up by songwriter Carole King and countless others: The earth moved.

We'll leave it to the art of the songwriter to describe the emotional aspects of the orgasmic experience. On a physiological level, here's what sex researchers tell us happens to male and female bodies when they reach orgasm.

THE MAN

Orgasm in the man is a two-stage process, although the length of time between the two stages is so brief we're usually not aware of it.

In the first stage, a series of rhythmic contractions brings sperm up from the testicles and mixes it with seminal fluid from the prostate gland. This process is tantamount to cocking your gun. It takes only a few seconds, but in those few seconds you will have the overwhelming feeling that you're going to have an orgasm. That feeling is correct: Unless you train yourself thoroughly to control your ejaculation (see "How to Have

Intensify Your Orgasm

• In general the longer you hold off having an orgasm, the more intense it will be. Practice getting close to orgasm during sex and then backing off just before you reach the point of no return.

• Some positions will afford your penis much greater stimulation than others. Experiment.

• Moan, groan, and yell: Expressing yourself verbally during orgasm will help you focus on the feelings—and intensify them.

• Strengthening your PC muscles (the same ones you use to stop your flow of urine) has lots of sexual benefits, including more powerful orgasms. See page 148 for the full story on Kegel exercises.

What Happens at Orgasm

During the first stage of orgasm, contractions bring sperm up from the testicles through the vas deferens to the base of the urethra, just below the prostate. It mixes there with fluid from the prostate to make semen. This is the stage Masters and Johnson called "ejaculatory inevitability"; it lasts only two or three seconds. A sphincter muscle closes off the bladder from the urethra, preventing semen from flowing into the bladder and urine from entering the urethra. In the second stage of orgasm, a powerful series of rhythmic contractions propels the semen along the length of the urethra and out the end of the penis.

▶ *At orgasm, sperm mixes with fluid from the prostate to form semen, which is forced out of the penis.*

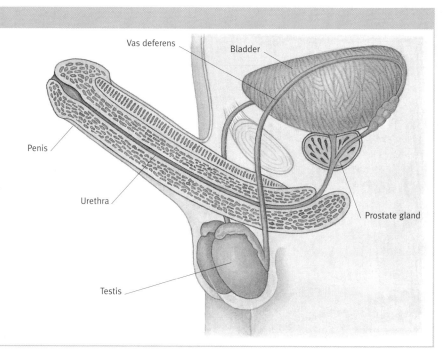

Vas deferens

Bladder

Penis

Urethra

Prostate gland

Testis

Multiple Orgasms" on page 148), once this stage is reached you have as much chance of stopping yourself from ejaculating as you have of holding back the tide.

The second stage of male orgasm is the ejaculation itself, which occurs between two and four seconds later. This is the explosive part. A second, more powerful series of rhythmic contractions begins convulsing the muscles along the entire length of the urethra, as well as the muscles at the base of the penis and along its shaft. These contractions pump the semen forward from its staging area just below the prostate until it comes spurting out the end of your penis.

Most of the ejaculate is ejected in the first three or four contractions, at which point the strength of the contractions and the amount of fluid ejected rapidly diminishes. You are, as the saying goes, spent.

THE WOMAN

The research by Masters and Johnson affirmed what Dr. Alfred C. Kinsey had discovered in the 1950s: that stimulation of the clitoris is almost always needed to bring on female orgasm. They also determined that women's and men's orgasms are far more similar than different physiologically. Add those two findings to their careful documentation of the fact that women are, if anything, more capable of enjoying sex than men—because women can have an indefinite number of orgasms—and you begin to see how far lab-coated sex researchers went in paving the way for the feminist revolution.

Once the clitoris has been stimulated enough, the woman's orgasmic contractions start in the lower portions of the vagina, where what's called a "penile-grasping" reflex often occurs. From there they spread to the uterus.

The woman's orgasmic contractions (which can resemble the early stages of labor during childbirth) occur at 0.8 second intervals, which is exactly the rate they occur in the man. Also like the man, after the first few contractions their intensity diminishes dramatically, although some orgasms are unusually powerful and long-lasting.

As with the man, the woman's orgasm is often accompanied by muscle clenching, both involuntary and voluntary, throughout the body, most obviously in the face.

Tips for Keeping Your Sperm Healthy

You can help keep your sperm happy and ready for parenthood if you:

• Quit smoking.

• Don't drink to excess (usually defined as more than two drinks a day).

• Wear loose-fitting underwear and avoid too many hot baths so your testicles stay cool.

• Keep plenty of antioxidant vitamins E, C, and beta-carotene coursing through your veins by eating five to nine servings of fruit and vegetables daily.

• Take a multivitamin supplement that will give you at least 20 milligrams of zinc a day.

• Reduce the amount of stress and anxiety in your life.

• Make sure your drinking water is free from contamination by lead.

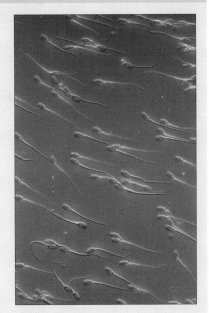

▲ *Seen under a microscope, healthy sperm swim vigorously.*

What Makes a Good Orgasm?

A lot of sex therapists will tell you we've become obsessed with the orgasm. Men are worried that they're climaxing too soon; women that they're not climaxing soon enough; both are worried that the fireworks they've been led to expect almost never materialize in their bedrooms.

Bernie Zilbergeld, Ph.D., sex therapist and author of *The New Male Sexuality*, says that men and women can both become so focused on giving their partners a great orgasmic experience that they neglect their own pleasure. The result is that millions of women habitually fake orgasms and millions of men are weighed down with fears of sexual inadequacy. Sometimes it looks as if nobody is enjoying sex anymore.

The answer, Dr. Zilbergeld believes, is for both partners to become assertive in asking for what they want in bed, and for both of them to stop obsessing about delivering their partners' orgasmic fireworks on demand.

Sex therapist Marilyn Volker, Ph.D., divides orgasms into two basic categories: those that are about physical release and those that combine physical release with a sense of emotional connection. "When you really have that sense of caring, love, and trust with a partner," she says, "then you have the potential for experiencing the most explosive type of orgasms, those where you reach a soul connection. Most people say that's the most powerful orgasm of all."

How to Have Multiple Orgasms

Some offers seem too good to be true. There's the salesman who phones to say you've won a free vacation in Hawaii, then there's the sex therapist who tells you that men don't have to be satisfied with just one measly orgasm, that they can reach the heights over and over again. Yeah, right. Read on.

Longer Lovemaking

All women are physically capable of having multiple orgasms, although surveys tell us that only about 50 percent have had the pleasure. As implausible as the *male* multiple orgasm sounds, some experts swear that with a little effort and dedication it can be achieved.

One of the more prominent proselytizers of the male multiple orgasm is sex therapist Barbara Keesling, Ph.D. Dr. Keesling contends that with enough practice, a man can experience the sensation of a true orgasm without actually ejaculating—and not ejaculating is what enables you to keep having orgasms again and again.

Dr. Keesling's program combines two components, one physical, the other mental. First, the man has to exercise his pubococcygeal (PC) muscles (the ones you use when you cut off the flow of urine) by contracting and releasing them several times a day. This is a simple process which should take between four and six weeks. For full details, see "Train Those Muscles."

The second part of the program is centered in the brain: You have to learn to identify stages of arousal during sex so that you'll know when to engage your beautifully toned PC muscles to head off ejaculation. During lovemaking or when masturbating, take notice of the different levels of arousal you pass through on the road to orgasm. Dr. Keesling suggests rating those levels on a scale of 1 to 10, from 1 for no arousal to 10 for orgasm.

THE MAIN EVENT

Once you've trained your PCs and are able to judge your arousal level, the next step is to teach yourself to pause at the various levels. Of great importance here is a cooperative and sensitive partner: If you haven't already, talk to her about the program before going any further.

When making love, start off by thrusting slowly to level 4, say, then stop, take a deep breath, and tighten your PCs. That should bring your level of excitement down at least a notch or two.

Now start thrusting again, and work your way up the arousal scale, pausing again and again using the PCs. At the high end of the scale,

---

The Allure of the Quickie

A lot of men would probably be surprised to learn that women don't mind the odd quickie—as long as it's not the only item on the sexual menu.

According to Joel D. Block, Ph.D., sex therapist and author of *Secrets of Better Sex*, you can enhance your chances of a brief encounter by encouraging your partner to seek you out after she's aroused herself through fantasy or masturbation. You can also learn to be flexible; many an opportunity slips by if you insist on waiting for the perfect moment.

Spontaneity is the key to the quickie's appeal, says Alex Comfort, M.D., sex expert and author of *The New Joy of Sex*. "The quickie is the equivalent of inspiration," he writes, "and you should let it strike in lightning fashion, any time and almost anywhere."

Train Those Muscles

Arnold Kegel was a gynecologist who in the 1950s devised a simple exercise to help women who'd just given birth get over their incontinence problems by strengthening their bladder control.

A Kegel exercise consists of tightening the pubococcygeal or PC muscles, which run in a band from your pubic bone to your tailbone. You clench your PCs when you try to squeeze off your flow of urine. That's a Kegel exercise.

The sexual value of Kegels is that the same muscles that squeeze off urine can also squeeze off an ejaculation, prolonging your time in the saddle and opening the way for multiple orgasms. They can also make your erection firmer and increase the intensity of your orgasm when you do let go.

You won't find a Kegel machine at the gym, but you don't need one. Start by trying a few "flicks." Simply contract and release your PC muscles 10 times in quick succession. Then try to contract your PCs and hold them for 15 seconds. Gradually increase your regimen so that you're doing 10 sets of flicks and 10 holds daily. Then try changing positions by practicing Kegels while lying on your stomach or your back.

It'll take about a month or six weeks to get your PCs in good condition. After that initial training period, the exercises will become almost automatic.

when you feel you're nearly at level 10, slam on your PCs as hard as you can, open your eyes (Dr. Keesling says this is essential, although she's not sure why), and take a very deep breath. You should be feeling all the blinding ecstasy of an orgasm without ejaculating.

Relax for a few minutes. You've earned yourself a break! So that's orgasm number one...

Is It Really for You?

Now, the downside. The fact is that a number of sex therapists are skeptical that a true multiple orgasm is possible for men.

Some experts are concerned that even the quest for a multiple orgasm is misguided, that it may put too much pressure on a man and actually lead to sexual difficulties. "Enough men are having enough problems with their first ejaculation," says Robert Birch, Ph.D., a sex therapist. "You set yourself up for disappointment by giving yourself scores."

Ejaculation and Orgasm: What's the Difference?

The key to achieving multiple orgasms is knowing that there's a difference between orgasm and ejaculation. Robert O. Hawkins Jr., Ph.D., a sex therapist, says that ejaculation is a local experience, the physical expulsion of semen, while orgasm is global, a whole-body experience.

That's essentially a more holistic explanation of the two stages of male orgasm identified years ago by sex researchers Masters and Johnson. They defined the first stage as the "initiation of emission," when the body gathers sperm from the testicles and seminal fluid from the prostate gland in preparation for ejaculation. The second stage was the ejaculation itself.

Masters and Johnson maintained that once a man reaches the first stage of orgasm, the second stage is inevitable. Other experts have subsequently disagreed. They argue that it's possible to experience the sensations that accompany the first stage of orgasm without actually ejaculating, even though those two points are only a few seconds apart. Any man who can separate orgasm and ejaculation, these sex therapists say, can have multiple orgasms.

No one argues that once a man ejaculates, he enters what's called a refractory period, in which his ability to get an erection is temporarily disengaged. How long that period lasts depends on several factors, including your age, how long it's been since you last had sex, and, no doubt, the persuasiveness of your partner.

We heartily agree that men don't need another performance demand in their sex lives. Still, there's no question that the techniques that Dr. Keesling and others recommend can be used effectively to prolong the enjoyment of sex. If that's one of your goals, why not give them a try? Just keep in mind that enjoyment is the operative word.

Afterplay

Millions of women will testify that afterplay is the least developed male sexual skill. Given that women are generally slower to become aroused and slower to reach orgasm than men, it stands to reason they're also slower to cool down. That, plus the high emotional component of sex for many women, means that afterplay—kissing, hugging, stroking, talking, cooing—often means much more to them than it does to us.

The British psychologist Glenn Wilson points out that the period after sex is an excellent time to offer words of support and appreciation for our partners. This is the sort of mutual esteem-building that often gets overlooked in the daily rush of events, he says.

▶ *Sex doesn't end with the fireworks of orgasm. Kissing, hugging, stroking—just being close—are fitting ways to bring proceedings to a close.*

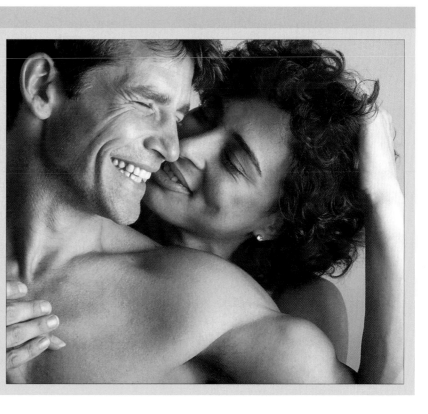

Positions for Play

The essence of intercourse is pretty basic. You take one penis, one vagina, and you get them together. End of story. But how you and your lover get them together can make the difference between a humdrum biological act and a sex life that sparkles with variety and excitement.

> **"I had a boyfriend once who said he learned a lot about women from watching his cat."**
> Linda Schneider, Ph.D., psychologist, Redwood City, California

Why Experiment?

The range of positions described in the *Kama Sutra*, the Indian love manual written some 2,000 years ago, demonstrates that the desire to add variety to sex is nothing new. Now no one expects you to work your way through every page of the *Kama Sutra*; that's a little obsessive. Creative lovemaking, though, demands an attitude that's open to variety and experimentation.

A lot of men like to fantasize about having an endless parade of sexual conquests, but the reality is that the majority of us end up having most of our sex with just one partner, our spouse. The monotonous potential of that can be downright depressing, unless we can find ways of keeping sex fun, vital, and interesting. Experimenting with different positions is a safer, more honest, and cheaper alternative to having affairs. And, anyway, the same problem would crop up with a mistress.

There's another reason to try new positions. Sexuality is one of the most deeply personal and highly expressive human attributes, so it stands to reason that certain people are going to find certain sexual positions far more satisfying than other positions. Some positions stimulate specific parts of the body, both male and female, more effectively than others. You and your partner owe it to yourselves to discover which positions scratch which itches.

Finally, it's good to try a range of positions to find ones that are more suited to your physical capabilities. The missionary position, for example, poses obvious problems when the man is overweight. If you've injured your knees playing football, squatting positions are not likely to be among your favorites.

Sampling the Smorgasbord

On the following pages, you'll find illustrations and descriptions of 19 different positions, some basic, some unusual, a few pretty exotic. It's not an exhaustive list, but it should give you plenty to work on.

Keep in mind, however, that sex is not an athletic competition. That may sound like stating the obvious, but it's true that some men become hooked on trying every possible permutation of every possible position. That risks missing the point.

Even sex expert Alex Comfort, M.D., whose book, *The Joy of Sex*, probably exposed more people to the myriad possibilities of human copulation than any book since the *Kama Sutra*, acknowledges that most couples start out by sampling a wide range of sexual delights, then wind up concentrating on one or two of them.

Sex should be fun. Variety is one way to get there, but it's not the main objective.

Contraception

Lest we forget, sex is not just about arousal and orgasms. It has something to do with making babies, too, unless you take precautionary measures.

For men, the single most effective form of contraception is a vasectomy. According to Kate Thomsen, M.D., M.P.H., medical director of the Planned Parenthood Federation of America, vasectomy has now been around long enough that many of the initial fears men had about its possible effect on potency have faded. Still, it's mainly popular among older men who have already had all the children they want to have.

Beyond that, the effectiveness of various contraceptive methods depends on how they're used. Planned Parenthood keeps statistics which show, for example, that condoms successfully prevent pregnancy 97 percent of the time—if they're used correctly and consistently. But in the real world of "typical use"— when they're occasionally put on improperly in the heat of the moment, or when they're occasionally skipped altogether—condoms fail to prevent pregnancy 14 percent of the time.

It's not surprising that the safest contraceptives are those that interrupt lovemaking least. Topping Planned Parenthood's list is Norplant, a synthetic hormone which is surgically implanted into the woman's arm. It lasts five years and has a failure rate of 0.05 percent. The Pill, which women have to remember to take daily, fails 5 percent of the time.

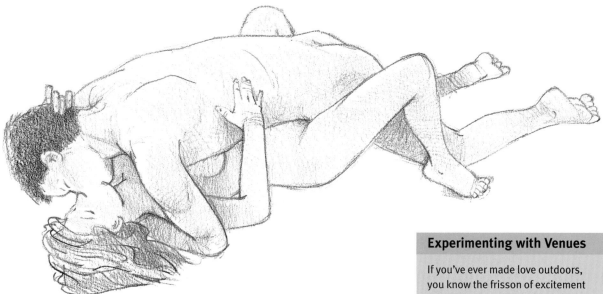

Missionary Position

This most basic of positions (in Western cultures, anyway) gets maligned more for the monotonous regularity with which many couples use it than for anything intrinsically boring about the position itself. In fact, its popularity probably derives as much from its effectiveness as from habit. The missionary position allows great face-to-face intimacy, deep penetration, and easy thrusting. The last can be a disadvantage for men who tend to ejaculate more quickly than they'd like.

The man dominates the action. Support your weight on your elbows—the position requires some strength and endurance—lest you pin your partner down. A deeper angle of entry will be provided by placing a pillow under the woman's hips. She can also vary the angle of penetration by wrapping her legs around you.

Seated Missionary

This variation on the missionary position isn't as strenuous for the man or as weighty on the woman. Thrusting isn't quite as easy, but that gives greater control over orgasm. Sit yourself between her legs. Your legs are spread wide, hers are slightly bent. You'll need to shimmy toward her till you make contact. This is a position in which couples can remain locked for a considerable period of exquisite time.

Experimenting with Venues

If you've ever made love outdoors, you know the frisson of excitement it provides, especially if you have a chance of being discovered. Boring it's not, which is pretty much the point, at least for adults. For teenagers, necessity is the mother of sexual invention.

The variety of venues that lend themselves to copulatory opportunity are limited only by the imagination. Alex Comfort, M.D., author of *The New Joy of Sex*, includes on his list bathtubs, showers, gardens, sand dunes, railroad cars, swings, rocking chairs, and swimming pools. All carry certain risks, he says, ranging from officious policemen to stinging insects. He's especially cautious when it comes to making love on motorcycles. "Has serious safety drawbacks," he writes. "Better not attempted on a public highway."

Knees to Chest

This position is sometimes called the "Rutting Deer." It's a more athletic variation on the standard missionary position, one that allows for the deepest possible penetration of the vagina. Obstetricians recommend it for hopeful parents, in fact, because the man's penis when he ejaculates is positioned right at the opening of the cervix.

She lifts her knees up to her chest, hooking them over your shoulders. Support your weight on your hands. From this position you're in a good spot to press your pubic bone against her, stimulating her clitoris.

Reverse Missionary

Here the woman takes control and the man literally lies back. This is the favored position for any guy who wants to delay orgasm. It's also great for those couples in which the woman is petite and the man is huge. For a switch you can spread your legs and she can lie between them, or you can both spread your legs in tandem. The latter position allows the woman to rub her clitoris against the man's body with particular directness, pushing her feet against the top of his feet for leverage.

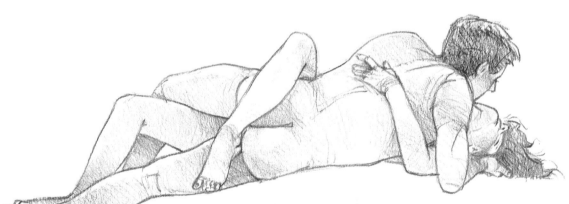

Cross Buttocks

You might call this a perpendicular missionary position. Both partners are in the same postures they would be in the classic missionary, but turned crosswise. The advantage is that the unusual angle of entry stimulates the sides of her vagina, which don't ordinarily get much attention. This position is also a good alternative if the man is considerably heavier than the woman.

Woman Astride

Among the numerous advantages of this position is the view afforded the man of his lover's body, particularly her breasts. Her clitoris is also available for manual stimulation (your hand or hers). The woman gains considerable control over the angle and depth of penetration, and it is she who most determines the rhythm and pace of the movement. The man gets to relax and enjoy.

As with all the woman-on-top positions, this one helps the man control his orgasm. The woman can take some of her weight off her partner by leaning back, supporting herself on his thighs.

Woman Astride, Facing Away

This position affords each partner a certain measure of privacy, if such a thing is possible during intercourse. Either is free to indulge in fantasy, although the male might prefer gazing at the view of his lover's backside. Meanwhile she can caress his testicles and her clitoris while he rubs her shoulders and buttocks. Again, the principal advantage of this position for the woman is the depth of penetration and freedom of movement it affords. For even greater mobility, the woman can rise up in a squat.

Classic Rear Entry, Kneeling

Rear entry is generally more popular with men than with women, partly because it reduces the sex act to a sort of primal level that isn't especially romantic. The "doggy-style" moniker is a crude but accurate indication of the animalistic fervor this position seems to embody.

The other reason women don't tend to favor rear entry is that it doesn't offer much in the way of clitoral stimulation, although manual assistance can easily be provided. The position does allow deep vaginal penetration at an angle which brings the penis into direct contact with the G spot, a supposed point of super-sensitivity on the foreground of the woman's vaginal wall. We say "supposed" because many experts think that the G spot is a myth. In any event, the man should be careful not to thrust so violently that his penis rams into the woman's cervix.

Rear Entry, Standing

This position takes the rawness of the classic rear entry a raunchy step further. It's an ideal position for quickies—try this in the kitchen with both your pants at half-mast—or for couples into domination fantasies. Big differences in height can be overcome by having the shorter partner stand on a pile of sex manuals or other weighty tomes. You might also try this on a flight of stairs, although having a banister to hold onto would be a good idea.

Seated Rear Entry

This is another position that's perfect for a quick sex session. It's probably best suited for chairs (or park benches, if you're into that sort of public danger), although it also works nicely sitting on the edge of a bed.

   The woman has plenty of freedom of movement, assuming her legs are in decent shape. The man can mostly relax, although he can gain some leverage for thrusting by putting his weight on his hands. As with all the rear-entry positions, the penis penetrates deeply, and each partner can simultaneously stimulate the other's erogenous zones by hand.

Spoon

One writer aptly described this as "the classic Sunday morning sex position." It's an intimate and effortless posture, perfect for long, loving, relaxing sex. Note the accessibility of the clitoris and breasts. Penetration can be a bit tricky to maintain— romantic though it may be, this is still a rear-entry position—but slight shifts in position can improve the angle. Thrusting isn't easy in the spoon position, either, but athleticism isn't the point here. Spooning is ideal for pregnant women or overweight men.

Facing Spoon

This may be the position that inspired the folk song refrain about "rollin' in my sweet baby's arms." It's intimate and restful. A lot of couples will wind up in the facing-spoon position temporarily on their way to or from other positions during lovemaking sessions. It's easy for the man to adjust the depth of his penetration by lifting his leg up or down.

Squatted Kneeling

Kneeling positions such as this combine intimacy with a certain degree of athleticism, although once the couple is in place they're not necessarily as strenuous as they look. Penetration is deep, yet the woman also enjoys direct stimulation of her clitoris. This is not a position for thrusting, but it affords an unusual degree of closeness between the lovers' bodies. Breast men, take particular note.

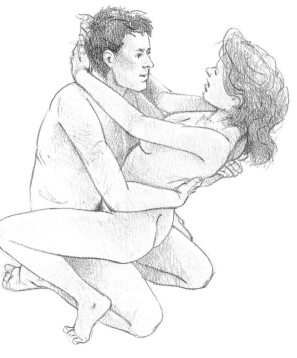

Rear Window

This is another rear-entry position that makes for deep vaginal penetration. The woman kneels down on the bed, supported on her elbows with hands clasped behind her head. The man then kneels behind and positions himself to enter her. Contact is made in a particularly raunchy manner when she hooks her legs around his and pulls him toward her. He supports himself by placing his hands on her shoulders.

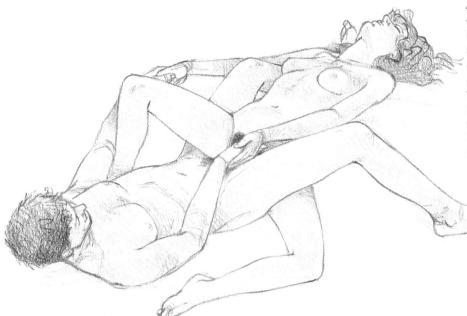

The X Position

A favorite of Alex Comfort, M.D., author of *The New Joy of Sex*, the X position is ideal for couples who want a session of slow, leisurely sex. Getting into it isn't as tricky as it looks. Start in the woman-astride position, then lean back, adjust your legs into a scissors position and grasp one another's hands. "Slow, coordinated wriggling movements will keep him erect and her close to orgasm for long periods," Dr. Comfort says.

Standing Wheelbarrow

For the athletic only: Both of you—especially her—should be in good shape to try this one. Start off in the standing rear entry position, then lift her up by the upper thighs or pelvis. For extra grip, she can wrap her legs around your waist. Don't expect to stay in this position very long, though.

   A word of caution is necessary here: Don't try this position unless you and your partner both have a good sense of humor.

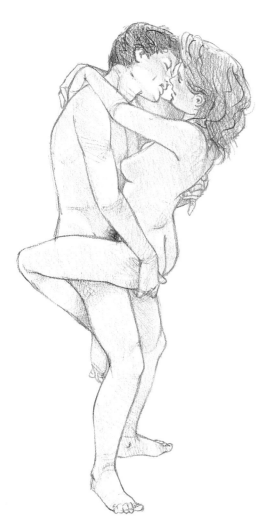

Standing

Like rear-entry positions, there's something inherently raunchy about having sex standing up. It's a favorite position for quickies, of course, especially outside the bedroom. Height differences can pose a problem; compensation can be made if the shorter partner stands on a stack of telephone directories or something similar. Bracing one partner against a wall or tree is helpful. For a lovely and less taxing variation, try a session of aquatic standing sex some warm summer evening at the lake.

Seated Wheelbarrow

You might call this the amateur version of the standing wheelbarrow, although the woman will still need to have some serious upper-body strength. Again, this is not a position you should expect to stay in for a very long time, but it's a fun alternative that offers an unusual angle of entry, not to mention a nice view of her hindquarters.

Woman on Top, Leaning Back

This variation on the woman-astride position—all she has to do is lean back—affords the man superb manual access to her clitoris. Or he can rise up on his elbows for a better view. There's a similar variation to the woman-on-top, facing-away position. Again, the woman simply leans back, in this case until she's lying with her back upon the man's chest. This puts her breasts within easy reach.

Alternatives to Intercourse

When it comes to sex, a lot of us modern guys think we're pretty liberated, but in fact many of us are still stuck on one of the oldest stereotypes there is: The idea that "sex" is defined as vaginal intercourse and only vaginal intercourse. In truth, there are lots of other satisfying ways of having sex.

Going Beyond Intercourse

The term sex therapists often use to describe alternatives to intercourse is "outercourse." They define outercourse as any type of sex play that doesn't involve the penis being inserted into a vagina, including masturbation, various types of body rubbing, oral sex, and fantasy games.

Sex experts list four major reasons why outercourse can sometimes be a better route to sexual satisfaction than intercourse.

• No babies. No one gets pregnant if sperm is kept out of the vagina. This form of birth control is organic, too: no hormones, no chemicals, no injections, no side effects.

• No diseases. If bodily fluids aren't exchanged, you won't catch any of the 20 or so sexually transmitted diseases, including AIDS.

• Great sex. Men who can take their focus off vaginal intercourse and put it onto other forms of stimulation find that they have stronger orgasms and more satisfied partners.

• No erection is required. Bernie Zilbergeld, Ph.D., a sex therapist in Oakland, California, and author of *The New Male Sexuality*, points out that men don't have to have an erection to enjoy sex. Stimulation of a soft penis feels good, too. Knowing that he doesn't have to get an erection to enjoy sex can take a lot of the pressure off a man, which is why sex therapists recommend outercourse as one of the principal treatments for performance anxiety. Outercourse works just as well for men who are impotent for physical reasons.

The advantages of outercourse are becoming more obvious because of AIDS, but the sexual frustrations of millions of teenagers could be alleviated by its pleasures as well. Michael Burnhill, M.D., vice president of medical affairs for the Planned Parenthood Federation of America, wishes outercourse had been more widely accepted when he was in high school. "I had my raging hormones as much as anybody else," he says. "If we'd been taught how to have orgasms in ways besides intercourse, and if we'd been allowed to, we could have avoided a lot of problems."

Ways and Means

Here's an overview of some of the better-known alternatives to vaginal intercourse. If you want to try them out, remember to talk it over with your partner first to make sure she's comfortable with the idea.

ANAL INTERCOURSE

Many sex experts wouldn't classify anal intercourse as outercourse because it involves penetration. It can also expose you to HIV, the virus that causes AIDS, and other sexually transmitted diseases (STDs). In fact, if practiced without protection, anal intercourse is one of the most likely ways to contract HIV. The tissues of the anus and lower colon are easily ruptured during sex, which opens a direct pathway for HIV to get into the bloodstream. Genital contact with fecal material can spread numerous other types of bacterial infection as well.

TRUE OR FALSE?

Masturbation is something mainly indulged in by adolescents and single people to relieve their sexual tensions.

False: A major sex survey found that married people were "significantly more likely" to masturbate than people who lived alone. Another major survey found that a majority of men continue to masturbate at least into their fifties.

A Proper Tool for Every Job

The well-equipped boudoir should have the following items on hand:

• Lubrication. Make sure it's a water-based product. Oil-based types can destroy condoms and damage delicate vaginal tissues.

• Condoms. Useful as sex toys as well as contraceptives.

• Massage oil. Natural blends of nut and vegetable oils are recommended.

• Cock ring. These wrap around the base of the penis (and sometimes the scrotum), making erections harder and longer-lasting. Make sure to take them off every 30 minutes or so to let your blood circulate.

• Dildo. Good for filling a woman up vaginally while you're simultaneously administering oral sex.

• Vibrator. This is the ultimate tool for clitoral stimulation.

Playing Games

One way to make sex more exciting is to play fantasy games. Games add variety and creativity to what can become an inhibited, boring routine. As leading sex expert Alex Comfort, M.D., put it in *The New Joy of Sex*, "Sex is the most important sort of adult play. Take off your shell along with your clothes."

The possibilities are infinite. "The Sultan and his favorite concubine" and "the burglar and the maiden" are two of Dr. Comfort's suggested role-plays. Masks and costumes can add to the fantasy. And the field of play isn't limited to the bedroom, either. Robert Birch, Ph.D., a sex therapist, suggests playing the pick-up game, which goes like this: While one partner sits at a bar, the other comes in, buys a drink, and plays the seducer.

Bondage games are among the most popular of all sexual diversions, partly because they enable a sort of unconditional surrender (the bonded partner has no choice but to lay back and let it happen) and partly because of the weighty psychological power (for both sexes) of sexual dominance and submission. Try tying your partner up some time, or let her tie you up. Use towels, bedsheets, the cloth belt from a bathrobe—anything softer than rope. The idea is to be effectively restrained, but not painfully so.

Whatever game you play, there are lines that shouldn't be crossed. "People should not do something that's so far out of character it causes shame," says Dr. Birch. "You should never do anything, or ask your partner to do anything, that feels degrading, for either one of you."

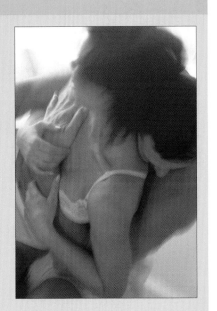

▲ *Sex games range from a bedroom tussle to bondage and role-play.*

These dangers may or may not be the explanation for why the thought of anal sex makes a lot of people so uneasy. A major survey of sexual attitudes in the United States found that 74 percent of the women surveyed and 69 percent of the men found it "unusual" or "kinky." The fact remains, however, that heterosexual as well as homosexual couples have enjoyed anal sex for centuries.

If you and your mate are among them, then a few precautions are definitely in order. Use a strong latex condom and lots of water-based lubrication; go gently to minimize damage to the anal tissues; and wash your hands and genitals thoroughly before and after. Be especially sure never to take your penis out of her anus and put it into her vagina.

BODY RUBBING

Another sexual practice that's been going on for centuries was in times past called "heavy petting"—foreplay that stopped short of intercourse, usually because of fears of pregnancy, or because the girl wanted to remain a virgin. Resourceful couples in that situation often looked for creative ways to relieve the man's sexual frustration (the woman was usually left to her own devices), leading to the discovery of several places on the woman's body where the penis could be rubbed with enough friction to achieve an orgasm.

Oral sex and masturbation have since become more acceptable and popular ways of dealing with this problem, but the old methods can still get the job done *and* add a *frisson* to couples' sex play.

Perhaps the most popular locale for penis rubbing has been between the breasts, which many men find exciting regardless of contraceptive concerns. Another alternative is femoral intercourse: The man rubs his penis between the woman's thighs, either from the front or from the rear. That's an area close enough to the vagina to warrant special care when ejaculating.

Self-Pleasuring

Woody Allen once described masturbation as "sex with someone I love." Jokes aside, for years now sex therapists have been waging a concerted campaign against masturbatory guilt. Not only is it okay to pleasure yourself, they insist, it's downright good for you.

We now know that what used to be called self-abuse helps keep a man's supply of sperm fresh and strong. It can also help stimulate the production of testosterone. Even more important, men can learn through masturbating how to postpone their orgasms, making them better, more considerate lovers.

It's an opportunity for self-improvement few men apparently miss. One survey reported that nearly a third of its male respondents said they masturbated once a week. Roughly another third said they did so between a few times a year to a couple of times a month.

Despite the therapists' best efforts, though, surveys show that most men who masturbate still feel a little embarrassed about it.

The Road to Safer Sex

Every year, one in 20 Americans catches one of the 20 or so sexually transmitted diseases. One night of unprotected ecstasy can leave you with a lifetime of regrets. It's a sad fact of life these days, but the truth is that you can't afford to let your guard down: Always practice safer sex.

Making Sex Safer

Sadly, experts say there is no safe sex today—*safer* sex is the best you can hope for. Unless you've been in a strictly monogamous relationship for at least six months, and both partners have been tested for HIV, protection from the range of sexually transmitted diseases is very definitely in order.

The basic rule of safer sex is to avoid sexual practices that involve sharing body fluids. That's because HIV and most other STDs are spread when the blood, semen, or vaginal secretions from an infected person come into contact with the blood or other body fluids of someone who's not infected.

Safe sex rule number one, therefore, is always—repeat, always—wear a lubricated condom. And it has to be a latex one: Lambskin condoms don't shield you from the HIV virus as effectively as latex. The lubrication helps prevent tearing of the condom. Using a spermicide along with the condom helps kill the HIV virus.

Anal sex is probably the single riskiest sex act for transferring HIV. Caution should also be exercised when practicing cunnilingus with new partners. Use a "dental dam," a sheet of latex used by dentists for oral surgery. Most drug stores carry them; they lay over the woman's vagina, preventing direct contact. It's not exactly romantic, but better than getting a dose of something nasty. Other acts that can put you at risk are oral–anal contact, sharing sex toys (condoms can be used to cover dildoes), and wet kissing.

All STDs can be treated (if not cured), especially if caught in the early stages. See a physician if you notice any symptoms described in the table opposite.

How to Use a Condom

To be an effective safer sex strategy—not to mention a reliable contraceptive—condoms have to be used correctly. We show you how.

In the heat of the moment it may be difficult, but put the condom on before the penis touches the vulva. Both pregnancy and transmission of STDs can occur before you ejaculate.

1 Unroll the condom onto your penis holding the tip of the condom with the fingers of one hand.

2 Leave a half-inch space at the tip of the condom to collect semen. Remember to smooth out any air bubbles once the condom is on— the bubbles can cause tears. Withdraw from the vagina before you lose your erection. Hold the condom against the base of your penis while you withdraw so that no semen is spilled.

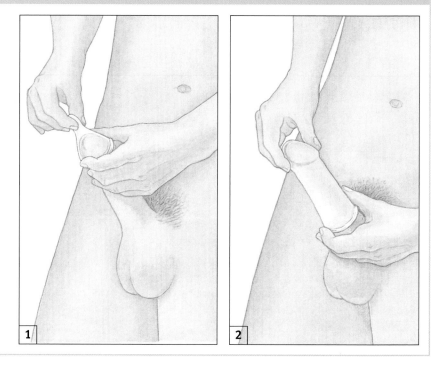

A Guide to Common Sexually Transmitted Diseases

Disease	How Acquired	Symptoms	Treatment	Complications if Not Treated
Chlamydia	Bacterial infection acquired primarily through vaginal or anal intercourse.	Many men and most women infected with chlamydia have no symptoms. Symptoms that do appear in infected men usually manifest themselves within one to six weeks after being exposed to the infection. They include a stinging sensation at the end of the penis, a watery discharge from the penis, swollen testicles, and painful urination.	Antibiotics.	For men, can lead to infections in the testicle area (epididymitis) and infertility. For women, can lead to severe pain and infertility.
Genital Herpes	Viral infection spread by contact with infected area (which may or may not show visible signs of infection).	Initial outbreak usually begins about a week after exposure with tingling and itching around genitals, followed by appearance of genital sores. Subsequent outbreaks usually produce milder symptoms.	Herpes is incurable. Severe outbreaks can be treated with medication to minimize symptoms.	Increases risk of HIV infection through open sores.
Gonorrhea	Bacterial infection of urethra, rectum, mouth, or throat, passed on by vaginal, anal, or oral sex.	Generally begins from one to seven days after infection. They include pain during urination, then yellow discharge from penis.	Antibiotics.	Untreated gonorrhea can cause infertility and infections of joints, heart valves, and brain.
Hepatitis B	Virus acquired through exposure to infected blood, semen, vaginal secretions, and saliva, usually via sexual contact.	One-third of carriers experience no symptoms; those who do experience them can have fever, headaches, muscle aches, fatigue, loss of appetite, vomiting, diarrhea. Advanced symptoms include dark urine, abdominal pain, and yellowing of the skin and whites of eyes.	Most infections clear up on their own in eight weeks, although some become chronic. Chronic infections can lead to cirrhosis and liver cancer.	A vaccine is available.
HIV/AIDS	Viral infection acquired by sexual contact and through exposure to contaminated blood; attacks immune systems.	Usually no symptoms appear in initial stages of HIV infection, although some people develop a short-lived illness that resembles mononucleosis. Antibodies can be detected in the blood within three to six months. Many HIV-infected men experience little disease progression for years. In full-blown AIDS the immune system breaks down, opening the way for numerous infections and certain cancers.	New antiviral drugs are available which slow development of HIV infection into full-blown AIDS.	Ultimately fatal.
Human Papilloma-virus (HPV)	Viral infection through vaginal, anal, or oral sex.	Sometimes there are none. Men often get genital warts on tip of penis. Warts vary from small bumps to larger growths resembling cauliflowers. Sometimes they are moist and itchy. They can appear anywhere from a few weeks to several years after exposure, although they are sometimes hard to see. Warts can also develop in the anus or throat.	If left untreated, warts may go away by themselves, remain unchanged, or grow larger. A doctor can remove them, although the virus which causes warts is incurable.	Cancers of penis and anus can occasionally develop. In women can lead to cancer of the cervix.
Syphilis	Bacterial infection acquired through vaginal, anal, or oral sex or by skin contact with open sores.	Between 9 and 90 days after exposure, a shallow, painless ulcer develops at the site of infection, usually on penis. It heals after a month or so. About 6 weeks later, a rash appears on palms or soles of feet, sometimes on mouth; swollen lymph nodes and wartlike growths on genitals may also appear. Symptoms can come and go for two years, after which disease enters a latent stage.	Penicillin will arrest disease, although existing damage won't be reversed.	During latent stage various tissues in body, including those in bones, heart, brain, eyes, nervous system, and joints, can be severely damaged.

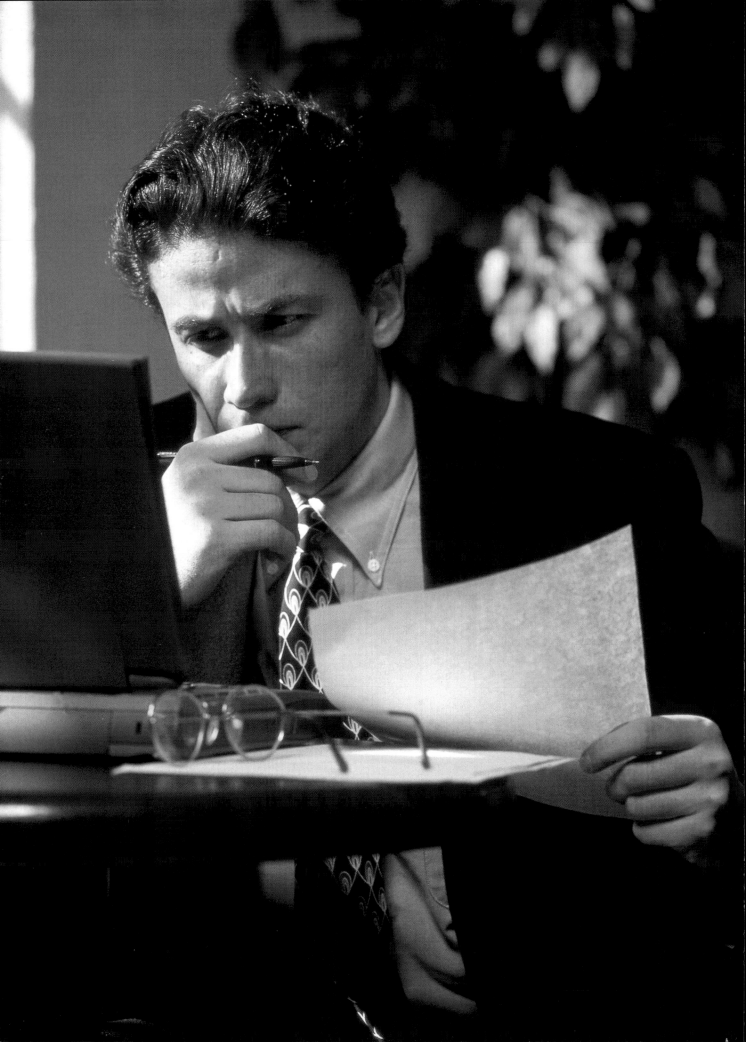

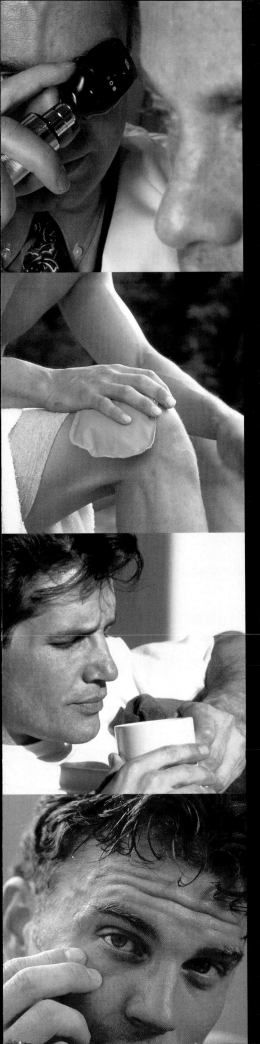

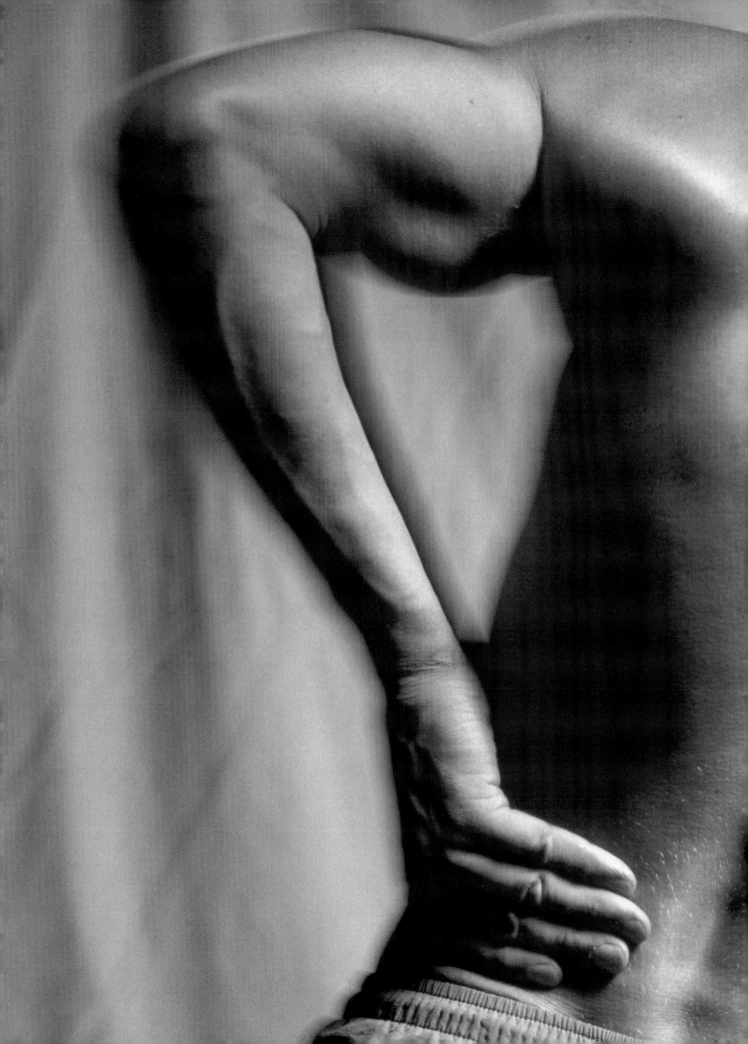

Symptoms, Causes, and Treatments

How Your Body Tells You What's Wrong

Men are perfectly capable of paying close attention to other things, but when it comes to our bodies we often seem to tune out completely. The fact is that your body is trying to get your attention all the time. Not in words, of course, but it's communicating nonetheless.

Your Body's Messages

"If I'd known I was going to live this long," said jazz great Eubie Blake at age 100, "I'd have taken better care of myself."

Not a bad thought to keep in mind when considering your own health. Sure, Eubie had already hit the century mark, but the point is to act like you're going to be around a long time. And the first step in doing that is simple: Listen up. It's a message you've heard countless times from parents, teachers, work colleagues, and partners. It's something even your own body is telling you.

Your body is constantly sending you messages, telling you when to eat and drink, for example. The body communicates in all the variations of pain you're able to feel, from a pinpoint prickling in your little toe to a major ache in your abdomen. And it sends messages in the cornucopia of other symptoms you can experience as well, things like fever, swelling, and bleeding.

Tune In for Good Health

Work hard, play hard is a man's credo, and that doesn't leave much room for physical problems. Fatigue, insomnia, a cough, or a sore throat are seen as inconveniences to be endured or at the very most treated with an over-the-counter remedy. "Men have this stoic sense," according to Lorraine Fitzpatrick, M.D., an associate professor of medicine at the Mayo Clinic in Rochester, Minnesota. "They tend to come in only for pain, like a fracture."

But instead of waiting for your body to shout at you with pain, why not try listening to the rest of what it has to say? What you stand to gain is a body that may serve you better in your quest to get the most out of life.

Once you begin listening to your body, you'll start to become familiar with its language. At times, the message will be obvious, but often you'll have to take some time to decipher it. Does feeling tired all the time mean that you're depressed or that you're not getting enough sleep? Consulting a medical reference book can help in these cases, but remember that books are no substitute for listening closely to your body. If you listen well, at the very least you'll be able to accurately describe what's going on to your doctor.

Taking Action

When you get a message from your body that something's not right, what can you do? You have a choice of four responses. Determining which one to follow depends on the circumstances, of course, but also on an ability to accurately hear what your body is saying.

The first option is to wait and see what happens. The body is an awesome healing machine, and you're often better off just letting it get the

Your 10-Point Health Check

Kenneth A. Goldberg, M.D., medical director of the Male Health Institute at Baylor Health Center, Irving-Coppell, Texas, offers the following checklist to self-monitor your health habits:

1 Do you smoke? Quitting is the best thing you can do for your health.

2 How's your diet? Avoid fats and load up on fruit, vegetables, and grains.

3 What about exercise? At a minimum, you need a 30-minute walk three times a week at a speed fast enough to get your heart rate up but not so fast that you can't carry on a conversation.

4 Do you limit sun exposure, especially between 10:00 A.M. and 4:00 P.M.? It's the main cause of skin cancer.

5 Sleep enough? Aim for eight or nine hours a night.

6 Do you know your body? Examine yourself every month for anything unusual. And find out your family's health history.

7 How's the alcohol intake? Limit yourself to one or two drinks a day.

8 Blood pressure under control? High blood pressure is a primary risk factor for heart attack.

9 Are you stressed out? Schedule some quiet time for yourself. And remember to laugh.

10 Got a doctor? If not, get one. The two of you are health partners.

10 Reasons to Go to the Emergency Room

When do you make a beeline for the ER? "The emergency room is there as a safety net," says Jonathan Hall, M.D., an assistant professor of emergency medicine at Washington University in St. Louis. "If you're worried about something that's going on, you should err on the side of safety and head to the ER."

In many cases—heart attack and stroke, for example—the quicker you get medical attention the better your chance of a swift and complete recovery. "Time can be your friend if you use it wisely," says Dr. Hall, "but it can hurt you if you don't." According to Dr. Hall and other experts, here are 10 reasons you should make a dash to the emergency room.

Trauma
The obvious emergencies—broken bones, deep cuts and wounds, bad burns, a nasty knock to the head.

Sudden Speech or Coordination Problems
Difficulty speaking or understanding statements, loss of coordination or vision, dizziness or loss of balance, or weakness or numbness of the face, arm, or leg—usually on one side of the body—are among the classic symptoms of a stroke.

Sudden Shortness of Breath
If it's not asthma and lasts for more than a half-hour, the suspects are heart attack, heart failure, angina, and pulmonary edema (an abnormal accumulation of fluid in the lungs).

Severe Abdominal Pain
Constant pain for more than an hour, especially when located in the lower right abdomen and accompanied by fever, may mean appendicitis.

Severe Chest Pain
It may be the sign of a heart attack, especially if it's located in the center of the chest, radiates to the neck or left arm, and is accompanied by dizziness, shortness of breath, sweating, nausea, or weakness.

Fever Above 103°F
According to Dr. Hall, even a fever of 102.5°F may merit a trip to the ER if you're experiencing other symptoms, like severe headache.

Sudden Change in Heart Rate
If there's no obvious reason, it's a danger signal for those over age 50. Other emergencies are a pulse that remains under 40 beats per minute and is accompanied by weakness or dizziness, and a pulse over 125 for no apparent reason, which can be life-threatening if it persists in an older person.

Nonmuscular Back Pain
If the pain isn't affected by movement or position—and especially if urination is frequent, painful, or bloody—you may have a kidney infection requiring immediate antibiotics.

Rectal Bleeding
A spot of bright red blood can be hemorrhoids, but black blood or stools that are tar-colored may indicate upper intestinal bleeding.

Sudden Testicular Pain
For adults, hernia and inflammation of the sperm ducts are two possibilities. More serious is testicular torsion, which cuts off blood to the testicle. It's rare past age 20, but if not corrected within a few hours the testicle may be lost.

job done on its own. If the symptom goes on for long, though, or if it's intense, you'll need to see a doctor.

The second response is to take action yourself. This can be as simple as popping some aspirin when your head hurts, or drinking plenty of water and fruit juice when you have a cold. As with option one, you should get medical attention if the symptoms persist or become intense.

Most minor symptoms you experience can be effectively dealt with by

one of these first two options. But there are times when none of us can be expected to know what's going on, much less treat the symptom. In those cases, a visit to the doctor—the third option—is in order.

The fourth response option—a trip to the emergency room—is called for when the body is sending you alarming messages that indicate something needs immediate attention. According to Jonathan Hall, M.D., an assistant professor of emergency

medicine at Washington University in St. Louis, things like sudden dizziness call for quick intervention, not a scheduled office visit.

A final word: Being a good listener is of vital importance, but there are many serious diseases that have virtually no symptoms, at least in their early stages. So supplement your listening with a doctor who knows you and your family health history and can periodically test for things your body can't alert you to.

Fatigue

We've all heard the term "energy crisis." It's when there's not enough fuel to run our cars, heat our homes, or power our factories and offices. But the human body can have its own energy crisis, when the batteries run flat. That's fatigue. Here's how to keep your batteries fully charged, day-in, day-out.

When You Run Out of Steam

Virtually all of us will experience fatigue at some point in our lives, and one study found that nearly 20 percent of men complain of major fatigue to their doctors. It affects men of every age, although it usually gets worse by the time we reach our thirties. Women are just as likely to experience fatigue, although men are less likely to deal with it until it becomes a serious problem.

To keep energized, our bodies need food and oxygen. If there's a deficiency in either fuel, the body's cells can't do their jobs properly and an energy crisis results. So does this mean that to avoid fatigue all you need to do is eat and breathe? Unfortunately, no. Fatigue is tricky. You can feel tired from too much physical exertion or not enough; from a lack of sleep or too much; from eating too little or from having to cart around excess weight. Fatigue sometimes occurs because you're ill. And what's more, it isn't always caused by physiological factors.

Head Off Your Energy Crisis

Fatigue is usually preventable. If you're feeling tired, the first step is to identify what's bringing your energy levels down.

Most of the time, you'll be able to correct the problem on your own by eating right, getting more rest, exercising, or reducing the stress in your life. If the fatigue persists, though, it could be a symptom of something more serious, and you'll need to see your doctor.

Symptom Sorter

Fatigue can be accompanied by symptoms other than tiredness. Your head may hurt, and you may have trouble concentrating. Over a period of time, you may experience depression or other changes in your personality.

If you need two alarms to wake in the morning, or if your energy level takes a nose dive between two and four o'clock in the afternoon, it's a good bet your body isn't getting the sleep, exercise, or fuel it needs. Another sign to watch for is always needing to "catch up" on your rest by sleeping a lot longer on weekends than on weekdays.

Unexplained muscle weakness that affects your ability to move is usually a symptom of something more serious—diabetes or stroke, for example. Make an appointment to see a doctor right away.

What Causes Fatigue?

A whole slew of factors can lead to fatigue. Stress, depression, mononucleosis, stroke, hepatitis, diabetes, anemia, heart disease, and cancer

Ingredients for a High-Energy Lifestyle

• Get physical. Sure, we all like to lump around from time to time, but a sedentary lifestyle is an energy killer. If your job isn't physical, moderate exercise will increase your body's ability to run at optimum levels.

• Focus on breakfast. Ditch the coffee and sugary roll, and try cereal with fruit and skim milk instead—the protein and complex carbohydrates will keep you going much longer.

• Know your energy cycle. Some of us are "morning people" and others zombies until noon. Schedule the day's more daunting tasks for your own peak energy period.

• Recharge your battery with sex. Not exactly a romantic reason for intimacy, but having regular, good sex—including a generous dose of cuddling—can energize and restore both you and your partner.

• Pursue your passion. You say that when you're bored you tire more easily? Welcome to the club. When you enjoy something, chances are you'll find the energy for it. If your job doesn't exactly push your joy button, leave time in your day for things that do.

• Take five. Our work days are often organized in large blocks of time, but we actually function better when taking periodic breaks. If your energy flags at work, stand and stretch for a few minutes, or go wash your face.

• Catch your Zzzs. A good night's sleep is an obvious but basic ingredient of a high-energy lifestyle. People's sleep differs, but the fact is that you can't teach yourself to need less sleep than you naturally require. Also, sleep should be as sound as possible to maximize its rejuvenating effects. Quality as well as quantity is important.

• Decline the drink. Alcohol is a depressant that can produce drowsiness. If you're having a fatigue problem, give up the booze for a while and see how you feel.

are some of the more serious conditions that may first manifest themselves by persistent fatigue. And that's just a partial list. "Fatigue can be a symptom of *any* severe, acute, or chronic disease," according to Paul Ellner, M.D., professor emeritus of microbiology, Columbia University .

Fortunately, though, most fatigue is brought on by easily rectifiable factors, chiefly lack of sleep, too little exercise, a bad diet, or stress.

SLEEP

Probably the most common and easily preventable cause of fatigue is a lack of sufficient sleep. Our slumber time has been decreasing over the past 15 years, and one study found that roughly half of all men sleep less than the 8 hours most of us need. While it's true that sleep needs among people do differ, and that some men can get by on as few as 6 hours a night while others need 10, you can't "teach" yourself to need less sleep than you naturally require.

EXERCISE

A desk-bound job eats away at your energy levels. Get out and do some moderate exercise at lunchtime (a 30-minute walk, say), and after hours take up an aerobic activity, such as running or swimming, to oxygenate muscles and revitalize your body.

DIET

We're all familiar with the mid-morning or mid-afternoon slump in energy levels at the office. That's often due to a sugary breakfast or lunch that's lacking in the protein and complex carbohydrates that give sustained energy. Eat a well-balanced diet to stock your body with all the nutrients it needs for its well-being. That also means eating fatty foods in moderation: Carrying around excess weight is energy-sapping.

STRESS

A man who hates his job—or is bored by it—may find himself fatigued no matter how well he eats, sleeps, or exercises. Why? Because he's a prime candidate for stress, and stress can lead to fatigue, according to Dr. Ellner. What's more, stress may be just the tip of the iceberg. "There's good evidence that stress affects the immune system and can increase susceptibility to viral and bacterial infections and perhaps even to cancer," Dr. Ellner says.

Strategies to Revitalize

To keep your batteries charged, aim for long-term results, not a quick fix. The following fatigue-fighters may remind you of the advice your Mom used to give you. But they work, according to Dr. Ellner "Everything your mom told you is 100 percent correct for fighting fatigue," he says.

• Quit smoking. Tobacco increases your body's need for oxygen while it decreases your ability to deliver it to cells. An energy drain is the result.

• Shed those excess pounds. Extra weight means extra effort, both physically and mentally. Avoid crash diets, though, which can slow your metabolism and make you feel even more tired.

• Retool your diet. Limit caffeine consumption and cut down on fatty, sugary food. Instead, load up on complex carbohydrates from grains and fruit. Drink plenty of water—six to eight 8-ounce glasses a day, experts say—and take some vitamins if you feel there's something lacking in your diet.

• Develop an exercise habit. "A workout in the morning gives you an energy boost for the rest of the day," according to Wes Myers, a Las Vegas personal trainer.

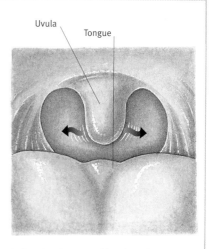
• Defuse the stress in your life. Stress is a reaction to the pressures of modern life. With time and effort you can control it.

How Snoring Wrecks Sleep

We men have gotten a bum rap from our bedmates for a lot of things over the ages, but one thing that's true is that we *do* snore. Between the ages of 30 and 55, about 20 percent of us produce that jarring midnight thunder, compared to just 5 percent of women. The gender gap narrows considerably after 60 years of age—60 percent of men and 40 percent of women—but by then the damage to our reputations is done.

Snoring happens when tissues in the upper airway that are taut during the day, such as the uvula—the dangling protuberance at the back of the throat—relax during sleep, and vibrate as air passes through the narrowed channel.

Snoring is sometimes so bad that medical intervention is warranted, possibly including surgery. In some cases, it's a symptom of more serious medical problems like nasal polyps or sleep apnea, a potentially dangerous condition in which a sleeper stops breathing—albeit temporarily—and snores loudly when he resumes.

If, however, you feel reasonably well-rested when you get up in the morning, and don't feel sleepy for long periods during the day, your snoring is probably harmless. Except, of course, for the effect it may have on your domestic tranquillity.

Headache

Have you ever felt like some sadist has your head clamped in a vise, or that an alien is trying to hack its way out of your skull, or maybe that a red-hot poker is being pushed into your brain? Join the club. A good 90 percent of Americans have at least one headache at some point during a year.

A Whole Heap of Headaches

As a general rule, headaches are just head aches. Some are very painful, of course, but usually there's no underlying serious problem.

Occasionally, though, there's a disease at the root of the problem. The usual symptoms of meningitis, for example, are a headache accompanied by fever, nausea, a stiff neck, and aversion to light. With stroke, there's a sudden, intense headache accompanied by speech and vision problems, and paralysis and numbness. And persistent head pain that comes on gradually over weeks or months might mean a brain tumor.

Headaches not caused by an underlying illness fall neatly into three categories: tension, migraine, and cluster headaches.

TENSION HEADACHES

Also known as stress or muscle-contraction headaches, tension headaches are the most common of the

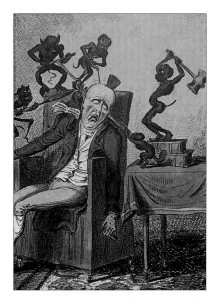

▲ *The torment of a headache, portrayed fancifully in a nineteenth-century cartoon.*

three types. They account for nearly 70 percent of all headaches and affect about 69 percent of men at some point in their lives.

Tension headaches are characterized by a dull pain that is mild to moderate in character, especially when compared with migraine or cluster headaches. The pain is steady rather than pounding or throbbing, and it can last anywhere from 15 minutes to a week.

A tension headache strikes on both sides of the head and it's usually impossible to pinpoint the exact center of pain. Frequently your jaw, upper back, and neck muscles will feel tense, and you might have a tight sensation around your scalp as well. Sometimes there's a lot of vise-like pressure. Tension headaches are brought on mainly by stress or fatigue. Eye strain, emotional problems, caffeine withdrawal, grinding your teeth, and even gum chewing can all provoke an attack, as can poor posture or sitting in front of your computer too long.

Who's at Risk?

• People experiencing prolonged bouts of stress: When you're emotionally stressed, you're often tense, and muscle tension is the source of many headaches. Purely physical stress on your body—bad posture, for example—can also play a role.

• Those with family history of migraine.

• People with a sensitivity to certain foods: Food may play a role in 10 to 40 percent of headaches, especially migraines; sensitivity varies among people, but most of the suspect foods (examples are red wine, chocolate, MSG, and aspartame, the artificial sweetener) contain substances that may cause blood vessels in the brain to constrict or dilate.

• People with disrupted eating or sleeping patterns: Fluctuations in your normal sleep and meal schedule can set off tension headaches.

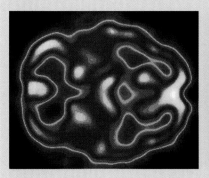

▲ *This scan shows the levels of electrical activity in a headache-free brain.*

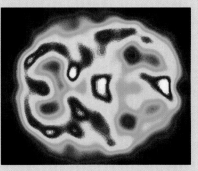

▲ *The green area, bottom right, shows reduced activity, indicating a migraine.*

The Headache Menu

According to the International Headache Society, the great majority of headaches not caused by some underlying disease— what doctors call "primary" headaches—are one of three types: tension, migraine, or cluster.

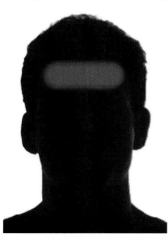

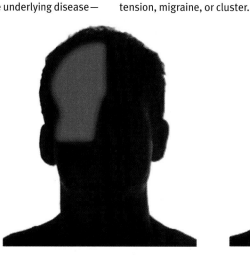

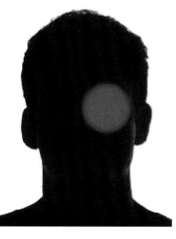

Tension Headache
• Strikes either on both sides of the head or throughout the head; there's no exact center of pain.

• Sometimes involves tension, pain, and pressure in the jaw, upper back, neck, and scalp.

• Head feels like it's in a vise.

Migraine Headache
• Typically involves excruciating pain on one side of the head only, usually from the eye socket upward.

• Pain often throbs in pace with the beating of the heart.

• There may also be numbness on one side of the face.

Cluster Headache
• Usually strikes on one side of the head only, either behind an eye or in the temple.

• Pain is steady and sharp.

• On the side that's affected, there may be nasal congestion and dripping, and the eye may start to water.

Headaches: His and Hers

Headaches are popularly—and erroneously—seen as a woman's complaint. In fact, the numbers are fairly close: 99 percent of women will have headaches at some point in their lives, compared with 93 percent of men.

While men and women are equally likely to suffer from tension headaches, statistics show that there's a significant difference between the sexes when it comes to the other two types of headache: migraine and cluster.

A woman is three times more likely to suffer from a migraine headache than a man, although medical researchers point out that migraines still affect 6 percent of American men. In the case of cluster headaches, men are far more likely to be afflicted—the ratio is about eight to one.

MIGRAINES

Migraines account for nearly one-quarter of all headaches, and most are experienced by women. There's a strong genetic factor: Studies show that between 70 and 80 percent of migraine sufferers have a family history of the complaint.

The word migraine comes from the Greek and means "half a skull," an apt name if ever there was one. Intense, incapacitating pain occurring in one side of the head is the typical scenario. The pain is usually described by sufferers as throbbing or pulsating, and it may be accompanied by other symptoms, including nausea, vomiting, numbness on one side of the face, cold hands, and sensitivity to light, noise, and movement. Migraines may last anywhere from four hours to three days and may recur from a few times each week to once every couple of years.

Migraines are sometimes called vascular headaches, because of the traditional belief that they're caused by the abnormal swelling and contracting of blood vessels in the head. Some researchers, though, believe that migraines have nothing to do with blood vessels and instead are caused by an abnormality in the brain's neurone circuits.

While migraines may come on like gangbusters with no warning whatsoever, about 40 percent of sufferers experience a preceding visual disturbance known as a migraine aura. The aura generally involves flashing lights, zigzagging or wavy lines,

Did You Know?

It's been estimated that headaches seriously interfere with the lives of perhaps 45 million Americans.

blind or dark spots, a temporary loss of peripheral vision, or splashes of color. It occurs about 10 to 30 minutes before the onset of pain, giving the quivering victim just a few moments to seek out a quiet, dark place.

CLUSTER HEADACHES

Cluster headaches often happen at night and are characterized by a sudden, excruciating pain on one side of the head, usually in the temple or behind an eye. On the side of the head that's affected, the nostril might plug up or run and the eye may start to water. The pain is steady and sharp rather than throbbing. Cluster headaches may occur a few times a day over a period of a few days, weeks, or months, and then disappear—only to return months or even years later.

This type of headache is relatively rare, and the exact cause is not clear. One researcher has noted a large

When to See a Doctor

If you experience migraine or cluster headaches, or think you do, see your doctor. A professional diagnosis is the first step toward a treatment plan.

While most tension headaches respond well to self-care, visit your doctor if they get in the way of your everyday life, or persist, according to Kenneth A. Goldberg, M.D., medical director of the Male Health Institute at Baylor Health Center, Irving-Coppell, Texas.

If headaches are recurring, it will help the doctor if you keep a written record of your symptoms. Note the date and time each headache started and stopped, the location, type, and severity of pain, factors that seem to trigger the headache such as food, bright light, or smoke, and any other

physical symptoms such as nausea or sensitivity to light and noise.

In a small number of cases, headaches are a sign of more serious conditions that may require medical intervention. So, Dr. Goldberg suggests you visit the doctor if you develop a new kind of headache, or if:

• Your headaches are getting worse.

• They aren't going away like they once did after the usual home treatment.

• They're accompanied by fever, a stiff neck, or explosive vomiting.

• They're accompanied by neurological symptoms like numbness, tingling, weakness, dizziness, visual impairment, or difficulty walking.

majority of cluster headache sufferers—more than 80 percent—have blue or hazel eyes. It's known that males are eight times more likely to be targets than females, with many

of the men who get them being heavy smokers and drinkers. Unfortunately, knocking off the booze and butts doesn't seem to make the headaches go away.

The Best Treatments for Headaches

If your headaches are persistent or interfere with your daily doings, you should seek medical help. A doctor can propose treatment plans you can't carry out on your own, such as the inhalation of oxygen from a mask. Otherwise, here are some antipain strategies suggested by the American Council for Headache Education, or ACHE.

Drugs
Headaches are most commonly attacked by taking an over-the-counter painkiller, usually what are known as nonsteroidal anti-inflammatory drugs (NSIADs), such as aspirin, ibuprofen, or acetaminophen. If these don't work and you have chronic or migraine headaches, your doctor can suggest prescription drugs—there are many available. Remember, though, that men who frequently take painkillers will need ever larger doses to get the same effects, and the drugs may actually cause "rebound" headaches. If possible, rely on nondrug treatments.

Exercise
A good workout will release brain chemicals called endorphins, which are powerful natural painkillers.

Relaxation
Do a mundane task to distract your mind. Meditate. Or learn specific relaxation and stress-reduction techniques. Anxiety and anger can aggravate a headache.

Ice
An ice pack, or a reusable frozen gel pack, on the part of your head that hurts is frequently effective.

Massage
For a tension headache, try rubbing the ridge between your neck and the back of your head for 10 minutes. Then rub your temples and the back of the neck where it meets the shoulders. Better yet, get a professional massage. It will reduce muscle tightness, alleviate the pain, and help you relax.

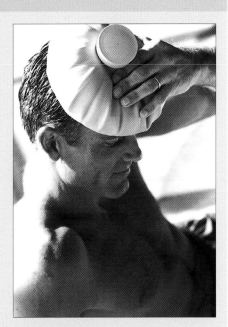

▲ Whenever possible, it's a good idea to soothe that aching head by using treatments that don't involve medications. Worth a try is the old-fashioned ice pack.

Dizziness and Fainting

Have you ever felt giddy or unsteady? A little light-headed? The world's in a spin? From the misery of motion sickness to the horrors of the drunken whirlies, dizziness, together with its close cousin fainting, seems designed to undermine our balanced view of a solid world.

A Bad Case of the Whirlies

Who among us hasn't been there? You've met some friends for a drink or two, and as the evening stretches on you imbibe a few more. By the time you make it home, the hour is late and you're dog tired. Thinking how wonderful it's going to be to finally get some sleep, you shed your clothes in a heap on the floor, hop into bed, close your eyes, and wait for the sandman to make his nightly run.

Only one problem, though. It feels like your bed is rotating, and you're beginning to get distinctly queasy. The whirling sensation doesn't go away unless you stare at the ceiling.

So you lie there, forcing your eyes to stay open as the lids get heavier and heavier. After a while, hoping you're past the worst of it, you lower your lids and begin to relax. Until the spinning starts again.

Virtually all of us recognize this as a case of the whirlies or spinnies or whatever they're called in your neck of the woods. An effect of drinking too much alcohol, they're a kind of dizziness doctors generally call vertigo—the sensation that your body or the world around you is spinning. In its most common form, vertigo is brought on when you change the position of your head, such as by leaning your head back to look up.

It can also be caused by an inflammation in the part of your inner ear that controls balance.

Why You Feel Dizzy

In medicine, dizziness is a general term used to describe one or more specific sensations—lack of balance, light-headedness, unsteadiness, disequilibrium, or that horrible feeling of spinning referred to above.

From a physiological point of view, you feel dizzy when your brain receives conflicting messages. If you're among those people who feel dizzy or queasy when they read in a moving car, for example, your eyes are telling the brain that you're sitting perfectly still while your inner ear is sensing the fact that you're actually barreling down the highway at a high speed. Your poor brain doesn't know what to believe until you finally put an end to the conflicting messages by closing your book and looking out the window.

The Best Treatments for Dizziness

If you don't have a history of imbalance and you find yourself suddenly feeling light-headed or unsteady, otolaryngologist Brian Blakley, M.D., advises that you keep your head as still as you can and lie down. "Trying to move around will make it worse," he says. "Rest for a little bit."

When you're ready to stand, first move your eyes, then your arms and legs, and then the rest of your body—slowly. If you're experiencing vertigo, sit up and avoid lying down.

Persistent or extreme dizziness should be treated by a doctor. But studies do show that tai chi can help your sense of balance. And, Dr. Blakley says, "Sometimes simple lifestyle things like getting a good night's sleep, avoiding stress, and making sure you're getting three square meals a day can do a lot for people who have general dizziness." For Ménière's disease—a condition caused by ear fluid accumulation with severe symptoms of a spinning sensation, ringing in the ears, ear pressure, and hearing loss—reduced salt intake and mild diuretics often help, according to Dr. Blakley.

For people who have traumatic or degenerative damage to the ear not caused by Ménière's disease, there are exercises to retrain your vestibular system. In one, you sit on the edge of a bed and do a side bend as far to the right as you can. Hold for 20 seconds, sit up, and then do the left side. Repeat three times on each side, three or four times per day.

Bringing Someone Round

We've all seen those movies where one character tries to revive another who has fainted by slapping and shaking the victim, and splashing cold water on her face—all the while yelling, "Wake up! Wake up!" When the poor woman finally begins to revive, she's propped up in a half-groggy state and urged to take a stiff drink.

Crude as they seem, those B-movie antics do serve a purpose, according to ontolaryngologist Brian Blakley, M.D., "They provide stimulation, and that can help," he says.

But there's a better plan of action. First, check if the person is breathing okay. Don't try to stand him up.

"One reason they probably fainted was there wasn't enough blood going to the head," Dr. Blakley says. "So lie him down on a flat surface." Elevate the feet above the head. "That helps get blood to the head," Dr. Blakley says.

▼ *If someone's fainted, lay him on the ground and raise his feet above his head. Keep monitoring his breathing and pulse.*

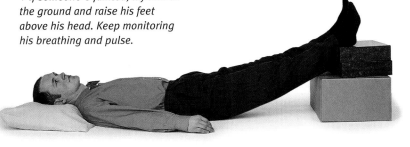

Loosen tight clothing, check for a pulse, and monitor breathing. If you suspect head, neck, or back injury, don't move the person but call for medical help. Also get help if the person doesn't revive within a couple of minutes.

There are many things that can send conflicting messages to the brain and end up making you dizzy. These include medications, stress, anxiety, alcohol, and illness. "Essentially, if you're sick for almost any reason you can get dizzy," says Brian Blakley, M.D., an otolaryngologist in private practice in Winnipeg, Manitoba. "Any time the body's not working well, one of the first things to go is our ability to maintain balance."

In older patients, poor blood flow to the brain and to the ear is a common cause of dizziness. Older folks also tend to get dizzy more often because of degeneration to their inner ears, nerves, and other parts of the vestibular system—the network that controls our sense of balance.

Occasionally, dizziness can be a sign that you're facing a serious problem. For example, having regular dizzy spells could be an early warning sign of a stroke.

Fainting: Not Just for Girls

Fainting is related to dizziness. It's a brief or partial loss of consciousness that's usually caused by a temporary dip in the amount of blood flowing to the brain.

Macho guys will tell you that women faint but men pass out—kind of like "men sweat, gentlemen perspire, ladies glow." Whatever you want to call it, though, men can and do briefly or partially lose consciousness. In fact, says Dr. Blakley, "Men tend to faint even more than women in a blood-test type of situation."

As with dizziness, there are many potential triggers for fainting, including sudden emotional stress or injury and heat exhaustion.

Seeing someone topple over in a faint can be alarming, even more so if you're that someone. But fainting's generally not a health threat. If you faint often, though, you need to visit your doctor. You also need to find immediate help for anyone who is unconscious for more than a minute or two. Prolonged lack of consciousness may indicate serious problems such as diabetic coma, concussion, stroke, shock, drug reaction, or epileptic seizure.

When to See a Doctor

Dizziness
There's usually no need to worry about an occasional dizzy spell that's neither persistent nor severe. But if dizziness is accompanied by other symptoms, see a doctor without delay. "The most ominous accompanying symptoms are numbness, an inability to speak, blindness in one eye, or double vision," warns otolaryngologist Brian Blakley, M.D. "They sometimes suggest a stroke." You also need to see a doctor if:

• The dizziness is accompanied by headache, loss of hearing, confusion, or weakness in the limbs.

• The dizziness is accompanied by a hangover-like feeling.

• You think medication might be causing the dizziness.

• Dizziness lasts more than a few days and interferes with your life.

• You have repeated dizzy spells over the course of a few days.

• You're experiencing severe or prolonged vertigo.

• You've completely or partially lost consciousness at any time.

• Your pulse when you're having a dizzy spell is less than 50 or more than 130 beats per minute.

Fainting
Repeated attacks of fainting need prompt investigation by a doctor.

Anxiety

"There's no need to worry," they tell you. That's fine for them; you're the one with the high-pressure job, a car that keeps breaking down, a big mortgage, a marriage under strain. Anxiety is a natural response to the pressures that surround us. It becomes a problem when it starts to rule your life.

Have You Got a Problem?

Anxiety is a normal emotion that engages our fight-or-flight response, says Madelynne Rigopoulos, Ph.D., a clinical psychologist in private practice in Long Beach, California. "It's almost like an instinct," says Dr. Rigopoulos, although the way we tend to think about things can heighten or dampen the degree to which the anxiety's felt.

Think of anxiety as an internal alarm system that alerts us to potential dangers lurking around the corner. Say you're feeling keyed up and on edge just before talking to your boss about that raise you think you deserve. Your hands may become clammy and your heart may race as adrenaline pumps into your system, but you're also focused on the potential dangers in asking for a 10 percent raise and that extra week of vacation. This is a natural and healthy response: You're getting ready for whatever the boss throws your way.

The problem with anxiety is that it can get out of hand, overwhelming you with the idea that something is more dangerous than it actually is. This happens because of illogical patterns of thinking—like seeing things only in terms of black and white, overgeneralizing, jumping to conclusions, and discounting positives and focusing on negatives. To return to our earlier example, if you're prevented from asking your boss for a raise because you focus on the one time he criticized your work and ignore all the times he praised it, you've got an anxiety problem.

An extreme anxiety problem may show itself in panic attacks. The attacks typically last a few minutes, and their symptoms can include hyperventilation, pounding of the heart, shaking, and feeling faint.

Keep the Lid on Anxiety

We know that advice is easy to give and hard to carry out, but here are a few techniques that experts say will keep anxiety to manageable levels.

• Make a conscious effort to breathe slowly and deeply and to relax your muscles; a written note to yourself will make a good reminder. You can practice your breathing during calm moments by putting one hand on your chest and the other on your stomach. If you're breathing from your diaphragm, which is the correct way, your lower hand should move out as you breathe in while your upper hand won't move at all.

• Face your fears a little at a time, but don't run; the only way to overcome them is to stay in the situation that makes you anxious.

• Try to examine the ways you typically think and react. Do you tend to be negative, for example, or do you ask too much of yourself? Try to sort out the good responses from the bad, and refocus on the positive.

• Get a physical release through exercise, and avoid caffeine and alcohol, which can disrupt an already precarious sleep pattern.

• Share your feelings of anxiety with friends and family members, or a professional, such as a doctor.

Develop a Winning Attitude

Part of successfully coping with anxiety is feeling positive about yourself and the world around you. There are lots of strategies to develop a positive, winning attitude. "Some may work better than others, depending on your proclivities," notes Alan Siegel, Ph.D., a clinical psychologist who practices in Berkeley and San Francisco, California. "But they can

---

Phobias and How to Fight Them

The thought of snakes makes you very uncomfortable. Do you have a phobia?

Phobias are persistent and irrational fears of particular things or situations. With a simple phobia, you may have an irrational fear of a specific object (snakes) or situation (flying). With a social phobia, the fear may be of parties or crowds. The most serious phobias are when you fear being in a strange or unfamiliar place or situation.

Those who find that a phobia severely restricts their life often find help with a therapist. One common professional treatment is to expose you to your fear in small doses in a controlled situation, so that your confidence and comfort level grow. By slowly and steadily increasing your exposure, the fear eventually recedes. A common example is a fear-of-flying program, in which participants often make initial visits to airports and planes on the ground to raise their comfort levels before taking a short flight.

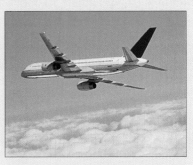
▲ An aerophobic's fears are usually at their peak during take-off and landing.

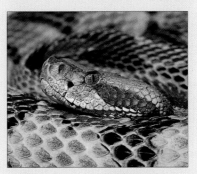
▲ Fear of snakes—ophidiophobia—is one of the most common phobias.

---

take you outside of your own problem and give you a positive role."

• Cultivate caring. Men who have no pride and no motivation often have stopped caring. Find things that interest you and pursue them. Try, try again. Pain and difficulty are givens in life, but our measure of success is if we try.

• Do good deeds. Something as simple as helping out an elderly neighbor with yard work can help you maintain a balanced, positive outlook. "Volunteer work can give you a sense of purpose," Dr. Siegel says.

• Focus on your greater purpose. We tend to become preoccupied with the minutia of daily life and lose sight of the larger picture. Think about why you're here and what you want out of life.

• Quiet the noise. With all the messages bombarding us day-in and day-out, it's hard to pick out the ones that really need listening to. Learn to focus on the messages that matter.

• Pick a positive path. There are many reasons to choose a course of action, but you need to look deep inside yourself and figure out the path that feels right and makes you the happiest.

• Sweat it out. Exercise allows you to think more clearly.

How Anxiety Can Harm Your Health

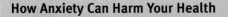

At root, anxiety may be psychological, but it's also been linked in some men to serious physiological problems.

Substance Abuse
Men, far more than women, are prone to use alcohol to gain relief from anxiety.

Heart Disease
One Harvard University study found that middle-age men who reported high levels of anxiety were 2½ times more likely to die from heart disease than those who reported lower levels.

Heart Attack
The same study determined that the risk of sudden death from heart attack was six times greater for the high-anxiety group.

High Blood Pressure
At the University of Alabama at Birmingham, researchers found that middle-age men who responded affirmatively to five of seven anxiety-related questions were more than twice as likely to develop high blood pressure than the less anxious group.

Depression

Life hits hard sometimes, and an occasional bout of the blues is pretty standard. Depression, though, is in a class of it own: It can be crippling, and in some cases, life-threatening. And it's not uncommon. Roughly 10 percent of men will be diagnosed with major depression at some point in their lives.

Men and Depression

Real men don't get depressed—we just feel blue from time to time. Right? Not right. While it's true that women are twice as likely than we are to experience major depression, don't start congratulating yourself quite yet.

Doctors estimate that about 1 in 10 men will be diagnosed with major depression, and that figure may not indicate the true severity of the problem since depression goes undetected and untreated more often in men than women. The reason for this, according to Madelynn Rigopoulos, Ph.D., a clinical psychologist in Long Beach, California, is that guys generally don't seek help for depression as readily as women and aren't as prone to exhibit easily identifiable symptoms, like sadness and crying. And because they're not getting the help they need, men more often than women turn to alcohol and drugs for relief.

The Types of Depression

Depression comes in many forms, causing problems that range in severity from a temporary lack of energy all the way to suicide.

One type is *dysthymia*, a chronically depressed mood that occurs most of the day, more days than not, for at least two years. A *depressive reaction*, which all of us have experienced, involves feelings of unhappiness in response to a specific, painful event like a divorce; the feelings are normal but may need treatment if they interfere with your life or go on for an unusually long time. Another kind of depression, *seasonal affective disorder* (SAD), affects a relatively small group of people who experience depressive symptoms during the fall and winter because of the lack of natural light. With *manic*

When to See a Doctor

If you're feeling bummed for a day or two, you don't need to run off to a shrink. "Anybody will have dark moments," says Alan Siegel, Ph.D., a California clinical psychologist. "But with depression, they're much more pronounced." So if you seem to be persistently plagued by symptoms of depression, and self-help measures haven't helped, get in touch with a professional. Start with your doctor, although you may need to be referred to a psychiatrist or psychologist.

True to form, men have a tendency to ignore depression. "Men are much less inclined to seek help for depression," Dr. Siegel says. "Socially, men are less trained to be expressive about their feelings." But while toughing it out on your own may work for the occasional "off" day, it could spell disaster if the depression is more serious. Left untreated, severe depression can be life-threatening. Another reason to have symptoms checked is that they can be signs of other serious diseases.

But depression can present a wide variety of symptoms, not every one of which may be present in any given case. So Dr. Siegel recommends that you see your physician if you're experiencing several of the following:

- A pervading feeling of sadness for most of each day
- Loss of interest in almost everything
- A changed appetite, weight gain, or weight loss
- Inability to sleep
- Agitation
- Fatigue
- Inappropriate guilt or feelings of worthlessness
- Inability to concentrate
- Suicidal thoughts

Drug Treatments for Depression

Therapy and self-help are invaluable aids in the treatment of depression, but sometimes those little prescription pills need to be called into action. A wide range of powerful antidepressant drugs is on the market these days. Like all drugs, even innocuous-seeming ones like aspirin, they can have side effects and should be taken only when the depression is severe. Here's a rundown on the three most commonly prescribed groups of antidepressants.

Drug Group	What They Do	Adverse Reactions/Side Effects	Names and Brands
Monoamine oxidase inhibitors (MAOIs)	Counteract enzymes that interfere with natural mood-lifting chemicals in the brain.	Sudden high blood pressure when used with alcohol, over-the-counter cold remedies, and foods containing caffeine. Severe reactions possible when taken with tyramine (a chemical in some wines and aged cheeses). Other side effects: dry mouth, blurred vision, dizziness, nausea, weight gain, sexual dysfunction, confusion, and constipation.	Phenelzine (Nardil), isocarboxazid (Marplan), tranylcpromine (Parnate).
Selective serotonin reuptake inhibitors (SSRIs)	Help prevent the dissipation of mood-lifting brain chemicals.	Gastrointestinal disturbances, anxiety, sleep problems, headache, dizziness, tremors, frequent urination, decreased sex drive, and delayed or inability to ejaculate.	Fluoxetine (Prozac), fluvoxamine (Floxyfral), paroxetine (Paxil), sertraline (Zoloft).
Tricyclic antidepressants (TCAs)	Help the brain retain the body's own pleasure-inducing chemicals, such as serotonin.	Dizziness, weight gain, sexual dysfunction, vision problems, dry mouth, fatigue, confusion, urine retention, constipation, and slight tremor. TCAs can also cause heart problems or exacerbate existing ones, and interfere with ulcer medications.	Imipramine (Tofranil), clomipramine (Anafranil), doxepin (Sinequan, Adapin), amitriptyline (Elavil, Endep).

depression, also known as bipolar affective disorder, mood swings are extreme—from energetic and elated to lethargic and despairing. And during periods of *major depression*, feelings of unhappiness are so painful and crushing that it's simply impossible to function.

Serious depression can run in families, and research suggests that it may be caused by an imbalance of the brain's chemical messengers, neurotransmitters. Heredity may also be accentuated by psychological factors like emotional strain when a loved one dies.

How to Bounce Back

It's important to remember that even severe depression is treatable. Professionals sometimes use prescription drugs and therapy quite successfully to treat depression.

For milder cases there are things you can do for yourself to get happy and functioning again. The key, according to Alan Siegel, Ph.D., a California clinical psychologist, is to stay connected with the world. "Not being isolated is a major healing factor," he says.

Here are some ways Dr. Siegel suggests to stay in the flow of things.

• Have realistic goals.
• Keep up your friendships and interests.
• Talk things through with people close to you.
• Don't be afraid to cry.
• Do some exercise.
• Get a good night's sleep.
• Keep alcohol, caffeine, and nicotine intake to a minimum.

The Prozac Generation

A group of drugs known as selective serotonin reuptake inhibitors (SSRIs for short) are known as the new-generation antidepressants. Their chemical compounds vary, but all SSRIs act by helping to prevent the dissipation ("reuptake") of serotonin, a mood-lifting chemical found in the brain.

Since its introduction in the United States in 1987, one SSRI has rapidly become the most widely prescribed of all antidepressants. Prozac (the brand name for fluoxetine) was controversial for a while because of anecdotal evidence linking it with a number of cases of suicide and violent behavior. After an investigation, however, the Food and Drug Administration eventually found that it was no more risky than other antidepressants.

Fever

As defense mechanisms go, it's pretty unpleasant. Up shoots body temperature, you feel like you've spent a couple of days in a sauna, and you're suddenly in need of tender loving care from your nearest and dearest. But a defense is exactly what fever is: Your body's way of dealing with harmful invaders.

Why a Fever Is on Your Side

We've all seen those Westerns where the pioneer family is carving out a life for itself on the untamed frontier. Between brief moments of peace and happiness they're subjected to all kinds of awful things—drought, locusts, marauding Apaches. Then the one thing they dread most happens—little Buck takes ill. He's put to bed, and after Ma lays a hand on his forehead, she whispers to the others the single scariest line in the entire movie: "He's got the fever."

In fact, though, Buck may have been far better off with his fever than without it.

Fever—an abnormally high body temperature—is not a disease. It's a symptom, and in many cases a beneficial one. "A slightly elevated body temperature enhances the work of your natural defense mechanisms," says Paul Ellner, Ph.D., professor emeritus of microbiology at Columbia University, "especially the action of antibodies and white blood cells." So a fever is your ally—it's cutting off bodily processes that would otherwise feed invading bugs and help them reproduce.

How does your body temperature go up? Normally, the hypothalamus, a natural thermostat in your brain, keeps your body at a relatively constant temperature. But when your immune system encounters an invader, such as a flu virus, it releases a protein called interleukin-1. This in turn starts a series of reactions causing the hypothalamus to bump up the body's thermostat setting and allow your temperature to rise.

What Causes a Fever?

Any number of things can trigger a fever. There are viral agents like flus and colds, of course, and bacterial ones like *Salmonella*. Fever may be a side effect of certain medications. It can even be the result of stress—the flush some people feel, for example, before giving a speech in front of a large group. While stress-induced fever hasn't been extensively studied, animal research indicates that it's similar to fever brought on by infection, in which levels of fever-registering hormones rise and cause the body's thermostat to be temporarily set higher. No one knows why it happens—it may be some primitive protective function kicking in—but it's not something that needs to be treated or worried about.

What You Should Do

What temperature constitutes having a fever? Since fever is defined as abnormally high body temperature, you have to first define "normal."

The most frequently cited temperature is 98.6°F, but some people have a slightly higher normal temperature than that. Also keep in mind that men tend to have a slightly lower normal temperature than women and that body temperatures tend to rise as the day goes on. In adults with an average normal body temperature, though, doctors generally consider a temperature of 100° to 101°F to be a fever.

So does that mean that you should start popping aspirin as soon as your

---

What's a Normal Temperature?

We're all taught that 98.6°F is the normal temperature. But is that always true?

Seems not. First, our temperature tends to rise throughout the day. Second, some people's bodies run a little hotter than others. The magical 98.6° number is only the average normal temperature, meaning that for any given person at varying times of the day, normal could be a bit higher or lower. If you'd like to find out what your own normal range is, take your temperature about every four hours during the day for three days in a row. Knowing your own range will help you determine whether you've got a fever.

Symptom Sorter

Fever can be accompanied by other symptoms that help to indicate exactly what's going on in your body. For example, microbiologist Paul Ellner, Ph.D., points out, "Chills accompanying fever often indicate that something foreign, like bacteria, has entered the bloodstream." Or with the flu virus, fever may be joined by chills, headache, fatigue, or muscle aches.

The list of potential accompanying symptoms is too long to memorize. Dr. Ellner suggests that you call a doctor if the fever doesn't go away on its own after a couple of days, or if it's accompanied by severe headache, pain while urinating, diarrhea, vomiting, or other serious symptoms.

The Best Treatments for Fever

The best-known way to lower the heat is also one of the fastest—popping an aspirin. Or any of its fellow pain relievers known as nonsteroidal anti-inflammatory drugs, such as ibuprofen or naproxen. "You can use Advil, Tylenol, or any of the others," says microbiologist Paul Ellner, Ph.D. "They all work."

They work by inhibiting the enzyme that causes your body's thermostat to click up a few notches. So to avoid swings in temperature take your over-the-counter meds on a regular schedule, following the directions on the package. And remember that children should never be given aspirin because of the danger of Reye's syndrome, a serious neurological condition.

Dr. Ellner advises drinking plenty of liquids if you have a fever. The additional sweating caused by the fever can be dehydrating, especially if you decide not to take medications to bring down the fever. "And get plenty of rest," he says.

Some other advice: Eat what you can without forcing food down. White rice, toast, juices, and fruit are often good choices. You can try to stay more comfortable by taking a lukewarm soak in the tub to make you feel cooler or by staying under a blanket to control the chills. Don't overdo either, though. A cold bath will only make your body struggle to maintain its elevated temperature, and piling on the blankets can lead to overheating.

---

temperature reaches 100°F? Not necessarily. For a healthy, adult male, fever is rarely dangerous. As long as your fever stays below 103°F, experts say, it probably isn't medically necessary to lower it; the high temperature, remember, may be helping your immune system. In fact, studies have shown that certain illnesses, including the flu and chickenpox, last longer and are sometimes more severe when fever associated with them is brought down with drugs.

That said, if the fever persists and you're experiencing other symptoms, or if it hits 103°F, you probably should consult your doctor. And while a mild fever may often best be left alone, there's another consideration. "Another reason to bring down a fever is for comfort," Dr. Ellner says. "Fever is very often accompanied by chills, and you may want to bring it down just to make yourself more comfortable."

So if chills—or headache or pain—make your fever too hot to handle, you may want to take steps to lower your body temperature, such as popping an aspirin or other pain reliever, or applying cool compresses (for details, see "The Best Treatments for Fever"). And be sure to drink lots of water, juice, or broth, since a fever will tend to dehydrate you.

MEASURING TEMPERATURE
Like Buck's mother in that old Western movie, many of us try to detect a fever by feeling the forehead. It's a very human gesture, and possibly of some psychological comfort to the patient—the cool, caring hand on the fevered brow sort of thing.

Unfortunately, it's also unreliable. A much more trustworthy way of detecting fever is to use a thermometer. Shake it down and rinse it with cool water before sticking it under the tongue for three minutes.

Danger Point

Your temperature has soared like a rocket to the moon and you can't remember ever being this hot in your entire life. Suddenly you recall a story you once heard about someone's brother's cousin who became brain-damaged because of an insanely high fever. You start to worry.

Relax. According to microbiologist Paul Ellner, Ph.D., you'd usually have to run an extremely high fever before risking major health problems. "However, when the temperature gets significantly high, say 104°F, then there is a possibility of brain damage and convulsions accompanying hyperthermia," he says. "Bringing the fever down then has to be considered an emergency procedure."

Since such a high fever is rare in a healthy adult male, you usually don't need to worry that your brain is going to soft-boil like a two-minute egg. But that doesn't mean you should ignore your fever. According to Jonathan Hall, M.D., an assistant professor of emergency medicine, a spiking temperature is unusual in adults. If the thermometer hits 103°F, or even 102.5°F when there are other symptoms, you should get it checked out right away. For some men—those with heart trouble—even a moderate fever can create problems, though. If a man's temperature rises from 98.6°F to 102°F, for example, his metabolic rate will increase by up to 25 percent. Additional strain on an already shaky heart is the potentially dangerous result.

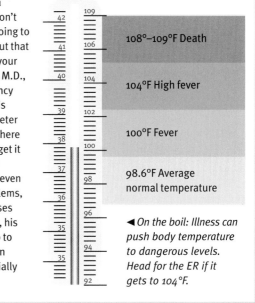

108°–109°F Death

104°F High fever

100°F Fever

98.6°F Average normal temperature

◄ On the boil: Illness can push body temperature to dangerous levels. Head for the ER if it gets to 104°F.

Rash

Rash. Just the word itself is enough to make you want to itch. And itch we do. There are 10,000 or so different rashes that can affect us, and virtually everyone can expect a nasty outbreak of something or other at least once in their lives. If you want to scratch the surface of this prickly subject, read on.

The Mother of All Rashes

Rashes are eruptions or breakouts on the skin. Sometimes they go under the name dermatitis, which is a very general term that's used for many types of skin inflammation, including eczema and psoriasis.

When your doctor refers to dermatitis, he's probably talking about either atopic dermatitis or about contact dermatitis, in which the skin reacts from contact with a specific substance, such as soap or a certain type of metal. Contact dermatitis is the most common dermatitis, and fortunately it usually gets better when the cause goes away.

ECZEMA

Eczema is a troublesome customer because of its longevity and intensity. It's often triggered by sensitivities to materials—like soap, dust, or wool—or by conditions like stress,

dry air, and cold weather. In many cases, a tendency to develop eczema seems to run in families.

PSORIASIS

We don't know for sure what causes this distressing form of dermatitis, but it does tend to run in families. During the natural process of skin renewal, something goes wrong: More skin is produced than needed, and the new growth accumulates under old skin, producing thick, red, scaly patches. For most people, psoriasis is a long-term condition with no permanent cure, but outbreaks can be relieved with appropriate treatment.

What Causes Dermatitis?

A truly baffling number of things can result in dermatitis, and your job is to find out what causes yours, if you get it. "The most important

thing in treating rashes is to determine what's triggering them off," says Victor Newcomer, M.D., clinical professor of dermatology at the University of California at Los Angeles School of Medicine. "Remove the cause and you're back to normal."

You have four general categories to choose from: illness, heat, allergy, and emotional stress. To help determine the cause of a rash, ask yourself these questions.

• Has my skin been in contact with anything new that could have irritated it, such as poison ivy, detergents, or soaps?

• Have I eaten anything new that I could be allergic to?

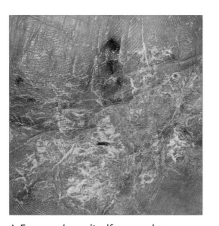

▲ *Eczema shows itself as a scaly, blistered rash that's intensely itchy.*

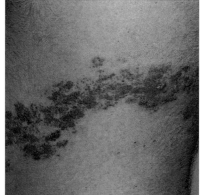

▲ *The beltlike rash of shingles, a condition caused by the chickenpox virus.*

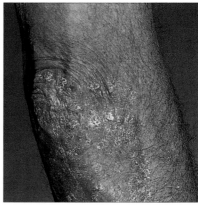

▲ *Psoriasis shows up as thickened patches of inflamed, scaly red skin.*

• Am I taking any medications that could be causing the rash?

• Have I been very stressed lately?

• Do I have joint pain or fever, too?

• Does the rash itch?

At the very least, your observations will help the doctor rule out various causes.

Shingles

Remember when you had that childhood bout of chickenpox? Well, it could come back to haunt you in the form of shingles.

Shingles is caused by a reactivation of the chickenpox virus, and it announces itself with a beltlike rash around one side of the chest, abdomen, or face. The rash, which is usually accompanied by pain and itching on the affected side of the body, and often fever and fatigue as

well, will blister and scab, and then clear up in a matter of a few weeks.

No one's sure why the virus comes alive again, and there's no way to either predict who will get shingles or prevent it—although it has been estimated that it strikes 40 percent of men who have had chickenpox. Shingles is most common in people over age 50, and half of 85-year-olds have had it. Shingles itself is not contagious, although exposure to the rash can cause chickenpox in a person who never had that disease.

See your doctor if you suspect shingles because there are drugs that can limit the rash and pain.

Prickly Heat

Prickly heat, or heat rash, happens when prolonged sweating clogs the sweat ducts, causing them to break open and leak sweat beneath the skin. The result: those red bumps.

Combat prickly heat with a few simple techniques, starting with the obvious: "Stay cool," Dr. Newcomer says. "Don't trigger off your sweat glands." For example, play sports during the cooler parts of the day, while avoiding tight-fitting clothes that trap sweat next to your skin. And build up slowly to any hot-weather activity. "If you're not used to heat, that's when prickly heat rash happens," he says.

If prickly heat hits, get cool right away and stay that way even after the rash subsides. "It takes at least four days for the pores to open up again, so you want to stay cool for that time," Dr. Newcomer advises.

To relieve the itching, take a tepid shower or pour a cup of white vinegar into tepid bath water and soak in it. Moisturizers that contain dimethicone can also help.

Sore Throats, Sneezes, and Coughs

Sore throat, coughing, and sneezing are an unholy trio if ever there was one. Like some package deal from hell, they frequently show up when you have allergies, a cold, or the flu—the banes of our upper respiratory system and the cause of untold human suffering since the dawn of time.

Sore Throats

Why do we get sore throats? The reasons vary, but think of your five-inch-long throat as an internal body part that also happens to be directly exposed to the outside world. All those little beasties floating in the air around us—germs and every sort of irritant—are sucked through the throat as we inhale.

You get a sore throat when there's an inflammation between the back of your tongue and your voice box. The inflammation is usually caused by a virus, bacterium, or allergen from outside the body, but at times it can be the result of stomach acid that refluxes—or flows backward—into the throat. You may also experience mild inflammation if your throat gets too dried out, which tends to happen if you breathe through your mouth or spend a lot of time in heated, indoor air.

When viruses cause your sore throat, there's not much you can do other than to soothe the symptoms and make the throat a less friendly place for the bugs. Sore throats caused by garden-variety cold and flu viruses are often accompanied by a runny or stuffy nose and possibly a cough, but that's not necessarily the case with those caused by other viral infections, such as mononucleosis (the "kissing disease").

A sore throat caused by bacteria is a very different situation. "It is important to determine if a sore

Every Breath You Take

Think of your respiratory system as an ingenious machine that delivers the oxygen your cells need, while getting rid of excess carbon dioxide.

Air enters the respiratory system when your diaphragm and its allied muscles contract, making the chest larger and allowing the lungs to expand; you exhale when the diaphragm and other muscles relax. The air can enter your body through either the nose or mouth. You normally breathe through your nose, though, with the nasal and sinus passages warming, moistening, and filtering the air.

Once inside, the air passes through the throat and trachea (windpipe), which is covered with mucus that traps particles. As the air reaches the lungs, the trachea divides into two bronchi—one per lung—and each of these then separates into ever smaller branches called bronchioles. The bronchioles terminate in alveoli, tiny sacs where oxygen is exchanged for carbon dioxide.

▶ *Lungs have to do two things: Extract oxygen from air, and rid the body of carbon dioxide. Fresh air, inhaled through the mouth and nose, is sucked down the trachea, or windpipe, to the bronchi and bronchioles. Stale air leaves the body by the same route.*

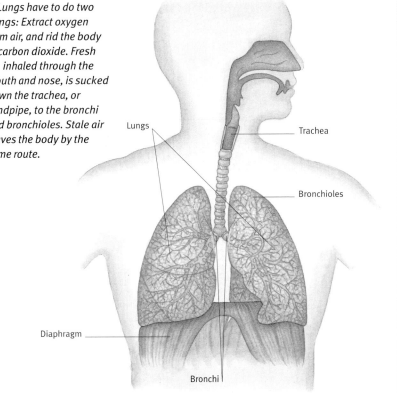

Lungs

Trachea

Bronchioles

Diaphragm

Bronchi

Allergies: Not to Be Sneezed At

Your immune system is in charge of defending the body against harmful invaders like bacteria and viruses, but sometimes it gets a little confused and launches an attack when confronted with perfectly harmless things—pollen, a particular kind of shampoo, or perhaps a peanut you've eaten. When the immune system gangs up on otherwise beneficial or neutral foreign substances, you've got yourself an allergy, and the imagined enemy is called an allergen.

Allergies are lumped into three categories based on what triggers them—contact allergies caused by things you touch, like wool or cosmetics; food allergies, in which eating something causes a reaction; and airborne or inhalant allergies, caused by, for example, dust and pollen. Most allergies entail mild,

annoying symptoms like sneezing, itching, and coughing, but they can mean serious problems as well. In some people, bee stings and food allergies, for example, may cause anaphylactic shock, an allergic reaction that's severe enough to result in suffocation.

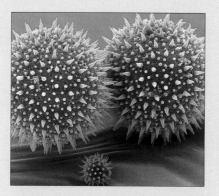

▲ *Certain pollen grains can trigger hay fever. This is hollyhock pollen.*

Inhalant allergies caused by house dust, pollen, pet dander, dust mites, and mold are by far the most common. If you suffer from them, try to identify the culprit, steer clear of it, and keep your indoor environment as clean as possible. Antihistamines may help.

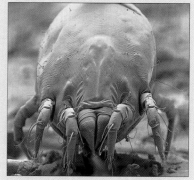

▲ *Inhaling the feces of dust mites can cause an allergic reaction.*

throat is caused by *Streptococcus pyogenes*, the strep throat bacterium, rather than by a virus," says Paul Ellner, Ph.D., professor emeritus of microbiology at Columbia University. "Strep throat should be treated with an antibiotic to reduce the risk of rheumatic fever and other complications." In addition to an often intensely painful throat, the signs of strep can be fever, bright red tonsils, a white or yellow coating on the tonsils, and swollen glands in the neck.

With allergens, there's nothing to kill off. An allergen is an otherwise harmless substance that your body mistakes for something threatening. If it gets caught in your throat when you breathe, the immune system attacks it there, generating mucus and soreness.

PREVENTION
"The best way to protect against colds and sore throats is to wash your hands frequently," Dr. Ellner says. "Most respiratory infections are transmitted hand-to-hand from

infected to susceptible persons. Kids continually exchange viruses at school and bring them home."

Here are some other strategies that might help to keep the pain out of your throat.

• If you're in heated rooms quite a bit, use a humidifier to make sure the air has moisture in it, and drink plenty of liquids.

• As much as you can, breathe through your nose.

• Stay away from irritants—cigarette smoke, especially—and from things you're allergic to, such as dust, and dog or cat dander.

When to See a Doctor

Sore Throats
A sore throat is usually traceable to a cold, an allergy, the flu, smoking, or some other obvious irritation. If even a mild sore throat persists for more than a week, you should see a doctor, advises Paul Ellner, Ph.D., professor emeritus of microbiology at Columbia University, because it could indicate mononucleosis (the kissing disease) or even something more serious. And, Dr. Ellner says, if you suspect you might have strep throat, get it treated with antibiotics right away to avoid developing other complications.

Sneezes
Frequent sneezing not associated with a cold or flu is probably hay fever. It

might be worthwhile being checked out by your doctor.

Coughs
If your sputum becomes thick, brown, or green, a call to your doctor might be in order. See a doctor if any cough lasts more than a week without improvement, says Alfred Munzer, M.D., past president of the American Lung Association. And definitely see a doctor if your cough is accompanied by other symptoms such as wheezing, shortness of breath, or tightness in the chest. "Once you bring up a lot of phlegm with chest pains and fever, you really have to seriously think of pneumonia," Dr. Munzer says. And see a doctor immediately if you cough up blood.

What Happens When You Sneeze?

You're shaking ground black pepper on your salad when a bit of it drifts up your nose and you sneeze. Physiologically speaking, what's just happened?

A sneeze is triggered when sensitive receptors in the nose are stimulated by inhaled particles or by the swelling of nasal membranes during a cold or a bout of hay fever. The stimulus travels along nerves to the brainstem, which relays it along the motor nerves to muscles in the chest. The chest muscles convulse and squeeze the lungs. Air rushes out of the lungs, and contracted throat muscles force most of it to exit your body via the nose.

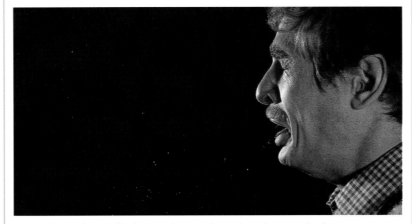

▲ A sneeze is the result of a complex set of reactions that start in the nose.

• If you have a problem with stomach-acid reflux, raise the head of your bed about four inches and eat dinner well before hitting the sack.

HOW TO SOOTHE THAT ACHE

"For viral sore throats, you can only treat the symptoms," Dr. Ellner says. Here are ways he suggests to do that.
• Mix aspirin or acetaminophen—either whole or else ground up—with six ounces of water; use as a gargle and then swallow.
• Gargle with warm salt water.
• Sip some lemon.
• Drink plenty of fluids.
• Take medicated throat lozenges.
• Take zinc gluconate tablets. One study found that when slowly dissolved in the mouth they help relieve sore throat and cold symptoms.

Sneezes

A sneeze is nothing to sneeze at. It's another of our body's beneficial reflexes, an involuntary attempt in most cases to clear the nose and upper respiratory tract of something irritating like pollen. In some people, though, sneezing can also be triggered by lots of other factors—sunlight, urination, shivering.

While you should welcome a sneeze as the body's way of evicting an undesirable tenant, anyone who suffers from hay fever is well aware that repeated sneezing can drive you nuts. Hay fever, or allergic rhinitis, is a respiratory allergy to airborne irritants like molds, dust, pollen, and dander, which are tiny bits of dried animal skin. Hay fever is one of the most common allergies, and in addition to sneezing it usually involves itchy or watery eyes, runny or stuffy nose, and a truly irritating itching sensation in the back of the throat.

PREVENTION

If you're prone to periodic hay fever, you can try to avoid the great outdoors. Or you can turn to over-the-counter or prescription antihistamines, which are designed to block the body's chemical that causes sneezing. Be aware that some antihistamines can make you drowsy.

Coughs

When you're hit with a coughing bout, you could do worse than to recall Glinda, the Witch of the North in *The Wizard of Oz*. You'll recall that

Which Cough Medicine?

Drugstore shelves are so full of cough preparations, you may worry you need a medical degree to figure out which one's for you. Relax. So long as you choose the right active ingredient, you'll do fine. And, by the way, experts say that generics are every bit as good as the pricey brand names.

There are two basic types of cough medicine: expectorants and suppressants. The active ingredient in an expectorant—guaifenesin—simply thins your mucus to make it easier to cough up, something you can also do by drinking lots of water, fruit juice, and tea. While guaifenesin has been approved by the Food and Drug Administration, its effectiveness hasn't

been conclusively demonstrated in clinical trials.

The active ingredient in a cough suppressant medicine is either codeine, diphenhydramine, or dextromethorphan. Each of these does the same thing—subdues your natural cough reflex—but there are significant differences in potential side effects. Codeine is a narcotic that acts directly on the brain; it's great at suppressing coughs but can upset your stomach. It also frequently causes constipation. Diphenhydramine is an antihistamine and so can make you drowsy. Dextromethorphan may be the best choice of the three since it doesn't have the side effects of the others.

The Best Treatments for Sore Throats, Sneezes, and Coughs

Sore throats, repeated sneezing, and excessive coughing can appear one at a time, in pairs, or all three at once. Doctors usually prescribe treatment based on what's causing the symptoms.

Your throat can be sore due to a virus or bacteria, or because of irritants and allergens. There's nothing you can do to kill a virus, says Paul Ellner, Ph.D., professor emeritus of microbiology at Columbia University, but in the case of bacteria, he says antibiotics usually do the trick. If allergens and irritants are the culprit, doctors often recommend antihistamines if you can't get away from the cause itself. With all sore throats, you may feel better when you gargle with warm salt water, suck on a lozenge, or indulge in other symptom-soothers, Dr. Ellner says.

With cold-related sneezing, there's nothing much you can do but wait it out, although sneezing caused by allergies usually can be controlled with antihistamines.

Coughing that's due to a cold can be a drag, but if it's productive—that is, bringing up phlegm—you don't need to treat it with a cough suppressant unless it's really bothering you.

This chart should help you better understand what doctors will look for and what they might prescribe.

Condition	Causes	Treatment
Sore throats		
Pain in throat accompanied by runny or stuffy nose or cough.	Cold or flu virus.	Symptom-soothers.
Severe pain in throat that comes on suddenly, accompanied by fever, red tonsils, or swollen neck glands.	Strep throat.	Antibiotics; symptom-soothers.
Throat pain accompanied by fatigue, aches, dizziness, swollen neck glands, and enlarged spleen.	Mononucleosis.	Rest, fluids, and over-the-counter painkillers for body aches.
Pain or itching sensation in throat.	Allergens or irritants, such as smoke, pollen, dust, overly dry air, prolonged shouting.	Antihistamines for allergens; symptom-soothers.
Sneezes		
Repeated sneezing.	Cold virus; allergies.	Colds—wait it out; allergies—antihistamines.
Coughs		
Cough that brings up phlegm and mucus; may be accompanied by runny or stuffed nose, fever, aches, sneezing, sore throat.	Cold or flu virus; bronchitis.	Cough suppressants and cough drops containing menthol, but only if cough prevents sleep or annoys others.
Dry cough; may be accompanied by sneezing, and sore or itchy throat.	Respiratory irritants, such as smoke, dust, pollen.	Cough suppressants; cough drops containing menthol.

Glinda wondered if Dorothy—newly arrived in Munchkinland—was a good or bad witch. The question you should pose in the case of a cough is equally direct: "Is it a good cough or a bad cough?"

Coughing is a natural reflex that kicks in to unblock the airways and keep irritants out of the lungs. The coughing action itself is actually a sudden explosion of air from your lungs, which can bring up phlegm and mucus. It can also clear your respiratory tract, from the lungs on up, of any foreign bodies.

A good, or productive, cough brings up phlegm. Often a feature of the flu or a cold, you should avoid suppressing such a cough with medications unless it keeps you awake at night. "A productive cough serves a definite purpose in expelling mucus," Dr. Ellner says. Bad, or unproductive, coughs are those dry hacks that just irritate your throat. They often develop at the end of a cold or when you've been exposed to an irritant, such as dust or smoke.

DEALING WITH COUGHS

Cough medicines are classed as either expectorants or suppressants. Expectorants simply make it easier for you to cough up phlegm. Cough suppressants are medicines that can subdue your body's cough reflex. "Use suppressants when a cough becomes constant and upsetting," Dr. Ellner says.

Breathing Problems and Chest Pain

The chest is home to two of our most vital organs, the heart and the lungs. Each usually goes about its job in a dependable, unspectacular fashion. When something goes wrong, you'll know it: Breathing problems and chest pain can range from a discomforting irritation to a life-threatening emergency.

A Great Pair of Lungs

Somebody with far too much time on his hands has estimated that if the many folds of tissue comprising a single human lung were spread out flat, they would cover almost half of a tennis court. No mention is made about how that would affect his serve, but this little factoid about the lung does underscore what an awesome organ it is.

The lungs—that's plural, because we're born with a pair—are the center of your respiratory system and one of the principal occupants of the chest, the area of your body that's enclosed by the rib cage. It's interesting to note that the left lung is somewhat smaller than the right so there's room for its important neighbor, the heart.

To understand what your lungs need, and what can cause breathing problems and chest pain, you have to know how the lungs work.

WHAT YOUR LUNGS DO

The lungs are the place where your body obtains the oxygen it needs to burn sugar and produce energy; they're also the place where you get rid of the carbon dioxide that's a by-product of energy production.

The air we inhale through the nose and mouth enters the lungs through two major passageways called the bronchi. Inside the lungs, the bronchi separate into 250,000 ever-smaller bronchioles, which divide into even smaller alveolar ducts. The ducts lead to 300 million cell-size air sacs called alveoli that are covered by a web of capillaries—tiny, thin-walled blood vessels. As dark, oxygen-depleted blood passes through the capillaries, it leaves the carbon dioxide it picked up from cells elsewhere in the body and takes on a fresh load of oxygen. The bright red, newly oxygenated blood then heads to the heart, which pumps it throughout the body. The carbon dioxide is eliminated when you exhale.

WHAT YOUR LUNGS NEED

So, what do your lungs need to do their job and not cause you any problems? Not much. They've got to have plenty of air, of course, and air that contains a sufficient supply of oxygen—that's one reason why the "thin" (reduced-oxygen) atmosphere

Something in the Air: Legionnaires' Disease

At a 1976 American Legion convention in Philadelphia, a group of Legionnaires and other guests mysteriously came down with similar symptoms—fever, chills, cough, abdominal pain, diarrhea, and, at times, confusion. Twenty-nine people died. At first, no one could figure out what was causing the problem, but eventually the culprit was tracked down to a bacterium that came to be called *Legionella*.

Legionnaires' disease is a form of bacterial pneumonia caused by *Legionella*. "Legionnaires' disease is not very contagious from person to person," says pulmonologist Alfred Munzer, M.D., who is past president of the American Lung Association, "but it's highly contagious from a common source, such as a contaminated air-conditioning system, for example."

Infection occurs when *Legionella*-contaminated water droplets are inhaled. The disease attacks the lungs, can hit anybody, and can be fatal, although older people who smoke or drink heavily are especially at risk. Antibiotics are usually effective in knocking it out.

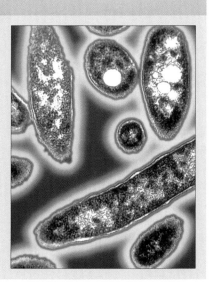

▶ *An electron microscope picks out the bacterial bodies of* Legionella, *the cause of Legionnaires' disease.*

What Happens during an Asthma Attack?

A couple of changes occur in the bronchial tubes when you're hit with an attack of asthma. First, the tubes go into spasm and contract, restricting the flow of air. At the same time, their linings swell and release excess mucus, blocking airflow even more.

Early in an asthma attack, the problem isn't so much with inhaling as exhaling. Your chest muscles are strong enough to draw in the fresh air, but they can't push out all the stale. With stale air remaining in the lungs, there's less space for a full breath of the fresh stuff. And as the attack continues, the bronchial tubes become more clogged and the muscles tire — making inhaling a struggle.

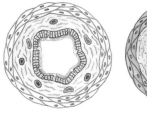

▲ *A cross-section of a normal bronchiole with a wide airway.*

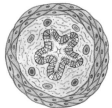

▲ *A bronchiole during an asthma attack — the airway narrows.*

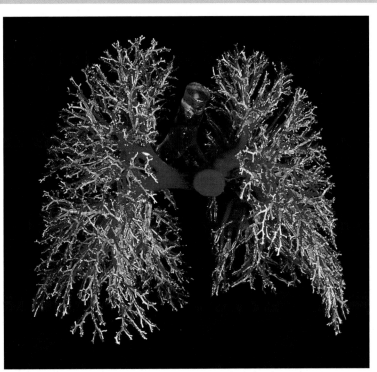

▲ *Asthma affects the smaller bronchial tubes, the bronchioles. They're the smallest "branches" of the bronchial "tree" in the picture above.*

---

at high elevations can cause breathing difficulties. Breathing deeper and longer, as well as regular aerobic exercise, will help get that oxygen to your lungs. Other ways to keep your lungs in shape include:

• Eating a healthy diet that includes the recommended daily allowances of iron and of vitamins A, E, and C.

• Breathing through your nose to warm, filter, and humidify the air.

• Not smoking, and avoiding smoky environments.

Did You Know?

As soon as you stop smoking, your lungs slowly start to repair themselves. After 10 years, your risk of lung cancer drops to 30 to 50 percent of that of smokers who didn't quit. And after 15 to 20 years, the risk becomes similar to someone who never took up the nasty habit at all.

• Using protective masks if your work or hobby entails paints, chemicals, or anything that produces a lot of airborne junk. Make sure ventilation is adequate, too.

Lung Problems

With all the junk floating around, it's inevitable that virtually every one of us, at some point in his life, is going to experience chest pain or breathing difficulties due to lung-related problems.

The deadliest problems your lungs can face—emphysema and cancer—are discussed in detail on pages 228 and 245 respectively. In summary, these two killers, unlike many minor lung disorders, are largely preventable. How? C'mon, you know the answer—don't smoke.

By now, most of us who are not brain-dead realize that the strapping, robust image of the Marlboro

Pleurisy

Pleurisy is a painful and common complication of pneumonia.

Each of your two cone-shaped lungs is suspended in a double membrane called the pleura, and between the membranes is pleural fluid that acts like a lubricant to let the lungs fill and empty more easily. When the membranes become inflamed, the result is the severe pleuritic pain that often accompanies pneumonia (and tuberculosis). The pain makes breathing and movement of the upper body difficult.

Pleurisy is sometimes accompanied by shortness of breath and possibly fever. It needs to be checked out right away by a doctor, says Kenneth A. Goldberg, M.D., medical director of the Male Health Institute at Baylor Health Center, Irving-Coppell, Texas. Once serious conditions are ruled out, your doctor will probably prescribe painkillers and rest.

man is a lie, but for some reason there are still men out there who continue to smoke. The best thing you can do for continued lung health—and for your health in general—is to lay off the butts.

ASTHMA

Asthma affects nearly 5 percent of Americans—about 13 million people—according to Francis V. Adams, M.D., an assistant professor of clinical medicine at New York University and author of *The Asthma Sourcebook*.

The condition is caused by hyperactive bronchial tubes that go into spasm and restrict the flow of air. What makes the bronchial tubes go haywire isn't always clear, although

there is typically a trigger such as smoke, pollen, dust, or air pollution. Anxiety and even exercise have also been known to spark attacks.

Asthma can be controlled with appropriate treatment—to such an extent that there are many world-class athletes who are asthmatics. If you do suffer from asthma, the first and best step to prevent an attack, according to the American Lung Association, is to avoid the particular "trigger" that sets you off. Most men with asthma, however, choose to see a doctor, and periodically control the condition with inhaled prescription medications.

BRONCHITIS

Perhaps the most common of all lung problems is bronchitis, an inflammation of the large tubes in the lung, the bronchi. It's caused by a germ—usually the same virus that causes a cold or the flu, but sometimes by bacteria.

When the germs penetrate your respiratory system as far as the bronchi and land there, the body protects itself by producing lots of gooey secretions of mucus along the airways. As the secretions build up, breathing becomes steadily more difficult, and you start to cough up the goo, usually in the form of green or yellow phlegm.

PNEUMONIA

When you get a dose of pneumonia, viruses (in most cases) or bacteria have penetrated to the smaller airways in the lungs, causing them to become clogged with phlegm, fluids, and other debris. Eventually, the lungs' tiny air sacs (the alveoli) fill with pus—disgusting thought, isn't it?—which hampers the transfer of oxygen to the blood.

Chest pain sometimes accompanies pneumonia, although it's not caused by the disease itself but by a condition called pleurisy, in which the lining of the lungs becomes inflamed. See page 189 for more information on pleurisy.

Pneumonia strikes about 1.8 million American men each year, often the elderly or people with weak immune systems caused by other conditions such as AIDS or alcoholism. Although it can kill you, pneumonia is generally not fatal if you get medical care in a timely fashion. For bacterial pneumonia, which is usually the more dangerous kind, that probably means a course of antibiotics; for viral pneumonia, often the best you can do is make yourself comfortable and drink lots of fluids while waiting it out.

OTHER CAUSES OF CHEST PAIN

The lungs are not the only inhabitants of your chest, and sometimes chest pain and breathing difficulties are caused by things other than the respiratory system.

Hyperventilation: A Hunger for Air

It's normal for breathing to speed up in response to physical or emotional stress. When you hyperventilate, however, you begin to breathe so fast and deep that the carbon dioxide level in your blood can drop too low.

Symptoms of hyperventilation include a numbness or tingling in the hands, feet, or mouth area, a heart that pounds or races, light-headedness, chest pain, and a feeling you're coming up short on air. If you hyperventilate long or severely enough, you may pass out.

Hyperventilation can occur during anxiety or panic attacks. To prevent hyperventilation, make an effort to slow your breaths to one every five seconds as soon as you notice your breathing has picked up speed. If an attack is underway, try breathing in and out of a paper bag held over your nose and mouth—this will help increase the amount of carbon dioxide in your blood.

▲ *If you feel you're hyperventilating, try breathing in and out of a paper bag. That should help your breathing return to normal.*

The Best Treatments for Chest Pain and Breathing Problems

Chest pain and breathing difficulty can show up simultaneously in a wide variety of conditions and diseases.

The problem with chest pain is that it's sometimes difficult to distinguish one kind from another. Asking yourself a few questions about the pain, though, will help you and the doctor figure out what's causing it.

• Is the pain sharp or dull, persistent, or sporadic?

• Does it occur only when you move, or when you're immobile?

• Does it occur only when you breathe?

• Is the pain localized to one spot?

• Does it radiate from the chest to adjacent areas?

• What were you doing when the pain hit?

Breathing difficulties, likewise, come in a variety of flavors. There can be wheezing, pain, or chest tightness when taking a breath, or shallow breathing. The breathing problem can be accompanied by chest pain or not. Even the classic catch-all symptom—"shortness of breath"—may come on suddenly or develop more slowly.

Condition	Symptoms	Treatment
Heart Attack	Crushing chest pain, possibly radiating to arms, neck, back, or jaw; shortness of breath; sweating; dizziness and nausea.	Get emergency medical help immediately.
Angina; Coronary Artery Disease	Dull pain or pressure in center of chest set off by physical or emotional stress; pain eases with rest.	Make appointment with the doctor right away; if symptoms last 10 minutes or more, get emergency medical help.
Collapsed Lung	Sudden chest pain or tightness when breathing, with increasing shortness of breath.	Get emergency medical help immediately.
Pleurisy	Sharp chest pain, especially when taking a breath; fever; headache; dry cough.	Make an appointment with the doctor right away.
Bronchitis	Tightness in chest; coughing up mucus; cold or flu symptoms.	Don't smoke; drink lots of fluids; breathe moist, warm air; use painkillers. See a doctor if symptoms persist or there's wheezing or shortness of breath.
Lung Cancer; Pneumonia; Tuberculosis	Cough producing yellow or red-brown sputum; chest pain; wheezing, shortness of breath; fatigue; weight loss; lack of appetite.	See your doctor right away.
Asthma	Wheezing; quick, shallow breathing; tightness in chest.	Get emergency help if victim's skin is turning blue or he's becoming confused; otherwise see a doctor soon.
Chronic Bronchitis ("Smoker's Cough"); Emphysema	Wheezing; shortness of breath; continuing cough, either dry or wet.	Get emergency help if skin turns blue; otherwise see a doctor soon.
Heartburn	Pressure or burning in chest or upper abdomen, especially when stomach is full.	Pop an antacid; avoid lying down. If symptoms persist or recur, see the doctor.
Anxiety; Panic Attack; Hyperventilation	Shortness of breath; tightness or pain in chest; fear; rapid heartbeat.	Deep-breathing and relaxation exercises; if symptoms recur, talk with the doctor.
Pulled Muscle; Injured Rib	Sharp chest pain that worsens with movement or deep breathing; pain felt when area is pressed; pain that suddenly appears after coughing, sneezing, or chest trauma.	Rest and apply ice. If pain persists, make a doctor's appointment.
Anaphylactic Shock (a severe allergic reaction to a food, insect sting etc.)	Tightening of chest or throat; wheezing; hives; itching; swollen eyes, lips, tongue; stomach cramps; vomiting.	Get emergency medical help right away.

Heading Off Heartburn

Heartburn occurs when strong acids in your stomach surge upward into the esophagus and scorch its tender tissue. The acids are normally kept within the tough lining of the stomach and out of the esophagus by a ring of muscle called the lower esophageal sphincter, but sometimes the muscle just can't do the job.

Smoking, alcohol, and being overweight can all contribute to a case of heartburn by weakening the muscle, but the main cause is overeating. The more you eat, the more your stomach needs to secrete the acids to deal with the food. And when you lie down while your stomach is busy breaking down food, you're asking for trouble.

To avoid heartburn, eat less and eat more slowly, and avoid hot and spicy food, says Kenneth A. Goldberg, M.D., medical director at the Male Health Institute of Baylor Health Center, Irving-Coppell, Texas. Also, watch out for things that might temporarily weaken the esophageal sphincter—chocolate, mints, alcohol, and fatty foods, for example. Reducing weight and quitting smoking will also help, as will staying off your back after you've eaten.

If you do manage to get an occasional case of heartburn, antacids are good for short-term relief. If it strikes more often, though, talk with your doctor.

▶ *Heartburn happens when stomach acid flows upward into the esophagus.*

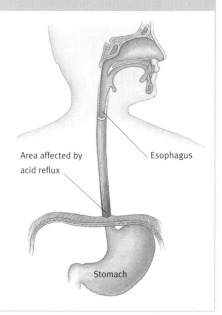

Area affected by acid reflux

Esophagus

Stomach

• A sharp pain might mean a pulled muscle, inflamed cartilage, or an injured rib.

• If you experience chest pain and pressure during physical exertion or emotional stress, the culprit may be angina—or clogged coronary arteries that deprive the heart of the oxygen-rich blood it needs.

• The pain of a heart attack can be close to that of angina, although it's frequently sharper, lasts longer, and may be accompanied by other symptoms, such as dizziness, nausea, shortness of breath, and sweating.

• A tightening or pain in the chest, sometimes accompanied by a rapid heartbeat and shortness of breath,

may be the sign of anxiety, a panic attack, or hyperventilation.

• Good old heartburn can cause what seems to be intense chest pain, so much so that some sufferers really believe that they're experiencing a heart attack or angina. If you suffer frequent bouts of heartburn, see "Heading Off Heartburn."

Angina's Painful Warning

Atherosclerosis. It's a fancy name for clogged arteries as well as the cause of the pain, pressure, and heaviness in the chest associated with an attack of angina.

Angina happens when your heart isn't getting the oxygen it needs because the arteries responsible for bringing it fresh, oxygenated blood are clogged with fatty deposits. Angina is frequently brought on by physical or emotional stress—situations when your heart demands more oxygen—and attacks are often relieved by rest. Typically, the pain will subside within 15 or 20 minutes.

Angina is a warning sign from your heart that you could be a candidate for a heart attack some time in the future. Anyone who experiences angina should see a doctor without delay.

Chest pain from angina typically spreads from the center of the chest.

Angina starts as a sensation of pressure in the central chest

Intense pain replaces feeling of pressure and starts to spread

The pain radiates up into the neck and down the back

The upper left arm becomes painful

Abdominal Pain

A pain in the guts is probably just a case of hot air or else indigestion, and can usually be dealt with by yourself. The problem, though, is that so many things can cause abdominal pain. So, never ignore pain in your guts, because it could be the sign of a serious illness or even a medical emergency.

The Guts of the Matter

"No guts, no glory." "Sure takes a lot of guts." "Gutsy move." How did our abdominal organs become associated with courage and determination? And then there's "intestinal fortitude" and "fire in the belly." What do intestines have to do with fortitude or bellies with the fire of determination?

The answer may lie in the feeling you get in your abdomen when you face a challenge—the butterflies in your stomach, to use one more expression naming an abdominal organ. Or it could lie in another meaning of "guts"—the inner essential parts of anything. In this sense, the association with the abdomen certainly is understandable. A lot of

your own body's inner essential parts are found there.

The abdomen is basically a cavity in your body located between the hips and chest, below the ribs. Its upper boundary is the diaphragm, a muscle that plays an important role in breathing.

The abdomen is home to the stomach, liver, intestines, gallbladder, and pancreas—digestive organs and glands which function like a food-processing plant to break food down into a form that your body can use, while at the same time getting rid of the waste. The abdomen also houses three other important organs: the spleen, which among other things helps keep the blood clean; the kidneys, which filter the blood and

excrete waste products and excess water in the form of urine; and the appendix, a small tube jutting out of the colon whose function is not entirely understood.

Symptom Sorter

Abdominal pain comes in all shapes and sizes. There's stabbing, dull, continuous, and sporadic pain. Pain can be high, low, or middle; right, left, or center; front or back. In terms of severity, it can increase, decrease, or remain constant.

While the location and type of pain are important clues as to what the problem might be, other symptoms may end up actually solving the case. The list of potential accompanying symptoms is long—nausea, vomiting, chills, bloody stools, watery stools, hard stools, swelling or bulge, fatigue, sweating, belching, loss of appetite, and clammy skin are only some of the possibilities.

While it's difficult even for a doctor to diagnose abdominal pain, noting your symptoms and reporting them will help tremendously.

Locating the Abdomen

Pancreas
Makes digestive enzymes and hormones such as insulin.

Liver
A powerhouse—it detoxifies blood, makes bile (a digestive chemical that breaks down fat), metabolizes alcohol, aids in blood clotting, and stores certain vitamins, minerals, and sugar.

Gallbladder
Stores bile after it's made by the liver.

Duodenum
Part of the small intestine where bile and enzymes break down food even more.

Appendix
Mystery organ whose purpose isn't known.

Spleen
Filters your blood and produces disease-fighting antibodies.

Stomach
Breaks down chewed-up food with acidic gastric juices.

Kidneys
Filter waste from every drop of blood.

Small intestines
Absorbs water and nutrients from digested food.

Colon
Also known as the large intestine; absorbs water and mineral salts to leave behind waste that forms into stool.

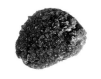
Why Does It Hurt?

Many different problems can cause abdominal pain, and while most of them are relatively minor, you should always pay attention when your guts hurt.

Some of the causes we all know and love. There's the gas produced as certain difficult-to-digest foods—like beans—are broken down in your intestine, for example, which can cause terrible pain in the lower abdomen, not to mention socially unacceptable emissions. Other common causes are heartburn, as well as stomach flu, mild food poisoning, diarrhea, and constipation.

Among the more serious abdominal problems that require medical attention are kidney stones. You should suspect them if it hurts like hell to urinate and you also have pain that starts on the side and moves toward the groin or abdomen. Gastritis, an inflammation of the stomach lining, will cause pain in the upper abdomen. The usual bulge or swelling of a hernia will often be accompanied by discomfort in the lower abdomen.

Ulcers—holes in the lining of the stomach or duodenum—and appendicitis—an infected and inflamed appendix—are two of the most common abdominal problems.

PINPOINTING PAIN

There are so many things going on in the abdomen that even doctors can have a hard time pinning down abdominal problems. "Diagnosing abdominal pain is tricky," admits Richard A. Cazen, M.D., a gastroenterologist in private practice in San Francisco. People can have what appear to be the classic symptoms of one abdominal problem—appendicitis, say—but it often turns out to be something else—kidney stones, for example. Your own observations often help in figuring out what's wrong.

When you do experience abdominal pain, the first thing to do is to figure out exactly where the pain is coming from. A good way of doing this is to think of your abdomen as divided into quarters by two lines— one horizontal and the other vertical—that intersect at your belly button. Ask yourself in which quadrant or quadrants it hurts, and whether the pain migrates from one quadrant to another.

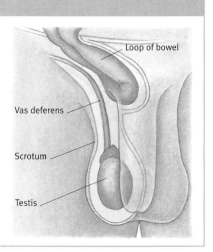

The Best Treatments for Abdominal Pain

Treatments for nonemergency causes of abdominal pain run the gamut from doing nothing to going under the surgeon's knife. There's not much you can do to actually prevent most of the following sources of abdominal pain, according to Arvey Rogers, M.D, gastroenterologist and University of Miami professor of medicine. But there are ways to take care of them if they do occur.

Gallstones

These hard deposits are usually found in the gallbladder, but sometimes one gets caught in a bile duct, in which case the pain is severe. For frequent attacks, the standard treatment is surgical removal of the gallbladder, although a nonsurgical approach using drugs or chemicals to dissolve the deposit may work with small stones.

Heartburn and Gas

These two usually occur as a result of something irritating that you ate or drank, according to Dr. Rogers, or from taking medicine such as aspirin. They usually eventually go away on their own, although an antacid may help with the heartburn. There are also medications to suppress gastric acid or soothe the stomach lining, he says. And, he adds, "To manage heartburn, minimize late-night, heavy meals, chocolate, cigarettes, and fatty foods." If you get gas and cramping every time you eat milk-based products, you may be intolerant to lactose, the sugar in milk, and the best treatment may be lactase pills or milk that's had lactose removed.

Hernias

While many hernias can be pushed back into place by you or your doctor, they can pop out again. "They may be managed by wearing a truss or be corrected surgically," Dr. Rogers says.

Kidney Stones

Kidney stones are usually treated with medication, fluids, and diet, although if a stone can't be passed, energy waves are often used to break it up. Only rarely is surgery involved. "Occasionally an underlying metabolic disorder is reponsible, such as a diseased lower intestine or gout," Dr. Rogers says. "In those cases, taking care of the disorder may dissolve the stones."

Ulcers and Gastritis

These can be caused by the bacterium *Helicobacter pylori*. "Once diagnosed, the infection should be treated with antibiotics and acid-suppressive treatments," Dr. Rogers says. "And it goes without saying that stomach irritants should be avoided."

Viral Stomach Flu

Usually, a bout of stomach flu will pass within a day or two. Because it's caused by a virus (and viruses don't respond to antibiotics), about the only thing you can do is make sure you replenish any liquids that may be lost due to diarrhea or vomiting.

ULCERS

An ulcer is simply a sore that forms when stomach acids begin burning through the lining of the digestive organs. Most ulcers occur in the duodenum, the part of the small intestine closest to the stomach, and the remainder—gastric ulcers—form in the lining of the stomach itself.

When to See a Doctor

In general, if you're unsure why you're experiencing abdominal pain, get in touch with a doctor right away. An immediate call is also recommended if the severity of the pain is causing you concern. "If the pain persists, worsens, or becomes increasingly severe, that's a red flag," says Arvey Rogers, M.D., gastroenterologist and University of Miami professor of medicine.

You need to seek medical help any time there are acute symptoms accompanying the pain—things like nausea, vomiting, or blood in the urine or stool.

Stress was once believed to be the main reason that ulcers formed. It's now been found, however, that the culprit in many cases is *Helicobacter pylori,* a bacterium. A doctor will prescribe antibiotics.

Most ulcers aren't life-threatening, although they can cause quite a bit of pain in your gut. In more severe cases, there can be internal bleeding, which typically turns your stool an ugly shade of black. That's a sign to get to a doctor without delay.

APPENDICITIS

Appendicitis happens when hardened bits of fecal matter clog the appendix. Left untreated, the organ can eventually burst, causing all sorts of internal problems.

There's no way to prevent appendicitis, but if it hits, you need treatment before the appendix bursts—usually 12 to 48 hours after the onset of the condition. The key symptom is general abdominal pain that localizes above the appendix, on the lower right side between your navel and hipbone.

Emergencies

Out-and-out emergencies that can cause abdominal pain—and that obviously require immediate medical attention—include heart attack, anaphylactic shock, diabetic emergency, and appendicitis.

Other emergencies that involve abdominal pain are a perforated ulcer, intestinal obstruction, pancreatitis—inflammation of the pancreas—and an initial attack of gallstones. This last condition frequently causes intense pain in the upper right or center of the abdomen that may spread to the back, chest, or right shoulder.

With all of these emergency conditions, the pain may be severe, and there may be other symptoms you can report to the emergency medical personnel to help them figure out what's going on.

Nausea and Vomiting

A dictionary doesn't do them justice: *Nausea*, a queasy feeling that may lead to vomiting; *Vomiting*, the involuntary, forceful ejection of stomach contents through the mouth. Throw up, barf, spew, toss your cookies: Only the visceral energy of slang can get across the sheer unpleasantness of this duo.

The Old Heave-Ho

Pity the poor carnival workers in charge of what have been dubbed—with only slight exaggeration—the "throw-up rides." You know the kind—the ones that whirl and spin until you're certain your stomach is permanently lodged somewhere near your throat. The rides are scary and fun, but the problem is they're also tailor-made to induce a few unlucky thrillseekers to toss their cookies—much to the dismay of fellow riders, spectators down below, and the hapless worker who, mop in hand, has to clean up the Giant Tilt-A-Whirl afterward.

We tend to think of nausea and vomiting purely as functions of our digestive tract. But as illustrated by the Giant Tilt-A-Whirl, both can be caused by things that, strictly speaking, don't have much to do with your digestive tract at all.

That's because your brain's vomit control center—known scientifically as the chemoreceptor trigger zone—can be set off by anything the body finds threatening, whether or not it actually is. And when the center is triggered, it sends a signal to the stomach that it's time to give the old heave-ho to whatever has most recently entered your digestive tract.

The list of things that can trigger nausea and vomiting is fairly extensive. There's eating too much and—especially—drinking more alcohol than your system can handle. Foul odors, emotional stress, and certain medications can cause you to retch, as can a whole variety of illnesses and conditions, ranging from ulcers, gallstones, and head injuries to migraine headaches and the good old stomach flu.

The Misery of Motion Sickness

The Giant Tilt-A-Whirl is a good example of one common cause of nausea and vomiting—motion sickness. It periodically afflicts up to 90 percent of us, but despite its prevalence the condition in a way remains a mystery. No one really knows why

Locating the Digestive Tract

About 30 feet long from mouth to rectum, the digestive tract breaks food into usable components and gets rid of whatever is left over.

In the mouth, food gets shredded by the teeth and soaked with saliva, whose enzymes break down starch. Esophageal muscles force the chewed food into the stomach, where it's churned by muscles and broken down by powerful acid. In the duodenum, enzymes and digestive chemicals from the pancreas, liver, and gallbladder are added to the now-soupy mixture, and during the trip through the small intestine most of the water and nutrients get absorbed.

The remaining mush moves through the colon to the rectum, and when enough accumulates, it's time to visit the john.

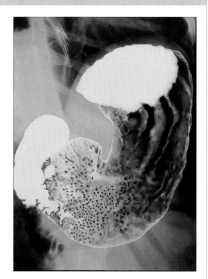

▲ *An x-ray shows the J-shaped curve of the stomach. This baglike organ is the first stop in the digestion process.*

some people seem naturally less susceptible to it and why the tendency to suffer from it can sometimes diminish with age.

Motion sickness happens when your body fails to properly adjust to movement. Your inner ear contains a sensitive network of fluid-filled canals and sacs called the vestibular system. The system's job is to help you maintain your balance by keeping track of your body's motion.

The problem is that sometimes—for example, when you're on a rocking boat at sea—your poor brain may be receiving conflicting messages from your eyes and your vestibular system. Your eyes may be intently focused on a fixed object, such as the 1,000-page novel you swore you'd get through on the cruise, but the fluid inside your inner ear is sloshing back and forth. The eyes signal the brain that your body isn't moving, while the inner ear is saying that it is. The resulting confusion in your brain can make you dizzy, which in turn can make you throw up.

PREVENTION

All types of travel have the potential to cause motion sickness, which can make vacation choices difficult if you're especially prone to this condition. There are, however, a number of things you can do to help prevent it. The principal strategy, according to Brian Blakley, M.D., an otolaryngologist in Winnipeg, Manitoba, is to "take maximum advantage of the senses, so your movements are reflective of the outside world."

Here are some ways Dr. Blakley suggests to do that.

• Try staring straight ahead at the horizon or a distant object rather than focusing on a close, fixed object. This means you should avoid reading while moving. If you're a passenger in a car, don't look out the side windows at the telephone poles and trees you pass.

• On all types of transportation, pick a seat where the effect of motion is minimized. In cars, this means sitting up front and sticking to routes that minimize the rocking of stop-and-go traffic. On a bus, sit a couple of seats behind the door. On a plane, train, or boat, a seat in the center is your best bet.

• If possible, try to hold your head as still as you can. "If you must look around, move your eyes, not your head," Dr. Blakley says.

• Don't obsess about whether you're going to get motion sickness. "If you can take your mind off it, you can at least forestall some of the dizziness," says Dr. Blakley. Anxiety can make the condition worse, and many people can actually think themselves into a bout.

• Be sure to get plenty of fresh air. Any unpleasant odor can trigger motion sickness, so stay on deck or open the car windows.

• A small, low-fat meal before a journey may help. But avoid heavy meals before traveling, Dr. Blakley warns. The last thing you want is having a giant vat of potential vomit when you embark.

• Whatever you do, stay away from nicotine and alcoholic drinks. They can upset your stomach and worsen your dizziness.

• Take some medication. There's dimenhydrinate (Dramamine), an over-the-counter antihistamine that stops

The Best Treatments for Nausea and Vomiting

There's no denying that nausea and vomiting are very unpleasant, but let's face it, sometimes it's just better to let loose, spill your guts, and get the whole thing over and done with.

Nausea

If you're feeling nauseated and can't seem to vomit—or would prefer not to—nibbling on crackers, dry toast, or some other bland and starchy food may help, as might sucking on ice chips or very slowly sipping a carbonated soft drink that's gone flat. A folk remedy many people swear by is Coca Cola that's been defizzed. The Coke remedy is so popular there's even an over-the-counter product called Emetrol that's made of more or less the same ingredients. Another product, Pepto-Bismol, will help with nausea from overdrinking; keep in mind, though, that it will turn your stool an unsettling shade of black.

Vomiting

If you do vomit, your stomach will probably tell you that it would just as soon you not eat for several hours.

Follow your stomach's advice. Taking sips of clear liquids like water or a sports drink, though, is fine. The liquids will help prevent dehydration, which can be a problem with vomiting. Sports drinks—like Gatorade—are particularly helpful since they contain sodium and potassium and can treat dehydration more efficiently than water or soda.

After you vomit, you will probably feel weak. Pay attention to this message from your body and take it easy. Climb into bed for a while, or stretch out on the sofa until you get some of your strength back.

When you do start to feel better after a bout of vomiting, slowly increase the amount of clear liquids you drink. Eventually, you can graduate from clear liquids to mild, easily digested foods. Dry toast and crackers—once again—are good choices, as are Jell-O and cooked cereal. Depending on how you feel, you may want to stay on this admittedly uninspiring diet for 12 to 48 hours following the disappearance of all your symptoms.

the inner ear from sending a chemical message to the brain that orders you to vomit. The prescription drug scopolamine works by depressing the body's central nervous system. It's available as an adhesive patch worn on the skin.

The Perils of Food Poisoning

When the food you eat contains harmful microbes, your body will act accordingly, ejecting it either through your mouth as vomit or through the other end as diarrhea.

Doctors make a distinction between food poisoning—in which the little bugs have already multiplied on the food before it's eaten—and food-borne infection—in which the bugs are on the food but bacterial growth happens in your body.

The kind of bug will determine the period of time between ingestion and the onset of symptoms, and the symptoms themselves can vary.

Depending on the bug, you may experience any combination of diarrhea, vomiting, abdominal cramps, and flulike symptoms, and if you're in generally good health the bout typically will end about six hours after it begins. For people whose health is compromised—by diabetes, AIDS, or liver disease, for example—the complications can be serious and you should see a doctor.

QUIZ

Q: What percentage of Americans each year are thought to get a dose of food poisoning?

A: Ten percent.

MICROBES YOU NEED TO AVOID
There are an estimated 42,000 cases of infection by the *Salmonella typhimurium* bacterium each year in the United States, in most cases linked to uncooked eggs and animal products. More than 1,400 varieties of *Salmonella* are known. It grows over a wide range of temperatures, and it's pretty tough, too, being able to live through both freezing and freeze-

Stay Out of the Danger Zone

Making sure your food stays safe is largely a numbers game. A good numerical trio to keep in mind is 2, 40, 140. Why? Because you should stay away from any meats, salads, dairy products, stuffings, or other perishable foods that have been kept for more than two hours anywhere between the temperatures of 40° and 140°F. That means you should either defrost meats slowly in the refrigerator or quickly in the microwave.

Easy, right? So here are a few more numbers. Your refrigerator should be at 40°F or below to make sure foodstuffs stay cold enough. For the freezer, the magic number is 0°F or below. Use a thermometer to check. Here are some other safety precautions.

• Keep your hands and all work surfaces clean when preparing food.

• Refrigerate all perishable foods right after you use them.

• Don't spread bacteria by cross-contamination—using the cutting board you've just cut up raw meat on, for example, to also cut up raw tomatoes for the salad.

• Be extra careful when using some of the foods most often associated with food poisoning and food-borne infection—chicken, milk (especially unpasteurized), hamburger meat, beef, eggs, and seafood.

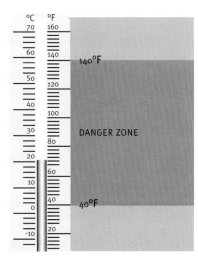

▲ *Bacteria that cause food poisoning grow best in temperatures above 40° and below 140°F, so keep food out of this danger zone as much as possible.*

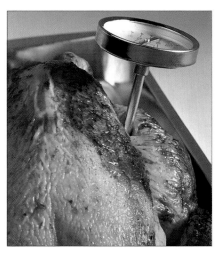

▲ *For safety's sake, always cook food to a high enough temperature to kill any bacteria that may be present. Use a thermometer to make sure.*

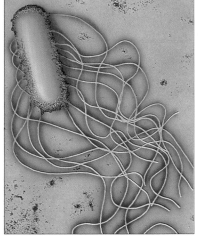

▲ Salmonella, *seen here under an electron microscope, is one of the most common causes of food poisoning. The whiplike tails are for movement.*

There's a bit of college fraternity folk wisdom to the effect that you can drink as much alcohol as you want without getting a hangover or feeling sick to your stomach as long as you stick with one kind of beverage per party. One twist on this dubious bit of handed-down wisdom even goes so far as to suggest that you'll be fine if you stick to drinking in alphabetical order—that's beer first, liquor second, and wine last of all.

Unfortunately, medical science doesn't appear to support either notion. "Alcohol is alcohol, and if you drink too much you'll feel ill," says Richard A. Cazen, M.D., a gastro-enterologist. Admittedly, there is a line of thinking that congeners—chemical compounds more prevalent in the darker-colored alcoholic drinks—will magnify the effects of a hangover, but at present it's nothing more than a theory.

---

drying. Keep in mind, though, that the one thing it can't survive is the heat of thorough cooking.

Infection by the bacterium *Listeria* can have nasty consequences, including meningitis and brain abscesses, although usually only in children, pregnant women, and elderly people whose health is compromised. The bug is linked to unpasteurized milk and unripened cheese.

Campylobacter jejuni is associated with poultry, beef, pigs, sheep, and water, and *Shigella* is a problem because a relatively few food preparers may pass it to food through poor handling practices.

Vibrio parahaemolyticus is another one to avoid. This bug grows in the ocean and is linked with raw seafood—like those oysters on the half-shell you like to slurp. Raw shellfish infected by the bacteria have been known to cause hepatitis in people with existing liver problems.

Clostridium botulinum (or botulism) is a very dangerous bug that produces a toxin which harms the central and peripheral nervous systems, and can cause death. It's linked to food that's not been properly sterilized during the canning process. And

Staphylococci, which causes vomiting, may get into food that's come into contact with a food handler's uncovered wound.

A microbe that's gotten a lot of press—because of people getting sick from contaminated beef that hasn't been cooked enough—is *Escherichia coli*, better known as *E. coli*. This is a variety of bug that lives in human and animal intestinal tracts, and it's easily spread. In some extreme cases, it can cause death—again, usually in the young and those with compromised health—and it can show up in foods other than the usual undercooked hamburgers.

PREVENTION

You should be properly impressed with the power of these little bugs to do you harm, but you should also know that by following a few, simple preventive measures it's possible to avoid them.

"Always wash fruit and vegetables thoroughly before eating," advises Arvey Rogers, M.D., professor of medicine and chief of the gastroenterology division at the University of Miami, "especially those that are imported during seasons when they're out of season here, like raspberries."

Cook food thoroughly, Dr. Rogers says. "Never eat hamburger meat or chicken which is pink after being heated," he warns. "This implies that the temperature has not been raised high enough to kill hemorrhagic *E. coli* or others." For most perishables, food temperatures of between 145° and 155°F will destroy most microbes. And, Dr. Rogers says, avoid drinking nonbottled water in countries where microbes are known to strike. That includes ice cubes and drinking from cool streams.

Diarrhea and Constipation

The media are filled with ads depicting the victims—the man with the runs who's trapped in a window seat on a long flight, or the husband at a party dying a slow death as his wife discusses how he uses Brand X laxative. Is the colon's operation really of that much concern to us? The answer is a resounding yes.

On and Off the Throne

When Dad explained the facts of life to you, he probably forgot to mention diarrhea and constipation. Virtually every one of us gets hit with a bout of diarrhea from time to time, and it can be horribly inconvenient to constantly excuse yourself to make a run for the throne.

As for constipation, it's the most common digestive complaint among American men, with about 7 percent reporting it as a chronic problem. The bottom line—so to speak—is that the colon, or large intestine, can be a real pain in the you-know-where if it doesn't do its job right.

The colon receives what's left of your food when the small intestine is done extracting nutrients from it. This undigested residue is pushed through the colon by means of muscle contractions that occur about twice each hour. The trip through the colon can take anywhere from 10 hours to several days, and along the way water and mineral salts are absorbed into the body through the colon's thin wall.

Harmless bacteria also devour any digestive enzymes left in your waste that could literally eat through the anus and surrounding skin if they passed out of the body.

Locating the Colon

The colon, or large intestine, is a five-foot-long, two-inch-wide muscular tube that's in charge of getting solid waste ready to exit the body. It begins in the lower right-hand side of your abdomen and makes the shape of an M as it winds through your gut—heading north and crossing to the left before descending back down to the rectum. It's made up of four sections: the ascending, transverse, descending, and sigmoid colon.

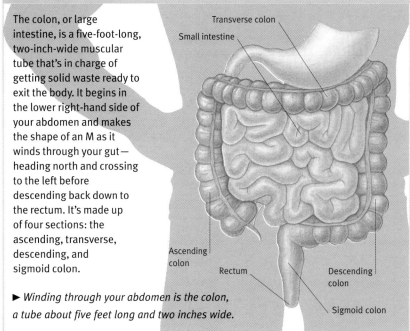

Transverse colon
Small intestine
Ascending colon
Rectum
Descending colon
Sigmoid colon

▶ *Winding through your abdomen is the colon, a tube about five feet long and two inches wide.*

By the time the undigested residue reaches the rectum—a five-inch-long tube for storing solid waste—it's been turned into stools, or feces. Ideally, the stools should be the consistency of heavy cottage cheese.

Keeping the Colon Happy

Maintaining your colon's health is a relatively easy proposition if you eat a healthy diet, drink plenty of water, and engage in regular exercise, according to Arvey Rogers, M.D., professor of medicine and chief of the gastroenterology division at the University of Miami.

A healthy diet means lots of fruit, vegetables, and grains. "They assure that the large intestine is provided bulk in the form of fiber," Dr. Rogers

Diverticulitis

Diverticula are small, saclike pouches that can form in the wall of the colon. The entrance to the pouch is in the colon itself, while the sac hangs outside the colon, protruding slightly into the abdomen. Diverticulosis—the existence of the pouches—is an extremely common condition in developed countries, and it may be linked to our diet, which is high in refined foods.

Normally, the diverticula don't cause many problems, but in some cases—

approximately 5 percent—they become infected and inflamed, causing a painful and potentially dangerous condition doctors call diverticulitis. An attack of diverticulitis usually entails diarrhea or constipation; and there's also severe pain, generally in the lower left part of the abdomen but sometimes elsewhere.

The condition needs to be treated by a doctor, who will usually prescribe antibiotics and a low-fiber diet for a while to let the colon rest.

Preventing future attacks of diverticulitis seems to be linked to a diet rich in fiber. One study found that 10 percent of patients who adopted a high-fiber diet after a bout of diverticulitis experienced a reduction in the frequency of symptoms.

Prevention also means staying away from food in particles that are big enough to lodge in the diverticula and cause infection. This means no seeds, popcorn, or nuts.

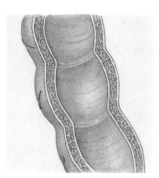

▲ *Normal colon with a wide passage and no pockets.*

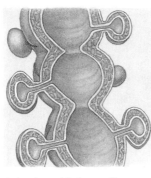

▲ *A colon with the saclike pockets called diverticula.*

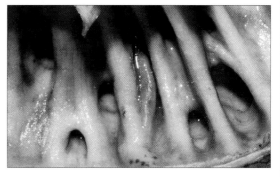

▲ *The inside view: A cross-section shows the characteristic pocketing of a colon affected by diverticulitis.*

says. Fiber—the indigestible part of plant foods—speeds the movement of food through the colon, absorbs water, and keeps your stool soft and pliable. Doctors recommend 20 to 30 grams of fiber per day. Get your daily dose through a balanced diet that includes at least five servings of fruit and vegetables, and six servings of breads, cereals, and grains.

Limit your intake of fat, which is more difficult to digest, but be wary of fat-free foods that are sometimes loaded with sugar, which also can be difficult to process.

Water and other liquids are important because they join with fiber in flushing food through the colon and keeping your stools soft, Dr. Rogers says. Drink six to eight eight-ounce glasses of fluids a day. Also, limit your coffee intake to a couple of cups per day since it contains oils that can irritate the colon's lining.

Finally, Dr. Rogers recommends regular exercise to stimulate the digestive tract, keeping food moving through the colon. It also may reduce the risk of some colon diseases.

Colon Problems

Given all the germs, stress, and hard-to-digest foods our colon has to deal with, it's not surprising that even a generally healthy and happy colon will act up from time to time. The most common symptoms of an unhappy colon are those two advertisers' delights already referred to, diarrhea and constipation.

DIARRHEA

Diarrhea—an increase in the frequency of bowel movements and the discharge of loose, watery stools—happens when the intestinal muscles go into spasms and move your food along too quickly for the body

to absorb nutrients and water. The spasms are often triggered by germs that reach your intestines—anything from a flu virus to microbes on contaminated food—and the resulting diarrhea is the body's way of quickly clearing out the invading bugs.

The spasms can also be triggered by a host of other things, including stress, anxiety, spicy food, and food allergies or intolerances, frequently to milk or milk-based products. Eating followed by physical activity can also bring on diarrhea.

CONSTIPATION

Stools may be hard and dry, and in really serious cases they can become stuck—or impacted—in the rectum. Constipation is usually caused by not eating enough fiber, getting inadequate exercise, and drinking too little water. Other causes include travel, stress, antidepressants and

Inflammatory Bowel Disease

This is a serious, chronic condition that takes in a number of ailments, the main ones being ulcerative colitis and Crohn's disease. Ulcerative colitis is characterized by microscopic sores that develop in the colon, resulting in diarrhea, abdominal pain, and rectal bleeding. With Crohn's disease, the entire digestive system from the esophagus to the colon can become inflamed, although the colon is the most common target.

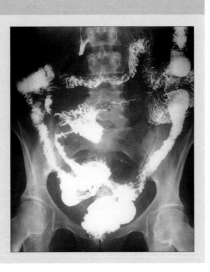

▶ *An x-ray of a patient with Crohn's disease, showing the inflamed colon.*

painkillers, and antacids that contain aluminum.

Yet another cause is, quite simply, not heeding nature's call. "Most constipation is the result of not defecating reasonably soon after a signal to do so," Dr. Rogers says. "The longer the stool is in the rectum, the greater the opportunity for the drying of that stool." In other words, if you delay having a bowel movement too long, your body starts to reabsorb water from the stool, making it hard, dry, and difficult to pass.

In advertisements for laxatives, constipation is always tied to the concept of regularity—that is, the frequent occurrence of bowel movements. Keep in mind that humans pass stools from three times each day to three times each week. If your movements happen only three or four times a week but they're fluffy and soft—like heavy cottage cheese—you aren't constipated.

DIVERTICULA

Diverticula are small pouches that form in the wall of the colon. It's estimated that a third of Americans develop the pouches by age 50.

Diverticulosis—or the existence of the pouches—is usually harmless, although the diverticula sometimes cause discomfort. In about 5 percent of cases, the pouches become infected and inflamed, leading to a painful and potentially dangerous condition called diverticulitis.

IRRITABLE BOWEL SYNDROME

Irritable bowel syndrome—a condition also known as spastic colon—afflicts an estimated 15 percent of Americans. It's basically a catch-all diagnosis that includes diarrhea, constipation, or stomach pain and cramping caused by an irritable or unpredictable digestive system.

COLON CANCER

Together with rectal cancer, colon cancer is the ninth top killer of men. Fortunately, it can be detected and stopped early.

Cancer of the colon is preceded by growths known as polyps. They're not cancerous at first but over time—typically about five years—some of them may turn malignant. Detecting polyps, and therefore cancer, is relatively easy with the use of a flexible sigmoidoscope—a thin, bendable tube with a light and lens that a doctor inserts through the rectum so that the lower third of the colon can be seen. That's where more than half of tumors occur. If polyps are found, the next step is a colonoscopy—using an instrument similar to a flexible sigmoidoscope but that sees farther

The Best Treatments for Diarrhea and Constipation

Diarrhea

Give your digestive system a rest until it settles down. Stick to mild foods like rice and bananas until you're better, advises gastroenterologist Arvey Rogers, M.D., and avoid dairy products, spicy foods, fruit, alcohol, and coffee for as long as you feel ill—but no longer. As with vomiting, dehydration can be a problem and you need to keep up your intake of clear liquids, Dr. Rogers says.

Since diarrhea is often your body's way of getting rid of a bug in your system, you shouldn't take antidiarrheal medications for the first six hours after an attack. There are three kinds of medications—thickeners that contain clay or fruit pectin (one brand is Kaopectate), antispasmodic products that slow the intestinal spasms (look for the ingredient loperamide), and products that contain both kinds of ingredients (brands include Donnagel and Parepectolin). But don't use any of these preparations if you have a fever.

Constipation

The best treatment for constant constipation is to prevent it in the first place through a fiber-rich, low-fat diet, plenty of water, and regular exercise. For occasional bouts of constipation, drink four extra glasses of water per day, especially in the morning. "More often than not, failure to simultaneously ingest more water with your increased fiber intake aggravates the problem," Dr. Rogers says.

Exercise a little more when constipation hits. "Increased physical activity may aid in relief," Dr. Rogers says. Using a laxative once in a while is fine, but keep in mind that bulk-forming products that draw water into the stool are preferable to stimulant laxatives.

Diarrhea, constipation, cramping, abdominal pain, and other symptoms of colon disorders are most frequently caused by unhealthy eating habits—such as insufficient fiber—or by viruses and other bugs that make it into the digestive tract. There are more serious diseases, however, that can strike the colon and that need to be treated by medical professionals. How can you tell when to see the doctor? In general, you should get a checkup if you've noticed a change in your bowel habits that's gone on for more than a week or ten days, according to gastroenterologist Arvery Rogers, M.D. "Fever or abdominal pain accompanying diarrhea is a concern," he says. "So is rectal bleeding, although it's usually the result of straining at the stool and provoking hemorrhoid bleeding."

Condition	Symptoms	Causes	Treatment
Irritable Bowel Syndrome	Diarrhea, constipation, or bouts of both; abdominal pain; gas and bloating; fatigue.	Unknown; stress and poor diet are suspected.	Dietary changes; exercise; stress management; psychological counseling.
Ulcerative Colitis	Diarrhea; abdominal pain; cramping; blood in stools; in rare cases can lead to malignant changes in the gut.	Unknown.	Change in diet; stress management; medication.
Crohn's Disease	Diarrhea or constipation; abdominal pain; cramping; blood in stools; weight loss; fever; skin irritations.	Unknown.	Change in diet; stress management; medication.
Diverticulitis	Pain, often in lower left part of abdomen but can be elsewhere; diarrhea or constipation; nausea; fever; chills.	Infection of diverticula, small pouches that develop in wall of colon.	Antibiotics; low-fiber diet to let colon rest.
Colon Cancer	Persistent diarrhea or constipation; black, tarry stools or bleeding from rectum; long, thin stools; persistent feeling of being unable to empty bowels; unexplained fatigue, weight loss, or lack of appetite.	Most commonly, polyps in colon that become cancerous. Ulcerative colitis (see above).	Surgical removal of cancerous section; possible colostomy, in which excreted wastes are collected in a bag or pouch; radiation and chemotherapy to prevent recurrence.

into the colon and has the ability to remove the polyps.

All men over age 50 should get a flexible sigmoidoscopy every two to three years; for men at high risk (a parent or sibling with colon cancer) testing should begin at 40. Doctors recommend a colonoscopy rather than sigmoidoscopy for this high-risk group, and also those with bloody, loose, and misshapen stools.

The Lowdown on Hemorrhoids

You've just finished straining to push a dry, hard stool out your anus. You stand up and it feels like you have a small egg tucked between your buns. Congratulations, you've got a hemorrhoid.

Hemorrhoids are swollen and inflamed veins around the anus. Virtually all of us have them, but usually they're neatly tucked inside the anus and we're not aware of them. Pressure—as when you strain to defecate—can cause them to pop outside.

Though they're rarely serious and will usually clear up after a few days, hemorrhoids are tender and can bleed. If a blood clot forms inside a hemorrhoid, a painful condition called thrombosis results.

Over-the-counter hemorrhoid treatments may help because they lubricate the anal area or contain soothing ingredients. But they won't shrink the hemorrhoids or make them go away sooner. You can also try hot baths.

Doctors say there's no reason you can't occasionally use laxatives. But you should keep in mind that they're addictive and can make constipation worse in the long term by weakening the muscles in your intestines. To avoid constipation, there's no substitute for a high-fiber diet, plenty of liquids, and regular exercise.

If you do need a blast to open your bowels, the bulk-forming laxatives—they contain an ingredient like psyllium to draw water into the stool and make it larger, softer, and easier to pass—are preferable to stimulant ones that contain phenolphthalein or senna, which speeds the passage of the stool by jolting the colon.

Weight Loss and Weight Gain

You reach for that favorite pair of jeans in your closet and slip them on. They feel a little different than usual—a bit snug around the rear and waist—and you find yourself inhaling to get the top button fastened. You don't need a bathroom scale to tell you that you've gained weight.

The Battle of the Pounds

Are you one of those people who keep a scale in the bathroom? As anyone who often weighs himself can tell you, most people's weight fluctuates slightly from day to day, even when there's no change in diet. You could lose a pound or two in a day, for example, if you've been sweating a lot; or you could gain a few pounds if you retain fluids because you've been eating salty foods.

Significant or long-term weight loss and weight gain, however, are almost always caused by the same three factors—diet, physical activity, and metabolism. Based on your level of physical activity and your metabolic rate, your body has certain energy requirements. If you eat more than needed to meet those requirements, you'll put on weight; eat less, and you'll lose weight.

Of the three, diet and physical activity are the most significant.

They also happen to be the two factors we can most easily control, although your metabolic rate will rise if you increase your proportion of muscle mass and lose fat.

Why Weight Fluctuates

Two of the most common causes of weight fluctuation are emotional/psychological factors—such as stress and anxiety—and a change in lifestyle, usually from a physically active one to a sedentary one.

Stress, anxiety, and depression—or, more specifically, your reaction to them—can trigger weight gain or weight loss. Some people turn to food for comfort during difficult times, and if your physical activity doesn't increase along with your intake of calories, you'll probably put on weight. For other people, stress, anxiety, and depression act as an appetite suppressant, and if calorie intake drops below the amount

Symptom Sorter

Clothes that don't fit like they used to are often your first clue that you've gained or lost weight. The reasons our weight changes can vary, but sometimes weight loss and weight gain are triggered by particular symptoms. Stress that leads to overeating, for example, may result in you putting on extra pounds, just as the digestive ailments associated with the stomach flu will frequently cause a loss of weight.

Medical disorders, ranging from diabetes to HIV infection, are occasionally the cause of weight gain or loss, although usually this type of fluctuation is accompanied by any number of other symptoms, which vary according to the disorder in question.

your body needs based on your level of physical activity and metabolism, you'll undoubtedly shed weight.

Either case can present problems if the over- or undereating goes on very long, and you need to find other ways to handle what's bothering you. Deal with the source of the problem, with professional help, if need be. And remember that exercise improves your state of mind, burns off extra calories if you're eating too much, and stimulates the appetite if you're eating too little.

Another common cause of weight fluctuation is a change in lifestyle. You might have noticed this when you got your first real job right out of school. As a student, your lifestyle was probably fairly active—playing sports, walking around campus between classes, and maybe working part-time in a bookstore unloading crates of textbooks. You also might not have had the income for a rich,

Are Medications Behind Your Problem?

Prescription drugs are designed to achieve particular results, but they may produce fluctuations in your weight as a side effect.

Diabetics who take insulin sometimes need to be placed on calorie-controlled diets to combat weight gain, and antidepressants can trigger either a gain or loss, depending on the drug in question. Medications taken to treat an underactive thyroid may result in

weight gain while those taken to treat an overactive thyroid may lead to rapid weight loss. And corticosteroids—used to treat rheumatoid arthritis, asthma, and other conditions—are one class of drugs that frequently causes gradual weight gain.

If you've been taking medication and have noticed that you've either lost or gained weight, be sure to let your doctor know.

The Best Treatments for Weight Loss and Weight Gain

In the vast majority of cases, treating an unwanted weight gain or loss boils down to altering your diet, altering your level of physical activity, or altering both.

Weight Loss

If the weight loss is caused by a temporary interruption in your regular eating habits—due to the stomach flu, for example, or a particularly stressful period at the office—you'll probably put the weight back on relatively quickly once you start eating normally. But Lawrence Cheskin, M.D., director of the Johns Hopkins Weight Management Center in Baltimore, says that if you suspect that your weight fluctuations are caused by underlying medical disorders or medications—or if you're not sure—it's best to consult your doctor.

Weight Gain

To treat unwanted weight gain, decrease your caloric intake while boosting your level of physical activity, Dr. Cheskin says. The way to do that, he says, is to keep your diet low in fat, include plenty of fruit, grains, and vegetables, and avoid "calorie-dense" foods such as cheese. And Dr. Cheskin suggests doing regular, moderate exercise that you enjoy enough to stick to, rather than occasional exercise binges.

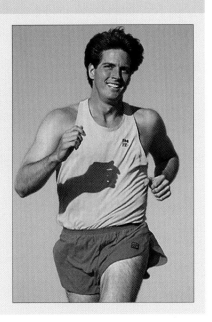

▶ *To take off weight, there's nothing like regular aerobic exercise, such as running. And keep your diet low in fats, too.*

---

high-calorie diet. With your first job, though, you're at a desk all day except for those nice, fattening business lunches, and now you just don't have the time for sports you used to love. Result? A gain in weight.

A change in lifestyle can also cause weight loss, such as when you switch to a job that demands more of you physically. In either case, to avoid unwanted weight gain or loss, you need to adjust your diet so the number of calories you take in matches your level of physical activity. And if you begin a job that's less physically demanding, even a moderate program of exercise will help to prevent weight gain.

OTHER CAUSES

Unexplained weight loss and weight gain are occasionally caused by an underlying medical disorder.

> ### "Diets are short-term changes in eating behavior and because they're short-term, all diets fail."
> Morton H. Shaevitz, Ph.D., associate clinical professor of psychiatry at the University of California, San Diego, School of Medicine

A rapid gain in weight is a symptom common to several health problems, such as congestive heart failure, kidney disease, hepatitis, cirrhosis—a disease of the liver caused by alcohol abuse—or a hereditary factor. Gradual weight gain can signal an underactive thyroid, the gland responsible for regulating how fast your body turns food into energy.

Unexplained weight loss is frequently one of the symptoms of cancer, HIV infection that can lead to AIDS, and malabsorption, a condition in which the intestines can't properly absorb the nutrients from food. Rapid loss of weight may signal diabetes or an overactive thyroid—or it could simply be that you've just had a bout of stomach flu that included diarrhea or vomiting and a loss of appetite.

Extreme loss of weight is characteristic of anorexia nervosa, in which a preoccupation with looking thin leads to compulsive dieting. Although it mostly affects younger women, this condition can hit anyone. It's estimated that 1 in every 2,000 teenage boys suffers from it, compared to 1 in 100 teenage girls.

When to See a Doctor

Fluctuation in weight usually doesn't require medical intervention because you'll have a good idea why the scale has gone up or down—a succession of rich meals, for example, or a bout of stomach flu that destroyed your appetite. "It's not uncommon for somebody on a diet to lose weight and then regain it," says Lawrence Cheskin, M.D., director of the Johns Hopkins Weight Management Center in Baltimore. "That kind of fluctuation is probably not harmful physically, though behaviorally it's probably not good for you." You may want to see a doctor, though, if your weight has gone up or down and you can't seem to get it back where you want it. At the very least, the doctor can rule out underlying medical problems and give you some ideas on how to achieve your weight goals.

You must check in with the doctor if you experience other symptoms with weight loss or weight gain, or an unexplained fluctuation in weight, or if your gain or loss happened rapidly. "If you unintentionally continue to lose weight, that's certainly a red flag," Dr. Cheskin says. "It can indicate a serious underlying problem. That's something you should run to your doctor about."

Muscle Soreness and Bruises

Does this sound familiar? You've been a weekend warrior. You've conquered the basketball court. But now it's Monday and your muscles are so sore you don't think you'll ever move again. It's happened to us all, and there's much you can do to ease the pain and head off future problems.

Sore and Sorry

Taking to heart all we've been saying about the rewards of exercise, you decide the time has finally come to get physical. After buying yourself a good pair of running shoes and joining a gym, you start on your new life of regular exercise. The first day, you run for a couple of miles around the neighborhood at a pretty quick pace, and since that went so well you head to the gym and pump iron for an hour. That night, you eat a healthy, balanced dinner and feel on top of the world. "This is going great," you tell yourself. "Tomorrow I'll crank it up a notch."

Only one problem: Tomorrow comes and your muscles are so sore you can barely get out of bed. You limp through the day in pain, wincing and moaning with every movement. So what do you do? You give the exercise regimen a break, of course, at least until you feel better. And then what? Two weeks later, you're back in action with the same enthusiasm—and back in pain the next day.

The moral of the story is that you have to start a new exercise program nice and slow. It may take you only a second to decide to start exercising again, but your muscles need time to adjust to your new-found resolve.

When a Muscle Gets Pulled

You haven't exercised since you won the tennis singles championship in high school. But the company's weekend tennis tournament is coming up and you aim to get that silver cup. If you're not careful, though, you may also cause yourself to have a pulled shoulder or hamstring, two of the most common—and painful—muscle strains there are. In either case, a proper warmup and some stretching will help prevent the problem.

Pulled Hamstring
The hamstring is the muscle on the back side of your thigh. A pulled one strikes most often during sports that rely on the sudden, powerful use of leg muscles—tennis, of course, but also basketball, running, and cycling.

Shoulder Pull
A pulled shoulder is more frequent in sports requiring shoulder power. These include baseball, tennis, golf, and swimming.

How Muscles Work

Our body's 639 named muscles give us strength and the ability to move—from running to smiling to the blink of an eye. Essentially a bundle of long, slender cells known as fibers, a muscle can be attached to another muscle, to bone, or to skin. And it can either act as an autonomous unit or as part of a larger system combining the effects of several muscles.

A muscle functions by contracting—or shortening itself—and then relaxing. Think of it as a spring that shortens when you push down on it and lengthens when you let go. The contraction of some slowly acting muscles is controlled at least in part by hormones circulating in the bloodstream, but when quicker control is needed, muscles contract in response to independent nerve impulses telling each fiber it needs to move. Some muscles move voluntarily, such as when you walk or throw a ball, while others move involuntarily, such as when the muscles in your stomach automatically churn food when you eat.

Muscles are the place where your body's chemical energy is converted into mechanical energy. As soon as a muscle gets the message to move, the fibers combine glycogen—a kind of carbohydrate stored in the muscle—with oxygen that's brought in by the circulating blood from the lungs. When the two are put together, a complex chemical reaction takes place which converts them into the mechanical energy that allows you to move. Carbon dioxide and other by-products of the chemical reaction are then carried away by the blood and exhaled through the lungs.

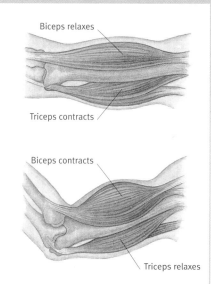

▲ *Moving an arm involves coordinated contraction and relaxation of the biceps and triceps muscles.*

Putting a Name to Your Aches and Pains

An ache is a pain is an ache, right? Not exactly. Muscles can hurt in a variety of ways, and so a whole slew of terms exists to describe what ails you. Here's a quick rundown on the most common muscle terms.

Delayed-Onset Muscle Soreness
Ordinary, all-day stiffness in a muscle that peaks a day or two after unaccustomed, strenuous exercise.

Muscle Tension
Pain from maintaining extremely taut muscles, often involuntarily, due to stress.

Cramp
A spasmodic contraction of a muscle; occurs most often in the calf or foot; harmless but often very painful.

Heat Cramp
Cramp caused by overexertion in hot weather; could result from dehydration, an overheated body, or an electrolyte imbalance.

Charley Horse
Slang for a painful, involuntary spasm in one of the calf muscles.

Muscle Fatigue
A state in which muscles are increasingly uncomfortable and decreasingly efficient because of extended exertion.

Bruised Ribs
An imprecise term that can refer to pulled or torn intercostal muscles, the thin sheets of muscle between each rib.

Sprain
Wrenching or twisting of a joint that could include tearing of a ligament.

Stitch
A pain in the side of the torso during running; "stitches" also sometimes refers to stomach cramps during exercise.

Strain
Overstretching or overexertion of a muscle that could include tearing of the muscle or a tendon connecting the muscle to a bone.

Sore Muscle
A pain that comes from anything, such as a bruise, overuse, or strain, for example.

Shinsplints
Pain along the shin caused by overworking the muscles and tendon around the shin bone; caused by running or walking.

"Whenever you do something you haven't done before, your body needs to adapt," says Edward R. Laskowski, M.D., co-director of the Mayo Clinic's Sports Medicine Center in Rochester, Minnesota. "Stressing and challenging your muscles in a different way can cause soreness."

That doesn't mean you should shirk the challenge; after all, stressing your muscles is a lot of what exercise is all about. But you can prevent soreness by understanding how your muscles are constructed and how they operate.

Why Does It Hurt?

Whenever one of your muscles becomes active and requires extra oxygen to produce motion, the blood vessels in the muscle open up to deliver greater flow. If you're really pushing your muscles, such as during a good workout, the cardiovascular system is going to have to compensate somehow to deliver the oxygen the muscular fibers need. It does this by closing down some blood vessels in the skin and internal organs and by causing the heart to beat faster and stronger so that more blood circulates. The active muscles produce extra carbon dioxide, and this in turn stimulates sensitive chemoreceptor cells in the brain that control your breathing. The result? Breathing becomes deeper and quicker so that the unwanted carbon dioxide is flushed out of the blood and more oxygen is absorbed.

During particularly intense exercise, the local blood circulation may not be enough to supply the muscles with oxygen. This leads to ischemic pain in the affected muscles—an example is the abdominal ache you feel when you do more sit ups than you're used to. Ischemic pain disappears when you stop exercising or reduce the intensity of the workout.

When there's not enough oxygen, the muscles get the energy they need from the glycogen in a different way—anaerobically, or without the use of oxygen. Lactic acid is created as a by-product, and any of it that's not carried away in the blood will accumulate in the muscles. And, Dr. Laskowski says, "When metabolic products like lactic acid build up in the muscle, that can cause soreness."

Soreness after physical activity can also be caused by the very process of

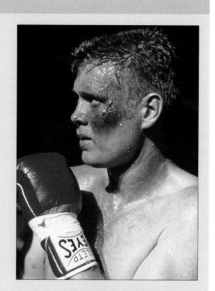
strengthening and building muscle that goes on during a workout. Muscles are made to stretch, but they do have limits. If you stretch a muscle more than it's used to, it strains. Keep straining it and you'll have a muscle tear. The worst tears are sudden and sharp, and the pain is usually immediate and located in a specific area. With strains, the soreness takes at least a couple of hours to show up and is more generalized.

If you had a microscope to look at one of your muscles as it strains, you'd see that the individual fibers are actually starting to pull apart. If the damage to the fibers is serious enough, the muscles may swell or turn stiff. But repeated straining of the fibers in moderation produces benefits. Muscles have a tremendous capacity to bounce back from injury, and in the hours and days after you strain them, they rebuild themselves with slightly greater size and capacity. Repeat your exercise regularly, and the strength and size of the muscle will grow.

The amount you increase in size, though, is limited largely by the length of your muscles, measured from tendon to tendon. The longer the muscle, the greater the potential for increase in size.

How to Prevent Soreness

The best way to prevent the muscle soreness that's associated with physical activity is to keep in shape through a regular program of exercise. Muscles that are used regularly have a greater capacity for exertion and are bound to cause you fewer aches and pains. Apart from that, there a number of preventive measures you can take.

WARM UP

Going full-bore into vigorous exercise without giving your muscles a chance to get used to the idea is a prescription for pain. "Warmup is key," Dr. Laskowski says. "It establishes bloodflow in the muscles, and that enables them to better handle the challenges you're going to impose on them."

That goes for any kind of physical activity. When you run, don't kick into a world-record pace until your heart rate is elevated to the point where you're warm. If you'll be doing heavy-duty work in the garden, such as turning soil, take it easy the first few minutes. Or, suggests Janet Sobel, a physical therapist and clinic manager at NRH/Suburban Regional Rehab in Chevy Chase, Maryland, "If you're going to be playing tennis, take the racket and just swing it through all the motions that you're going to be using in your game."

You can find a full discussion on how to warm up on pages 86 and 87.

Remember that the key word is "warm." Says Dr. Laskowski, "Tissue is more extensible when it's warmer, so the threshold for it to feel irritated will be higher."

COOL DOWN

Rather than stopping your physical activity abruptly to plunk yourself down in front of the television, let your muscles ease gradually out of their exercise mode. Consider a cooldown period of less intense exercise as a cleansing operation. "Low-level activity keeps up an increased bloodflow in the muscle," Dr. Laskowski says. "That can help wash out some of those toxic metabolic products." A gradual slowdown also allows the muscles to more efficiently return to their normal elasticity without stiffness setting in.

You don't have to cool your muscles down very long to reap the benefit. A 5- or 10-minute walk is enough, according to Dr. Laskowski, or simply continue your workout activity at a slower pace for a few minutes. "It doesn't have to be intense," he says. "If you've been lifting weights, maybe take a spin on the stationary bike."

DRINK, DRINK, DRINK

Your muscles are mostly water so they need plenty of it before, after, and during a strenuous workout.

"It's important for your muscles to be hydrated while you're exercising," Dr. Laskowski says. Muscle dehydration is a major cause of cramps and spasms, so at the very least drink a glass or two of water before you begin and after you're done. And remember, caffeine and alcohol act as diuretics, boosting fluid loss by making you urinate more often.

TRY SOME ANTIOXIDANTS

To help protect your muscles, some experts recommend taking reasonable doses of antioxidants such as vitamin C, vitamin E, and beta-carotene. These active compounds protect your muscles from damage by combating what are known as free radicals. "The jury is still out on whether they are indeed protective," Dr. Laskowski says. "But a lot of body-builders use them."

STRETCH FOR SUPPLENESS

The increased flexibility that comes with regular stretching exercises can help keep your muscle tissue pliable and injury-free, Sobel says. But you should keep in mind that stretching isn't a substitute for a warmup. In fact, you should always warm up before you start to stretch, according to Barbara Sanders, Ph.D., P.T., chairman of the physical therapy department at Southwest Texas State University. "You don't want to jump right out of bed and stretch," she says. "You can get sore from stretching."

What Are Bruised Ribs?

We've all heard football and ice hockey players proudly announce they suffered bruised ribs in the latest contest. A badge of manly honor, perhaps, but what exactly does it mean?

The term "bruised ribs" can actually refer to three different injuries. First, unlike other bones, your ribs can be bruised through direct contact. Second, you may pull or tear your intercostal muscles, which are the muscles between two ribs. Finally, there's a separated or strained joint between a rib and the sternum.

So the next time an ornery, 300-pound linebacker says he's bruised his ribs, be sure to let him know the phrase doesn't mean much unless he specifies which of the three injuries he's talking about. And then run.

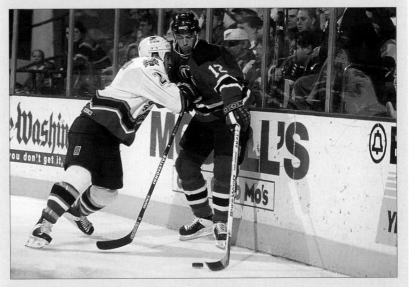

▲ A cross-check, where one player slams into another when he's against the wall, is a common cause of bruised ribs. Other contact sports risk the same type of injury.

Since getting sore is exactly what we are all trying to avoid, many sports-medicine experts actually recommend doing your stretching *after* your workout, rather than doing it before. "That's when the bloodflow has heated up the muscles and you're more likely to gain the benefit from the stretch," advises Dr. Laskowski.

Both Sobel and Dr. Sanders recommend that you don't bounce as you stretch, and don't overdo it. "Move to the point where you're beginning to feel discomfort and no further," Dr. Sanders says.

PROGRESS SLOWLY

Try not to get overambitious, either at the start of a new program or well into it, because pushing yourself too hard leads inevitably to muscle soreness. "Doing more than you're used to doing, or using different muscle groups, can contribute to sore muscles," Dr. Laskowski says. "The key is to introduce changes slowly and in progressive fashion."

Do You Need a Support Belt?

You see them on the guys delivering beer to the bar, on furniture movers, on professional and amateur weight lifters and even on people who are stocking shelves in the corner grocery store. They're back support belts and they sure look macho. The question is, do they do anything to head off muscle soreness in the back? According to the National Institute for Occupational Safety and Health, the answer is probably not. Some medical professionals, though, believe the belts can be helpful psychologically: They work as a kind of alarm, warning people who wear them that they need to be on guard when engaging in activities that put a lot of stress on a back.

Joint Pain; Numbness and Tingling

Ever seen a photo of a ballerina's bare feet? It's not a pretty sight. Years of dancing give the feet a battered look. Think of the strain placed on the joints in a dancer's foot and it's easy to see why the inevitable fate of many of those joints is arthritis. Joints can take a lot of abuse, but they do have their limits.

Joints and What They Do

You've got joints all over your body, wherever any two bones meet. Joints come in several varieties. There are fixed joints whose job is to hold bones together, like those in your skull that fuse and become immovable during childhood. Among the joints that move, there's the pivot type, such as the neck, that allows rotation on a plane. There's also the hinge type—in places like knees and elbows—that swings back and forth, again primarily in one plane. Joints in your spinal column have very limited motion, but since there are so many individual ones all in a row, your back is pretty flexible.

Ball-and-socket joints in your hips and shoulders are the most versatile. Allowing movement in different directions, these joints are held together in part by large muscles that provide the power to move so many ways while remaining stable. The joints also have powerful tendons, which connect muscle to bone, and strong ligaments, which connect one bone to another.

Movable joints are complicated structures made of varying types and amount of ligament, muscle, and cartilage—a strong elastic tissue which covers the ends of bones that would otherwise touch. There are also specialized membranes and fluids that will lubricate each joint and provide a cushion against stress.

Preventing Joint Problems

Keeping your joints healthy is a matter of exercising, taking a few precautions, and keeping to a reasonable body weight so that excess poundage doesn't put added pressure on them. Physical activity that makes your muscles stronger will lessen the stress on joints. One caveat, though: "Try not to abuse the joints," advises Joel Press, M.D., medical director of the Center for Spine, Sports, and Occupational Rehabilitation at the Rehabilitation Institute in Chicago. "Don't do a lot of exercise where there's high impact and a lot of pounding. Swim, ride a bike, or use a NordicTrack."

Stretching your joints frequently will keep them loose and healthy. When exercising or playing a sport, get in shape before you go at it full bore. And if your joints start to hurt during one type of activity, try switching to something that puts less strain on them. Drinking six to

---

Symptom Sorter

The common denominator in most joint problems is pain in the affected area. Symptoms vary according to the the cause and location.

Sprains
Swelling of the joint, often muscle spasms, and sometimes some bruising. Mainly affects the ankles and wrists.

Tendinitis
Tendon inflammation causes tenderness and restriction in muscle movement. Affects the shoulders (raising the arm in some angles causes pain), fingers, knees.

Cartilage Damage
Causes restricted movement. Mainly affects knees.

Bursitis
Inflammation of the bursa causes a fluid-filled swelling in the area. Affects the knees, elbows, hips, and shoulders.

Temporomandibular Disorder
Clenching and grinding of teeth leads to jaw pain that can radiate to the head, face, ear, neck, or shoulder. A popping or clicking sound in the jaw joints often occurs when you open or close your mouth; there may also be a locking of the jaw.

Arthritis
Osteoarthritis: Stiffness in the morning with pain ranging from a dull ache to excruciating. Pain can be referred (from a place other than the affected joint). Sometimes swelling. *Rheumatoid arthritis*: May cause the joints that hurt to become red, swollen, and warm to the touch. A low fever, loss of appetite and weight, a dry mouth or eyes may also occur. Affects the hands, feet, wrists, knees, elbows, shoulders, and hips. There's also stiffness in the morning. *Gout*: Joint pain is usually in the big toe, or else in the wrist or knee, and it comes on suddenly and severely. Redness and swelling around the affected joint and sometimes fever.

eight glasses of water a day helps keep the ligaments at joints fluid, and the joints lubricated.

Joint Problems

Why do joints go bad? A lot of it is normal wear and tear over time. But there are also specific problems that happen to the joints' components.

SPRAINS

One common problem is a sprain, which is the stretching or tearing of a ligament. It's possible to sprain any ligament in your body, but the usual victims are those that come under the greatest stress—the ones in your ankles, knees, and fingers.

TENDINITIS

Another relatively common problem is tendinitis, the damaging or tearing of a tendon attaching muscle to bone. It's usually the result of trauma or overuse, and it most frequently develops in the shoulders, ankles, and elbows, as any of you who've suffered the type of tendinitis called "tennis elbow" can attest.

TEMPOROMANDIBULAR DISORDER

This disorder, whose complicated name is usually shortened to TMD, affects the temporomandibular

What Happens When Good Joints Go Bad?

When your joints are healthy, you're able to use their full range of motion without feeling any pain. The cartilage on the end of each bone acts as a nice cushion so the bones don't touch and rub together. And the entire joint is encased in a lining or membrane called the synovium, which contains inside it a thick, egg-whitelike lubricant called synovial fluid.

But when a joint isn't healthy, it turns swollen, tender, and stiff. The range of motion is drastically reduced, and whatever motion you can make is accompanied by pain.

With rheumatoid arthritis, the inflammation causing the problem is actually in the synovium. As the synovium swells, it invades and damages both cartilage and bone. Eventually, the condition causes the breakdown of cartilage and the unprotected ends of each bone begin to rub against one another.

Gout, a form of arthritis, affects 10 times more men than women. The cause is a buildup of crystals of uric acid, a by-product of digestion, in the joint space and nearby tissues. The result is inflammation and intense pain.

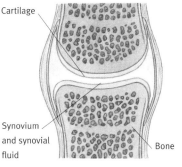

Cartilage

Synovium and synovial fluid

Bone

▲ *A joint is a complex arrangement of bone, cartilage, and synovium.*

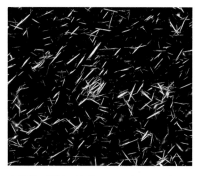

▲ *Uric acid crystals—seen here under a microscope—are the cause of gout.*

joints, which connect your lower jaw bone to bones on either side of the head, allowing the jaw to open, close, move backward and forward, and from side to side. When the

joints are jarred, such as during a car accident, or when there's gradual deterioration from tooth grinding, bad posture, or even stress-induced clenching of the teeth, TMD sets in. The condition causes the joints to pop, creak, grind, and shoot pain through your head, neck, and shoulders. This condition is estimated to afflict 1 in 10 men.

BURSITIS

With bursitis, there's an irritation of the bursas—the tiny sacs surrounding tendons—which allow the tendons to slide around moving parts of a joint. The bursal sacs normally resemble empty, plastic sandwich bags, but when you repeatedly apply too much pressure to them—think of a carpet installer constantly on his knees—they can become inflamed

Who's at Risk for Arthritis?

There are more than 100 conditions grouped together under the heading arthritis, ranging from mild to terribly disabling. While doctors don't know the exact causes of most of these conditions, they have identified a number of risk factors.

Your chance of getting osteoarthritis increases with age. According to orthopedic surgeon Robert Martin, M.D., if you're over 40 there's a good chance your joints already show some signs of it, especially if your job is physically demanding. It's just part of the aging process, affecting men and

women equally. With rheumatoid arthritis, however, younger people tend to be affected—in men, it usually hits between the ages of 20 and 40—and women are more often the victim.

Gout afflicts men more often than women, and the primary target is a sedentary, middle-age man who eats and drinks too much and whose weight and blood pressure are on the rise.

With most kinds of arthritis, obesity, lack of exercise, and injuries to joints at an early age are risk factors, and heredity seems to play a role as well.

and filled with fluid. Bursitis occurs most often in the aforementioned knees and in elbows, hips, and shoulders, and it frequently goes hand-in-hand with a bout of tendinitis.

DAMAGED OR TORN CARTILAGE

If you constantly apply pressure to cartilage, the normally smooth and marblelike tissue will sometimes flake off, leading to grinding pain. Cartilage damage can also be caused by twisting injuries.

ARTHRITIS

Of all the conditions that can affect joints, arthritis frequently is the most disabling. It's actually a collection of more than 100 different conditions—including gout, rheumatoid arthritis and, most common of all, osteoarthritis—that can cause swelling, pain, and loss of motion in the joints. Osteoarthritis is the form that is most closely linked to age, and it results from the breakdown of cartilage. Rheumatoid arthritis is potentially the most severe and debilitating, and it's known to be an immune system disorder although doctors aren't sure what causes it.

Gout is one of the few forms of arthritis that affects men more than women. It's a metabolic disorder in which uric acid crystallizes in a joint, often the big toe. Although diet alone doesn't cause gout, an attack can be triggered by eating foods like mussels and most organ meats that are high in purines—chemicals that turn into uric acid in the blood. Alcohol consumption can also be a trigger.

Numbness and Tingling

As any sportsman knows, when a joint goes bad, it can cause you a great deal of pain and, sometimes, that discomforting duo, numbness

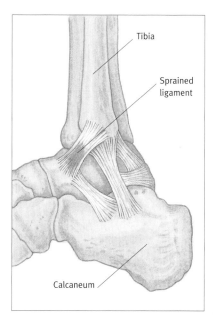

▲ A sprain is the stretching or tearing of a ligament holding bones together. The ankle is a common injury site.

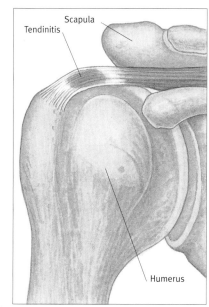

▲ Tendinitis of the shoulder often hits tennis players. It happens when a tendon is damaged or torn by overuse.

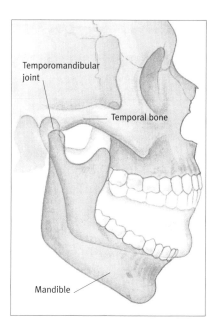

▲ The temporomandibular joints allow the jaw to move. Jarring or deterioration lead to temporomandibular disorder (or TMD).

The Best Treatments for Joint Problems

Sprains
Mild sprains should be iced. Hold an ice pack—or a bag of frozen vegetables wrapped in a washcloth—on the affected area for 15 minutes several times a day for a couple of days. If possible, keep the area elevated above the heart while applying ice. Try not to put any weight on the sprain for a day or two. Severe sprains—those that cause a lot of pain and swelling—should be checked out by your doctor.

Tendinitis and Bursitis
Apply ice as for sprains, but after a few days, moist heat might help relieve the pain. You can use a heat pack or a towel soaked in hot water and wrung out. Anti-inflammatory medications like aspirin and ibuprofen will decrease the pain by reducing the inflammation and swelling. As with sprains, rest the affected area until it's better, and then start to exercise it very gently.

Cartilage Damage
Cartilage won't heal on its own, so see a doctor, who can give you noninjectable medicine to regenerate cartilage.

Temporomandibular Disorder
Take an anti-inflammatory, massage the muscles around the jaw joints, and use hot and cold packs. If the disorder recurs, you should probably go to see the doctor.

Arthritis
Doctors treat arthritis with a combination of anti-inflammatory drugs, physical therapy, and recommendations for lifestyle changes. Some health professionals and arthritis sufferers, though, believe that a combination of Western medicine and alternative therapies works best. There are many dubious treatments out there—ranging from cow manure to copper bracelets—but there is some medical support for juice therapy, acupressure, and aromatherapy.

To relieve pain from osteoarthritis, rheumatoid arthritis, and gout, you can take an anti-inflammatory pain reliever, but stay away from aspirin if you have gout. Warm baths as well as heat and cold packs applied to your aching or stiff joints can help, as can an over-the-counter cream or lotion containing capsaicin—the chemical that puts the hot in hot peppers.

and tingling. A dislocated shoulder, for example, usually means severe pain in the shoulder itself as well as numbness and tingling in the arm. Numbness and tingling in the thumb and first three fingers often accompany the pain of carpal tunnel syndrome—a condition where the nerve that runs through a narrow channel between wrist bones and ligaments is squeezed.

Numbness and tingling happen when there's some problem in the working of the sensory nerves. If the nerve is interfered with—such as by being pressed or pinched in one of your joints—the sensory message from the affected area of your body can't reach the brain, resulting in numbness, a loss of feeling. With tingling, also called "pins and needles," the loss of feeling is only partial because the sensory message isn't entirely blocked.

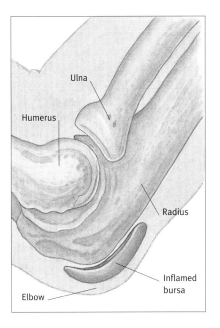

▲ When the bursa at the tip of the elbow becomes inflamed from constant pressure, you've got bursitis.

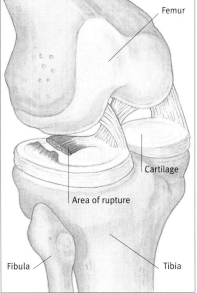

▲ The cartilage in this knee joint has been ruptured by a twisting impact— a football tackle, for example.

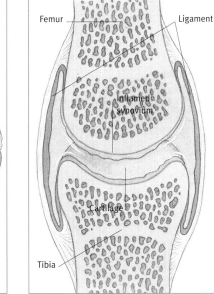

▲ Rheumatoid arthritis can cripple. Inflammation starts with the synovium and spreads to the cartilage and bone.

Back Pain

Back pain is one of the most common ailments there is. Almost all of us will experience it at some point in our lives. And apart from sore throats and colds, back pain is the single most common condition that doctors treat. The good news is that treatment is usually successful.

Sit Up Straight!

Our poor mothers did their best to make sure we developed good posture habits as we grew up. For Mom, good posture wasn't so much an issue of health as one of character. When she said, "Sit up straight" and "Don't slouch," she seemed to be implying that the slouchers of this world don't get ahead in life. With a straight back, though, you'll be able to go straight to the top.

Now, far be it from us to say that Mom was full of it. Better to say that our mothers were on the right track in getting us to think about our backs and how important they are to our overall well-being.

According to Leon Root, M.D., author of *No More Aching Back* and co-author of *Oh, My Aching Back*, back pain is not a new phenomenon. We know for certain that it's been around for centuries, and it seems only logical that it's been an occasional and inevitable part of life ever since we humans first stood up and started walking around. Virtually every one of us will experience it at some point, although 9 out of 10 people with lower back problems—the most common kind—recover within a month. As for the chronic and debilitating variety, it will hit only about 5 percent of back pain sufferers.

Them Bones, Them Bones

To prevent back pain, it helps to understand how your intricate spinal system works and what can cause it to get out of whack.

The spine is made up of a series of ringlike bones called vertebrae. There's a total of 33 of them stacked on top of each other; 24 are separated by joints and the others are fused together. In the little tunnel created by the vertebrae runs your spinal cord, the superhighway of nerves. Impulses from the brain travel to the far reaches of the body via the 31 pairs of major nerves that branch off the spinal cord, and the same route is used for messages sent back to the brain from nerves as far away as your toes and fingers.

Sandwiched between the vertebrae are little shock absorbers made of tough fibers and cartilage with a soft center. These are called disks, and their job is to prevent the vertebrae from grinding against each other and to cushion the spine against pounding motions, such as when you jump off a wall and land on your feet. Together, the disks and the vertebrae help protect the spinal cord and allow for a great deal of

---

The Best Treatments for Your Aching Back

The standard treatments for back pain used to be bed rest for prolonged periods, muscle-relaxing drugs, heavy-duty painkillers, and even surgery. But many medical professionals now believe that you can sometimes make matters worse by relying too heavily on these options. To be sure, they're still used, but all of them tend to be limited to more severe or chronic cases.

The first order of business is to listen to your pain. If it comes while you're moving boxes, say, or doing some other physical activity, stop what you're doing. Then consider the following treatments suggested by Joel Press, M.D., medical director of the Center for Spine, Sports, and Occupational Rehabilitation at the Rehabilitation Institute in Chicago.

• Take a pain reliever. Aspirin, acetaminophen, or ibuprofen will reduce the pain.

• Rest, but not too much. If your back hurts, you'll want to take it easy for a while. But how long is a while? Studies have found that more than four days of bed rest can actually interfere with recovery by weakening your muscles. "You should do a little bit of gentle activity to get things moving," Dr. Press advises. "You don't want to stiffen up too much."

• Get it cold. "Ice is a very good anti-inflammatory," Dr. Press says. So wrap ice cubes or a bag of frozen vegetables in a towel and apply the towel to the sore spot. "Doing it 15 to 20 minutes twice a day decreases the spasms and it can block your pain," Dr. Press says.

• Get it hot. Applying a heat pack will also reduce pain, according to Dr. Press, but heat doesn't have the anti-inflammatory properties of ice. "So you might want to try cold first," Dr. Press advises.

The spine that runs down the middle of your back is divided into five distinct regions. There's the cervical or neck region, the thoracic region of the middle back, and the lumbar region, which roughly corresponds to the small of your back. Down at the end of the spine are the sacral and coccygeal (tailbone) regions.

Pain can strike in any of these regions, although problems in the lumbar area are most common.

The lumbar region seems to bear the brunt of back pain because it's located at the body's halfway point and acts as a sort of fulcrum.

Most back ache is the result of garden-variety muscle strain, and only 1 in 200 cases of back pain has a serious cause, such as a tumor or an infection of the spinal column. Here's a quick rundown of some possible causes of back pain and the symptoms they present.

Arthritis
Often there's a steady ache, rather than sharp pain, accompanied by stiffness in the back that may extend to your buttocks and thighs. The ache can show up anywhere along the spine.

Osteoporosis
Bones become brittle and can break. The back may ache and posture may become round-shouldered, stooped, or hunched. There can also be a loss of height, although this usually doesn't happen until after age 70. It is not only a women's disease; in men it relates to a decrease in testosterone.

Injured Disk
When an injured disk presses on a nerve, pain is severe, often located in the lumbar region, and made worse when you cough, lift, twist, or bend. If the pain runs from the lower back through the buttocks and to the feet, the sciatic nerve may be involved. In severe cases, there may be loss of bladder or bowel control.

Ankylosing Spondylitis
This is a rare form of inflammatory arthritis that usually affects men under age 40. Symptoms are lower back pain that's either periodic or frequent, morning stiffness in the back of hips that improves as the day goes on, stiffness around the ribs, and rib, chest, or neck pain. There can also be weight loss, fever, eye pain and blurred vision, fatigue, and loss of appetite.

Spinal Tumor
The pain is persistent, can be felt in any region of the spine and is frequently bad at night. There's often numbness, tingling, and muscle weakness that becomes progressively worse, and in some cases a loss of bladder or bowel control.

Strain or Sprain
There's soreness, stiffness, and periodic sharp pain if you move the wrong way. The pain is often in the lumbar region. It can either come on suddenly after an injury or physical exertion, or develop gradually.

Spinal Stenosis
The pain in the back and legs may be mild, but it frequently worsens when you walk and gets better when you sit. Numbness and muscle weakness may also occur.

flexibility. But to hold the spine in place and provide movement, your back also needs a complex set of muscles, tendons, and ligaments.

Any component of the spinal system can cause back pain. Your disks can dry out and rupture, muscles can cramp, ligaments can get inflamed, tendons can strain, vertebrae can chip, and nerves can get pinched or pressed. Although you hear a lot of talk about ruptured disks—also called herniated disks—they account for only a small portion of back pain. The prime cause is actually muscle strain, although identifying the exact source of an aching back is often difficult.

Caring for Your Back

You've heard this before in other contexts, but it's true all the same: The first step in keeping your back in good shape is to stay in good physical condition. "There's no question that people who are more fit will probably have fewer episodes of back pain," says Joel Press, M.D., medical director of the Center for Spine, Sports, and Occupational Rehabilitation at the Rehabilitation Institute in Chicago.

Thirty minutes of aerobic exercise three times a week—particularly low-impact activities such as walking, swimming, and cycling—keeps your back muscles, ligaments, and joints strong and flexible, as well as keeping your cardiovascular system in great shape. One caveat: Make sure you warm up thoroughly for 10 minutes before each session.

You also need to pay proper attention to muscles that provide crucial support for your spine, the most important of which are to be found in the abdomen and buttocks. "The stronger the muscles are, the more stress they can take off your back

during twisting and turning motions," Dr. Press says.

Here are a few other simple measures that should keep you and your back away from the doctor.
• Stay off the cigarettes. Medical researchers have discovered a definite statistical link between smoking and back pain. Nobody's sure why, but Dr. Press suggests two possible links. "If you smoke, you might not be getting a good supply of blood to the spine," he says. "Another possibility is that you might be coughing more,

and coughing increases pressure on the disks of the back."
• Remember to stretch. "Flexibility in certain muscle groups can have a protective effect," Dr. Press says. If you find you don't have a great deal of flexibility, you may want to join the increasing number of men who do yoga. After even just a few weeks, you will be amazed at how far you can stretch.
• Sit up straight. Take your Mom's advice to heart, and don't slouch. This is especially important if you have a job that involves a lot of sitting. "Bad posture, especially at the work site, is not uncommon," Dr. Press says. "With better posture, your muscles don't have to work as hard to hold up your back."
• Lift things right. Lifting a heavy load the wrong way is a real back-killer. "The most common way to hurt your back is to twist and bend at the same time as you lift something," Dr. Press says. "You should lift the weight close to your body while bending your knees." The same precautions apply to exercise. "If you're doing weight lifting, make sure you're doing it with the proper technique," Dr. Press says.
• Shed excess pounds. Flab, especially in the belly, isn't doing your back any good.

How to Protect Your Back

Lifting

When you lift a heavy load, always bend at your knees, keep your back as vertical as possible, and let your leg muscles do the work. And be sure to use the same technique when it's time to put down that same load. Guys who insist on bending at the waist when picking up or putting down something heavy put a lot of strain on the vulnerable muscles of the lower back. They also provide a lot of business for chiropractors and physical therapists.

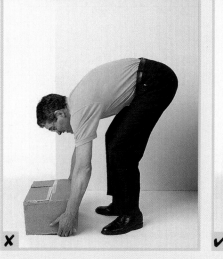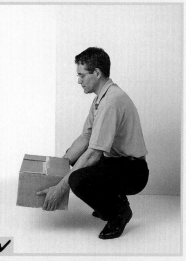

Carrying

You've correctly lifted a heavy box without bending at the waist, and now it's time to carry it across the warehouse. The way to protect your back is to carry the box as close to your body as possible. If you hold it away from your body even a slight amount, the strain on your lower back muscles increases dramatically. Also, avoid any twisting of your torso while you're holding something heavy.

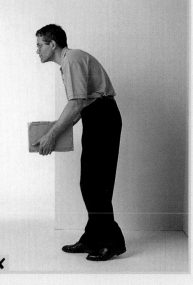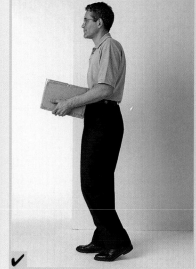

Sleeping

Protecting your back is one of the few things you can do in your sleep. Sleeping on your stomach exaggerates the curve of the lower back and twists the neck, so the best slumber position is on your back or side. It's important to have a firm mattress that can support your weight and keep your spine straight whether you're a back- or side-sleeper. And for side-sleepers, having a pillow of proper height will also help maintain a straight spine.

Sitting

The ideal is to be comfortably erect. Sit back in your chair so that your buttocks are aimed at the point where the seat and backrest meet, and keep your feet flat on the floor. Armrests are a good idea because they help decrease the load on your lower spine, and if you're in a straight-back chair, you may want to use a pillow in the small of your back for extra support. If you use a computer, position your chair so that you look at it straight on without having to twist or bend your neck.

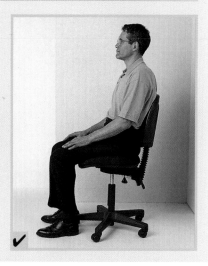

Sports Injuries

Our playing fields often sound like the fields of war. Teams "do battle," players "fight" for control of the ball, and coaches "plot" their strategies. There are blitzes, sudden-death play-offs, and sneak attacks. Sport isn't war, of course, but there is one resemblance: In sport, as in war, too many people get hurt.

What Causes Injuries?

Sure, the bang-'em-up team sports like football and rugby exact an injury toll. But the truth is, most sports injuries aren't caused by contact. More likely you'll get hurt on your own—often while you're cutting, pivoting, stopping short, or landing from a jump. "Those are the kinds of high-velocity movements that make your body susceptible to overload and strain injuries," according to Edward R. Laskowski, M.D., co-director of the Mayo Clinic's Sports Medicine Center in Rochester, Minnesota.

No wonder, then, that sports injuries often occur around particularly vulnerable areas of the body, especially the joints in your back, knees, ankles, hips, shoulders, and elbows. In each of these spots, there's a complex meeting of bone, muscle, cartilage, tendon, and ligament, any one of which can cause you problems if injured.

So if you overwork a part of your body, use improper technique, or fail to train sufficiently, you're asking for injury.

How to Head Off Problems

While sport and war both involve injury, in sport, at least, much of it is preventable. How can you prevent sports injuries? Simply pay attention to five things: muscle strength, flexibility through stretching, a proper routine, equipment, and alertness.

STRENGTH

You need to make sure that the muscles you use in your sport are strong. One of the best ways to do that is by lifting weights, even if your chosen activity is golfing, cycling, running, tennis, or something else that you don't always associate with pumping iron. "Strength training is very important for preventing injury," Dr. Laskowski says.

When sports medicine professionals recommend lifting weights, they're not talking about becoming the next Mr. Universe. Rather, Dr. Laskowski says, "You'd like to have a good base of strength in each isolated muscle group that you're going to be using in your sport. And you want what we call 'integrated' strength, which comes from, for example, leg presses, which use all the lower-extremity muscles the way they're used in walking or running or jumping."

Three moderately paced workouts per week—using the proper amount

10 Rules of Injury Prevention

1 Warm up properly.

2 Stretch slowly and thoroughly after you warm up and before you exercise.

3 Wear shoes that are right for your sport and that fit correctly.

4 Wear clothing that's appropriate to the weather and protective gear that's appropriate to the sport.

5 Start your workout slowly.

6 Learn and use the proper form and technique for whatever sport you choose to play.

7 Stop immediately if you feel dizzy, get abnormally short of breath, feel pain, or break into a cold sweat.

8 Cool down gradually after your workout or sport.

9 Stretch again.

10 Be alert to your body and your surroundings.

Stamping on Cramps

Muscle cramps, or spasms, are involuntary contractions of muscle: The muscle fibers contract and then freeze in that locked position, causing intense pain. Cramps may strike in any muscle, but the calf and foot are the usual victims. They can hit while you're exercising, in many cases because of dehydration or lack of flexibility. They're also common at night in bed, often caused by a sudden pointing of the toes.

The most important thing to do to prevent cramps is to drink lots of water, according to Edward R. Laskowski, M.D., co-director of the Mayo Clinic's Sports Medicine Center. "Dehydration is probably the number-one cause of muscle cramps." he advises. Also, he says, be sure to properly stretch your muscles. "If your muscles are really tight, it doesn't take much to set off a cramp," he says. You may decrease your chances of suffering night cramps by not tucking in your top sheet and blanket too tightly, sleeping on your side, and trying not to point your toes. If a cramp hits, stretching and massage usually help.

Sports injuries can happen to virtually any part of your body, but each sport seems to specialize in specific areas. With running, of course, most injuries are to the legs, ankles, knees, and feet, and other leg-injury-prone sports include aerobics, tennis, basketball, rugby, football, and soccer. Injuries to the hands and fingers, predictably, are common in handball, volleyball, and basketball. And baseball and tennis have more than their fair share of arm injuries—think of "pitcher's elbow" and "tennis elbow," different names for the condition medically known as elbow tendinitis. The chart below gives a quick view of the symptoms and causes of the ten most common sports injuries affecting men.

Back Strain
Pain, swelling and possibly bruising, frequently in the lower back, caused by a tear or stretch of a muscle or tendon. Often triggered by inadequate stretching and warming up and weak abdominal muscles.

Groin Pull
Pain, swelling, and possibly bruising on the upper, inside thigh. The cause is a tear or stretching of a muscle or tendon, and it often occurs during sudden lateral moves in basketball, running, and skating.

Knee Strain
Pain, swelling, and possibly bruising in the knee area, caused by a tear or stretch in a muscle or tendon. Sports of relatively frequent occurrence: running, cycling, and swimming.

Achilles Tendinitis
Pain and tenderness around the heel. The cause is inflammation of the Achilles tendon, which runs from the calf to the heel. It's often brought on by overuse, an inadequate warmup or stretch, and shoes with poor arch support or heel cushioning.

Foot Swelling
The symptom is self-explanatory and a common cause is running, playing basketball, or doing some other foot-intensive physical activity while wearing shoes that are worn out or don't provide enough support.

Shoulder Pull
Pain, swelling, and possibly bruising in the shoulder area. The cause is a tear or stretch of muscle or tendon, and the injury frequently pops up in baseball, racket sports, golf, and swimming.

Elbow Tendinitis
Pain and tenderness around the elbow that often becomes worse with movement. The cause is a tendon that's become inflamed because of overuse, but inadequate warming up and stretching can contribute to the problem.

Shinsplints
Pain in the front or side of the lower leg, caused by inflammation of bone, tendon, or muscle in the calf. Frequently the result of excessive running on a hard surface.

Pulled Hamstring
Pain, swelling, and possibly bruising around the hamstring muscles, which run along the back side of the thigh between the knee and buttocks. Inadequate stretching and warming up are often the trigger.

Ankle Sprain
Pain, swelling, and possibly bruising around the ankle are the symptoms, and the medical cause is a tearing or stretching of a ligament. Basketball, running, and racket sports are the usual suspect activities.

---

of weight, good technique, the right number of repetitions, and a day off between sessions—is plenty to accomplish those goals.

For full details on strength training, see "Exercises for Improving Strength" on page 92.

With strength training through weights, your muscles—as well as your tendons, ligaments, joints, and bones—won't feel the effects of physical activity anywhere near as much. And weight lifting may also help to prevent the gradual loss of bone mass called osteoporosis and the fractures that sometimes go with it.

STRETCHING
Proper stretching is vital to keeping your muscles and joints as flexible as possible. Together, the strength

from lifting weights and the flexibility from stretching let you move more easily and efficiently, thereby reducing the chance of injury and decreasing or eliminating altogether any postexercise soreness.

Unlike weight lifting, stretching is something you can do every day to maximize your range of motion. But don't rush into it. "If you stretch before exercise, warm up first," Dr. Laskowski advises. "You shouldn't stretch a cold muscle."

And when you stretch you'll want to work all the major joint–muscle connections in your body from the neck down through the shoulders, elbows, wrists, waist area, lower back, hips, knees, and ankles. Be sure to stretch slowly, until you feel a healthy tension, and then hold still for 30 seconds. And avoid tugging or bouncing motions.

For full details, including a complete stretching routine, see "Exercises for Improving Flexibility" on page 98.

THE RIGHT ROUTINE

Always start an exercise routine by warming up, regardless of the sport or activity. "Warmed-up muscles are going to be less likely to tear," says Tom Baechle, Ed.D., chairman of the exercise science department at Creighton University in Omaha, Nebraska. "Plus, warmed-up muscles pick up oxygen a little more effectively and therefore ward off fatigue."

Between 5 and 10 minutes of light exercise, such as walking or easy cycling, should get the blood flowing through your muscles, making them warmer and more flexible. See "Warming Up" on page 86 for the details.

Once you're properly warmed up, you can get into your main activity. Be sure to be fluid in your technique and to avoid short, jerky motions that cause unnecessary wear and tear to your body, particularly to your joints and connective tissues. If you've chosen a sport that's new to you, or you're uncertain about proper form and technique, get some instruction before you throw yourself into it. Not only will you protect yourself from injury, you'll perform better over the long haul.

Following the main activity, give yourself a cooldown period of easy, gentle movements to let your body slowly return to a relaxed, stable level of exertion. To end the entire session, you'll want to stretch one more time to help keep your muscles from tightening and aching. Do the same stretches you did before exercising, only briefly this time, and give special emphasis to the parts of your body that were used most during your workout.

EQUIPMENT

Make sure you use the right gear. "Equipment plays a role in injury prevention," Dr. Laskowski says. "For example, if you're going to ride a bike you better wear a bike helmet. Making sure the gears shift easily and the brakes are in good shape will help keep you out of trouble." Another good idea are the plastic safety glasses worn in sports with a high incidence of eye injuries, such as squash, badminton, football, soccer, racketball, and hockey.

As well, your clothes also should be right for both the weather and activity. In hot, humid weather, for example, wear clothing that's loose and light—both in terms of color and heaviness—and keep your head covered. When it's cold, Dr. Laskowski recommends keeping your skin covered and dressing in layers. Do that by putting on a polypropylene garment next to your skin to wick away sweat and prevent rapid cooling. The outer layer should protect against wind, although runners and cross-country skiers need venting to release heat. A hat will prevent heat loss through the head, and mittens will keep your hands warm.

Wearing the right shoes is essential to guarding your health during a workout. You don't need fancy shoes with a lot of gimmicks like pump-up action. Instead, focus mainly on shock absorption and support, the two things that are going to protect you most from injury. If you're a runner, for example, your shoes need to have good shock absorption and tread. If you play basketball, volleyball, or another sport that involves a lot of stopping and starting, your shoes should be able to absorb shock well but also provide support. High-tops are a good way to give your ankle support.

When it comes to footwear, it's absolutely crucial to find a good fit. Make sure that your toes have about a thumb-width's space at the front, that the ball of the foot fits into the shoe's widest point, and that your heel is snug and doesn't slip. If you wear the shoes often, they should be replaced regularly—as often as every four months. While they may look fine, the shock absorbing material in the shoes will have broken down.

ALERTNESS

Stay mentally alert during any physical activity. That may sound insultingly obvious, but injuries happen when you least expect them. Pay attention to your surroundings to avoid potential hazards, and tune in to your body to monitor your performance, watching for any warning signals, such as tightness or pain. The immediate benefits of staying mentally alert are twofold: You'll prevent self-caused injuries while improving performance.

The Best Treatments for Sports Injuries

Remember RICE: rest, ice, compression, and elevation.

Soft-tissue injuries
Following any soft-tissue sports injury, you should use the RICE formula for the first two days. Avoid unnecessary movements—that's the "rest" part of the equation—and apply an ice pack to the injured area for 10 minutes every three hours. If you don't have an official ice pack, ice cubes or a bag of frozen vegetables wrapped in a towel will do just as well. Compress the area by wrapping it with an elastic bandage that extends well above and below the injury. Be careful not to make it so tight that circulation is cut off. Finally, keep the injured area elevated—above the heart, if possible.

Fractures
Any sort of bone fracture—the classic "broken bone" or the microscopic breaks known as stress fractures—require treatment by a medical professional. If you have an obvious fracture, or if what appear to be soft-tissue-injury symptoms don't go away after 48 hours of RICE, see a doctor right away.

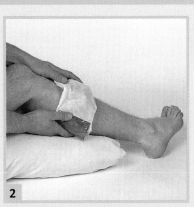

▲ Remove tight clothing and rest the injured leg on a soft pillow or cushion. Keep the limb still.

▲ About every three hours, place an ice pack wrapped in a cloth over the injured area, and leave it there for 10 minutes.

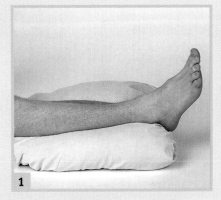

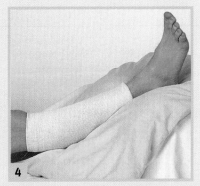

▲ Apply an elastic, compression bandage that extends well above and below the injury. Make sure it's not too tight.

▲ Elevate the leg to reduce swelling and speed up fluid drainage. The injured area should be above the heart.

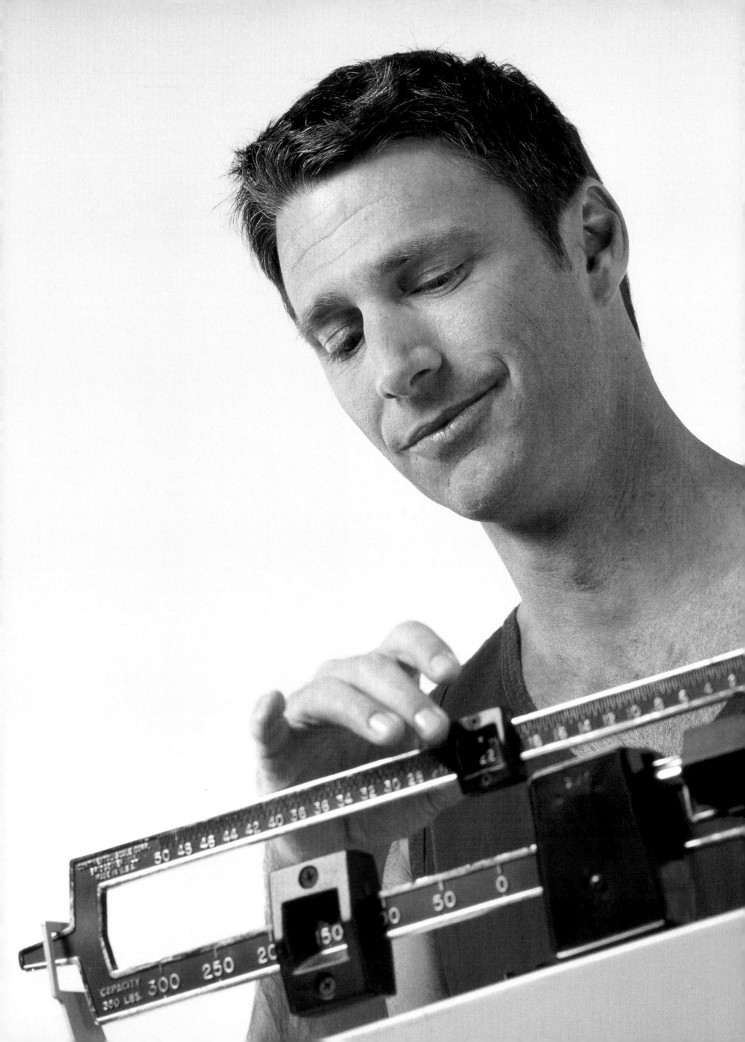

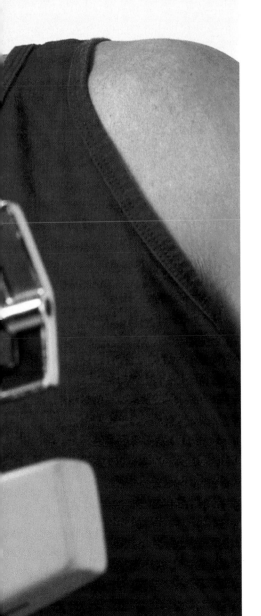

Major
Diseases
of Men

How to Be a Death Defier

Lifestyle factors are among the root causes of the big killers of men. Simply put, the choices are these: Stop smoking, exercise regularly, eat a healthy diet, don't get stressed out, and don't drink to excess. Follow that basic roadmap and you'll not only be alive longer, you'll live better while you're alive.

The Road to Wellville

When women are sitting around talking about men, one of the things they often laugh about is how guys would rather drive the streets aimlessly for hours rather than stop and ask directions. We have to admit there's some truth to that characterization, but we also like to think it stems from a basic male strength: We men prefer taking care of business on our own. We pride ourselves on our independence.

Top 10 Killers of Men

The World Health Organization keeps statistics on worldwide causes of death and disease. Medical researchers and health authorities use them to discover and promote preventive health strategies. Here are the 10 leading causes of death for men in developed countries of the world, in order.

1 Heart attack

2 Stroke

3 Cancers of the lung, trachea, and bronchial tubes

4 Emphysema and chronic bronchitis

5 Pneumonia

6 Traffic accidents

7 Suicide

8 Stomach cancer

9 Colon and rectal cancers

10 Cirrhosis of the liver

When it comes to our health, in many ways that's good, because even a cursory glance at the top 10 killers of men will tell you that any man who wants to take care of himself—and the fact that you're reading this suggests that you're in this category—can substantially reduce his risk of dying young.

If you put accidents to one side, a long, healthy life basically comes down to this:
• Sensible eating choices
• Regular exercise
• Avoiding harmful stresses
• Drinking alcohol only in moderation (about two glasses a day)
• Not smoking

Your health, in other words, is largely in your control, which is just the way most men like it. That said, there is at least one element of men's cherished independence that works against their health: They tend not to seek a doctor's help as often or as soon as they should. It just seems to be part of the male ethic to grin and bear it when you hurt. But while "working through the pain" may be a great attitude when you're on the third leg of a triathlon, it's a terrible way to manage your health.

RUNNING FROM THE DOCTOR

The fact that men are less likely than women to pay a visit to the doctor may be due to two factors. First, men like to think of themselves as being

"bullet-proof," according to Kenneth A. Goldberg, M.D., medical director of the Male Health Institute at Baylor Health Center, Irving-Coppell, Texas. They see going to a doctor as a sign of weakness.

Lisa Capaldini, M.D., an internist in San Francisco agrees, adding, "Sometimes there's a macho mind-set with men." In other words, for some men, admitting to pain or discomfort strikes at their masculinity.

The other factor that keeps men away from the doctor is fear. "Older men especially aren't as used to seeing doctors for regular maintenance as women. So there's a lot of worry and apprehension connected with an office visit," says Dr. Capaldini.

THE WAY AHEAD

But seeing the doctor is not a sign of weakness, nor should it be a prospect to dread. Note that in our table of basic preventive measures on the page opposite, getting checkups on a regular basis is a piece of advice that appears often, especially for men who are into middle age.

Think of it this way: You wouldn't let your car go for years without a mechanical checkup. Have the same respect for your body and it, too, will get you where you want to go. Even if you're not always precisely sure just where that is.

How to Avoid the Major Killers

Problem Area	Serious Problems	Risk Factors	Prevention
Heart and Circulatory System	Heart attack, stroke, angina, impotence.	Being male; having high blood pressure, diabetes, or high cholesterol; obesity; age; lifestyle (especially smoking, a bad diet, and lack of exercise); genetic predisposition.	• Stop smoking; eat a low-fat, high-fiber diet which includes lots of fruit and vegetables; lose weight; reduce salt in your diet; have a glass of alcohol or two a day (but not more); exercise regularly; reduce stress in your life; consider taking aspirin (but check with your doctor first). • Have checkups to keep track of your blood pressure and cholesterol levels.
Respiratory System	Chronic bronchitis, lung cancer, emphysema, pneumonia.	Being male; age; lifestyle (especially smoking); urban living; genetic predisposition.	• Stop smoking; avoid pollution, including radon and second-hand smoke; avoid contact with people who have colds or the flu; exercise regularly; eat lots of fruit and vegetables; avoid stress. • Check with the doctor if you have a chronic cough, if you consistently have trouble breathing, or if you spit up blood. • Get an annual flu shot.
Digestive Tract	Stomach, colon, rectal cancers.	Age; lifestyle (especially a high-fat, low-fiber diet); genetic predisposition; inflammatory bowel disease.	• Eat a low-fat, high-fiber diet; avoid salty, smoked, or pickled foods; drink moderately; exercise regularly. • Get regular checkups after age 40.
Prostate	Enlarged prostate, prostate cancer, prostatitis.	Being male; age; lifestyle (especially a diet high in red meat and high in fat); genetic predisposition.	• There is no known way of preventing enlarged prostate. You may be able to reduce your risk of prostate cancer by exercising regularly and eating a low-fat, high-fiber diet that includes lots of fruit and vegetables (red tomatoes and soy products such as tofu are thought to be especially helpful). Cut down on caffeine and alcohol. • Have regular checkups after age 50, or after age 40 or 45 if you are black or have a family history of prostate cancer.
Mental/ Emotional Fitness	Depression, suicide, and car accidents.	Stress; alcohol abuse; being young; having a risk-taking personality; irrational thinking; ignoring emotional problems.	• Recognize and deal effectively with stress; drink moderately; obey common sense; learn to think rationally; be willing to admit when something's wrong emotionally and take steps to deal with it.

Respiratory Disorders

Our lungs supply each cell in our body with the oxygen it needs to live and function. But increasingly, we are also breathing in anything from automobile pollution and cigarette smoke to bacteria and dog hair. So how do you stay well when you're surrounded by that junk?

Breathing Easy?

It's through our lungs that we have our most intimate, most consistent interaction with the outside world. We breathe in air once every five seconds or so, about 17,000 times a day, and our lungs carry the oxygen we inhale into the deepest parts of our inner selves.

But in today's world there's a price to be paid: A large number of pollutants—many of them man-made—get inhaled, as well as the life-giving oxygen. It's enough to make you want to hold your breath.

Keep Your Lungs Healthy

You can stay healthy by taking good care of your lungs. Breathing deeply, doing regular aerobic exercise, and avoiding the major pollutants (including cigarette smoke) are three simple ways to do it.

TAKE A DEEP BREATH

Most of us take shallow breaths, which are simply not as efficient as deeper ones at bringing fresh air into the system and getting rid of stale air. That makes our lungs work harder than they ideally should; it also increases stress.

Physiologists and yoga instructors recommend that you regularly practice deep breathing, concentrating on using the strong muscles of your upper abdomen—your diaphragm—to suck the air in, rather than relying on the weaker muscles of the upper chest.

Who's at Risk?

• Men who smoke: They increase their risk of death from lung cancer by more than 22 times, and from bronchitis and emphysema by nearly 10 times.

• City dwellers: Living in a city where there are significant levels of air pollution, and high concentrations of dust, molds, animal waste, and other allergenic substances, will increase your risk of many lung diseases, especially asthma. Stress may also be a factor. City dwellers are also more likely to be exposed to flu and cold viruses, which can lead to bronchitis or pneumonia.

• Second-hand smokers: A non-smoker who is married to a smoker stands a 30 percent better chance of developing lung cancer than one who isn't.

• Older men: As you age, your lungs gradually lose some of their natural elasticity, making you more vulnerable to lung disease.

• Heredity: In some cases of lung disease heredity is a factor.

What Happens When You Breathe?

The air you breathe passes through filters in the nose, throat, trachea, and bronchial tubes before it reaches the lungs. The lungs depend on the chest muscles and the contraction of the diaphragm to pull them in and out.

The bronchial tubes branch into smaller airways called bronchioles. Each of these in turn ends in a cluster of tiny air sacs called alveoli—there are millions of them. Oxygen passes through the walls of the alveoli and is absorbed by the capillaries which surround them, where it attaches to hemoglobin molecules in the blood. Oxygenated blood is carried to the heart, which circulates it through the body.

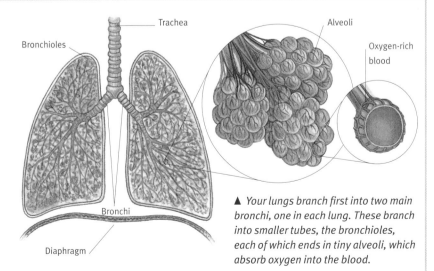

▲ Your lungs branch first into two main bronchi, one in each lung. These branch into smaller tubes, the bronchioles, each of which ends in tiny alveoli, which absorb oxygen into the blood.

Counting the Cost of Smoking

How does smoking damage your lungs? Let's count the ways.

Cigarette (or cigar) smoke contains tar, which is made up of over 4,000 chemicals, at least 43 of which are known to cause cancer. Another ingredient of cigarette smoke is carbon monoxide, a toxic gas which reduces the amount of oxygen the lungs carry to the blood. Smokers have been found to have 10 times more carbon monoxide in their blood than nonsmokers.

The chemicals in cigarette and cigar smoke irritate the bronchial tubes which carry air to the lungs, leading to chronic bronchitis, otherwise known as "smoker's cough." These same chemical irritants inhibit the immune system in your lungs, which makes you more susceptible to various types of lung disease, such as pneumonia.

There's more. The airways of the lungs are lined with tiny fibers called cilia. Normally, the cilia move rhythmically to sweep harmful material out of the lungs, but smoking destroys them. Hence, the lungs are less able to rid themselves of poisons, including the carcinogens in tobacco smoke. Smoking also gradually destroys the elasticity of the alveoli, the tiny air sacs which pass oxygen from the lungs to the blood. Eventually, the alveoli rupture, which starts a progressive, irreversible, and fatal condition called emphysema.

▶ *A cross-section through a healthy airway (top) shows numerous cilia, which keep the lungs clean. A smoker's lung (bottom) has few cilia and lots of mucus.*

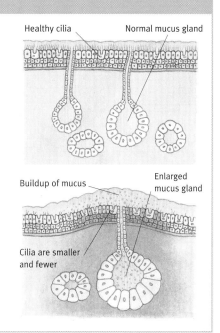

Healthy cilia   Normal mucus gland

Buildup of mucus   Enlarged mucus gland

Cilia are smaller and fewer

GET AEROBIC EXERCISE

According to Jay T. Kearney, Ph.D., senior sports physiologist with the United States Olympic Committee, aerobic exercise won't do much for your lungs themselves—they're built to have much more breathing capacity than we'll ever need—but it will increase the efficiency of the network of muscles that makes the lungs breathe in and out.

Aerobic exercise also will enable your body to process the oxygen your lungs take in more effectively.

AVOID POLLUTANTS

It's a dirty world out there, particularly in our big cities, and your lungs are paying for it.

Outside on any given day, you're likely to be inhaling a sickening combination of carbon monoxide, lead, ozone, and nitrogen dioxide; inside, you may be breathing doses of pollen, dust mites, viruses, radon (a natural form of radioactive gas which can seep from the ground into homes), formaldehyde, second-hand tobacco smoke, and asbestos, among other things.

To protect your lungs, you need to minimize your exposure to hazardous materials. That means:
• Stopping smoking.
• Paying attention to air-pollution reports and avoiding strenuous outside activity on days when pollution is at peak levels.
• Exercising early in the morning or at night, when ozone and other forms of air pollution are lowest.
• Making sure your home and your office are well-ventilated.

Ventilation is vital. Viruses, bacteria, fungi, and molds can flourish in air ducts, air conditioners, humidifiers, and carpets. Other sources of indoor air pollution include the glue compounds used in furniture, second-hand cigarette smoke, cleaning solvents, deodorizers, copy machine chemicals, and paint. Unless fresh air is circulating, these hazards can create a toxic environment that is dangerous to your health.

Lung Disorders

Unlike cancer, most lung problems are easy to recognize. You tend to notice when you can't breathe.

"We don't advise routine lung check-ups," says Norman H. Edelman, M.D., a medical consultant to the American Lung Association, "but we do advise seeing a doctor if you develop symptoms of lung disease. Those would include chronic coughing, coughing up blood, shortness of breath that seems out of proportion to exertion, or any chest pain that persists."

If you do need to be seen by a doctor, he or she will most likely give you a physical examination, listening to your breathing through a stethoscope. A breathing test may also be administered with a device called a spirometer, which measures your lung capacity by gauging the forcefulness with which you're able to blow into a tube. A chest x-ray is the other common diagnostic tool. Depending on the results, blood tests, sputum analysis, and other procedures may be called for.

On the following pages, you'll find an overview of the most common lung diseases. For more on asthma and on lung cancer, see pages 190 and 245, respectively.

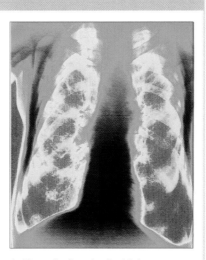

▲ *The red coloration in this lung x-ray indicates emphysema. There's no cure for this devastating disease.*

EMPHYSEMA

This disease results from a breakdown of the most basic process of breathing. Inside the lungs there are millions of air sacs called alveoli. Oxygen molecules from the air you inhale are emitted through the walls of the alveoli and into the blood carried by capillaries around them. Emphysema occurs when the alveoli lose their elasticity, become overstretched, and rupture. These ruptures, usually caused by smoking, are irreversible. If enough alveoli are damaged, you'll feel as if you're suffocating, which, in fact, you are.

PLEURISY

Each of your lungs is encompassed in a sac called the pleura which keeps it from rubbing up against your rib cage. The pleura consists of two layers of tissue separated by fluid. Sometimes infections in the lung, such as pneumonia, can cause either the pleura or the pleural fluid to become inflamed. This results in breathing or movement of the upper body becoming very painful.

BRONCHITIS

The bronchi are the large tubes in the lung. When they get inflamed, bronchitis results. Irritation causes the bronchia to thicken, which reduces the amount of air that can pass through them, making it more difficult to breathe. That difficulty is made worse by the mucus the lungs produce to help soothe the irritated bronchial tissues. People with bronchitis cough a lot, because breathing irritates the bronchi, and because they are coughing up phlegm.

Many people have a bout of bronchitis when they get a bad cold or the flu. The problem becomes more serious when it's chronic. Chronic bronchitis is medically defined as the presence of a mucus-producing

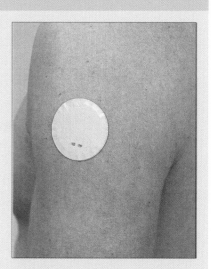

Threats to Your Lungs' Health

Believe it or not, it's likely that you'll breathe in and out at least six million times this year. That adds up to a lot of work for your lungs, but taken care of, they are more than equal to the task. "We're vastly overadapted in the lungs," according to Jay T. Kearney, Ph.D., a senior sports physiologist with the United States Olympic Committee. "We have a huge amount of pulmonary capacity devoted to getting oxygen to the system." Learning how to breathe deeply can help your body process oxygen more efficiently, but the real key to maintaining maximum lung capacity is not mucking up the works with disease and pollution. The table below gives you an overview of the six most common lung problems.

Condition	Symptoms	Causes	Treatment
Asthma	Difficulty breathing, tightness in chest, dry cough, wheezing. Symptoms manifest periodically in asthma attacks.	Colds, allergies (to pollen, dust mites, molds, fungi, pets, insects, foods, etc.), hay fever, stress.	Avoiding source or sources of allergies; drugs (often breathed in through hand-held inhaling devices called bronchodilators).
Bronchitis	Persistent coughing, phlegm.	Smoking, colds.	Stopping smoking; avoiding pollution; antibiotics; vaccination against flu.
Emphysema	Shortness of breath; coughing.	Smoking, air pollution, genetic predisposition.	Emphysema damages lungs irreversibly. Goal of treatment is to provide relief of symptoms (drugs, oxygen) and to prevent further damage (stop smoking).
Lung Cancer	Chronic cough, spitting up blood, wheezing, chest pain.	Smoking. In far rarer cases, exposure to radon gas or industrial carcinogens such as asbestos.	Surgery; radiation; chemotherapy.
Pleurisy	Painful breathing, chest pain.	Pleurisy is a symptom of other lung diseases, such as pneumonia.	Treat original cause; drain fluid.
Pneumonia	Symptoms vary, and include shaking, chills, chest pain, coughing (sometimes violent), difficulty breathing, mucus, muscle pain, weakness.	Bacterial or viral infection, sometimes precipitated by weakness of the immune system due to other illnesses or conditions.	Antibiotics (for bacterial pneumonia); rest.

cough most days of the month, three months of the year for two years in a row. Another name for the condition is smoker's cough.

PNEUMONIA

Pneumonia is not a single disease but a catch-all term for a wide variety of diseases that range in severity from discomfort to life-threatening illness. What they share in common is that the microscopic air sacs in the lungs (the alveoli) become inflamed and produce fluid, which makes it difficult for oxygen to reach the blood. The infection may be confined to one part of the lungs or it can spread throughout them.

Pneumonia is often a complication of a cold or the flu, and for that reason many doctors recommend a flu shot as a way of preventing pneumonia, especially for the elderly and those who have chronic diseases. A vaccine is available for the most common bacterial pneumonia, for those in the higher-risk groups.

Heart Disease

It's not hard to understand why the featured event in pagan sacrifices was the moment when the high priest ripped some poor guy's still-beating heart from his chest and held it aloft. Beating hearts have an undeniable mystical power: More than any other organ, the heart is the essence of the life force.

Your Most Important Muscle

A normal heart is a strong muscular pump a little larger than a clenched fist. Each and every day it will beat, meaning expand and contract, about 100,000 times, pumping the equivalent of some 2,000 gallons of blood through your circulatory system. When you're at rest, the entire circuit around the body takes only about a minute.

Each beat is sparked by an electrical charge from a bundle of nerve cells located in the upper right chamber of the heart. Called the sinoatrial node, it sends a jolt of electricity that makes your heart contract, pump blood, and relax, all in the space of about a second.

We tend to think of it sentimentally, but the heart is a workhorse. If you live to be 70, your heart will beat more than 2.5 billion times. Since your blood carries nutrients and oxygen to all the tissues of your body, from your brain to your little toe, it's important to keep the flow moving briskly along. Blood goes out from the heart through the arteries, and comes back, depleted of its oxygen and nutrients, via the veins. Your heart beats faster when you exercise in order to speed delivery of needed reinforcements to the cells which are doing the extra work: It's a case of supply and demand.

Like any hydraulic system, there's pressure involved in pumping blood through your body. The arteries expand and contract as the heart pumps blood through them. When you put your fingers on your wrist or touch your girlfriend's neck, the rhythm you feel is the pulsing of the arteries just beneath the surface of the skin. In and out, in and out: The body's pulse is an undeniably sensuous thing. No wonder vampires are attracted to it.

Keeping Your Heart Healthy

The most important thing to remember about keeping your heart in good condition is that it's a muscle, and like any other muscle it needs exercise to stay in shape. Also like other muscles, the heart needs a steady supply of nutrients and oxygen if it is to perform at its best.

The heart pumps blood to itself through a series of coronary arteries, which wrap like fingers around its surface. Blockage of the coronary arteries is the most common cause of heart disease.

Who's at Risk?

- Smokers

- People with high cholesterol

- People with high blood pressure (African-Americans and Hispanics are more likely to have high blood pressure than whites due to heredity and lifestyle factors)

- The physically inactive

- Men from adulthood to early middle age: They are more likely to have heart attacks than females of the same age group

- Older people: Studies show that about four out of five people who die of a heart attack are age 65 or older

- Those with a history of heart disease in the family

- Obese people

- Diabetics

- Those who drink more than two glasses of beer or wine a day

- Highly stressed people

Should You Have a Checkup?

As vital as the heart is to our health, we should keep track of how healthy it is by getting checkups on a regular basis, beginning in your twenties.

That seems pretty straightforward. The problem is that every doctor seems to have a different opinion of what the most sensible checkup regimen is.

Kenneth A. Goldberg, M.D., medical director of the Male Health Institute at Baylor Health Center, Irving-Coppell, Texas, came up with the following list. These may vary depending on your family and medical history.

- History and physical exam: Every 3 years; at 40, switch to every 2 years; at 50, annually

- Complete blood count: Every 3 years; at 40, switch to every 2 years

- Blood glucose: As needed to monitor diabetes; otherwise, every 3 years; at 40 switch to every 2 years

- Cholesterol: Every 3 years; at 40 switch to every 2 years

- Blood pressure: Every 3 years; at 40, switch to every 2 years

- EKG: Baseline once per decade

How the Heart Works

The heart is a hollow, muscular bag which in most adults weighs between seven and ten ounces. It's enclosed in a sack of tough tissue (called the pericardium) which holds the heart in place and protects it from rubbing against the lungs or the walls of the chest.

The heart is divided into four chambers: two atria on top and two ventricles on the bottom. Depleted blood returns from fueling the body and feeds into the right atrium. From there it's pumped down into the right ventricle, then up and out through the pulmonary artery into the lungs. There it's restocked with oxygen before being returned, via the pulmonary vein, to the left atrium. Finally it passes into the left ventricle and out through the aorta, where once more it begins its circulatory rounds. One-way valves keep the blood going from chamber to chamber without back-washing. When your doctor puts a stethoscope to your chest, it's the sound of those valves opening and closing that he or she is listening to.

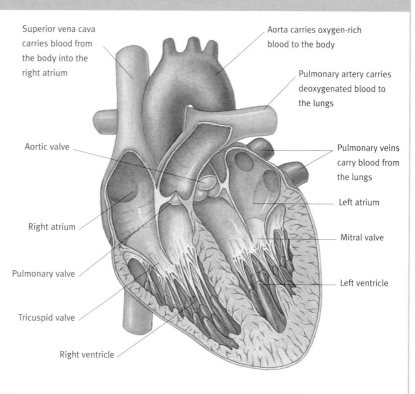

Superior vena cava carries blood from the body into the right atrium

Aorta carries oxygen-rich blood to the body

Pulmonary artery carries deoxygenated blood to the lungs

Aortic valve

Pulmonary veins carry blood from the lungs

Right atrium

Left atrium

Mitral valve

Pulmonary valve

Left ventricle

Tricuspid valve

Right ventricle

The Circulatory System

To maintain a continuous supply of oxygen and nutrients, and to remove carbon dioxide and other waste products, the blood circulates through the body along an ever-smaller network of arteries and veins like the root system of a tree.

Oxygen-rich blood starts its journey from the heart's aorta, the body's main artery. Once the blood has passed around the body, it is returned via a system of veins to the right side of the heart where it is oxygenated before it starts on its arterial passage once again.

Linking arteries and veins are capillaries. These tiny blood vessels have walls so thin that oxygen and other nutrients can pass easily into the tissues, and carbon dioxide and other waste products can pass in the opposite direction.

▶ *Blood is carried around the body by a system of arteries and veins. From the left side of the heart, oxygen-rich blood is pumped through arteries (shown in red) to tissues. Oxygen-poor blood returns through veins (blue).*

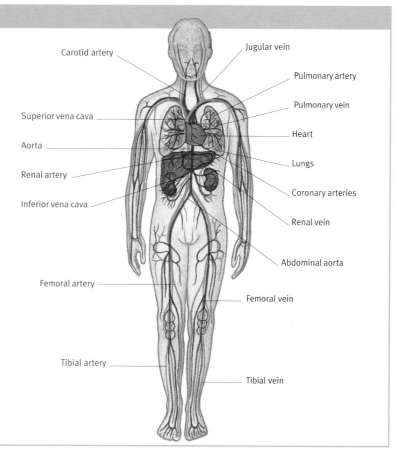

Carotid artery

Jugular vein

Pulmonary artery

Pulmonary vein

Superior vena cava

Heart

Aorta

Lungs

Renal artery

Coronary arteries

Inferior vena cava

Renal vein

Abdominal aorta

Femoral artery

Femoral vein

Tibial artery

Tibial vein

What happens is that fatty deposits of cholesterol and waste material build up and harden on the artery walls. The flow of blood becomes clogged—much as a buildup of hair and other gunk slows down the drainage of water from a shower—and the heart is deprived of oxygen and nutrients. Eventually, the arteries can become completely blocked, which causes a heart attack.

The buildup of fat deposits on the arteries is related to lots of other heart problems, which we'll discuss in more detail later.

FOOD FOR THOUGHT

Heart disease is not something you want to fool around with. We're not trying to scare you, but here are a few statistics to keep in mind.
- Heart disease is the leading cause of death in the world, accountable for some 7.2 million fatalities a year. Many more people are disabled.
- Various forms of heart disease account for about half of all deaths in industrialized countries, compared to only a quarter of the deaths in developing countries.

Hold the Salt

Some of us can't get enough salt. Popcorn, french fries, steak...we love to pour it on. But we're probably not doing our blood pressure any good when we do.

Salt is 40 percent sodium, and sodium can help raise your blood pressure by drawing fluid into the circulatory system. Doctors recommend that you limit your sodium intake to about 2,400 milligrams a day, but many people eat double that or more.

The salt shaker isn't the only place sodium gets into the diet. There's lots of salt hidden in many packaged and prepared foods, and in many over-the-counter medications, like antacids. Read the labels.

When a Good Artery Goes Bad

Clogged arteries cause heart attacks. Step by step, here's what cardiologists believe happens when an artery becomes clogged.

1 Somehow the protective lining of the artery wall gets damaged, possibly by high levels of cholesterol in the blood, by high blood pressure, or by smoking.

2 A buildup of fats, cholesterol and other substances begins to collect on the exposed artery wall. This buildup, called plaque, is accelerated by high levels of cholesterol and by smoking.

3 Fat continues to build in and around these cells, increasing the size of the plaque deposit. Plaque consists of a fatty core topped by a fibrous cap.

4 The plaque deposit causes the lining of the artery to thicken and harden, eventually restricting the flow of blood through the artery. The hardened artery also becomes more prone to cracking, which can create dangerous blood clots.

- Heart attacks, stroke, and other circulatory diseases kill a total of more than 15 million people a year, or 30 percent of the annual total of deaths worldwide.
- Almost twice as many men die from heart disease as from all types of cancer.
- You're seven times as likely to die from heart disease as you are from an accident.

HEADING OFF TROUBLE

Some people are genetically more inclined to developing heart disease than others, but bad habits are by far the greater danger. One major study found that men who smoked cigarettes and who had high levels of cholesterol were more than twice as likely to have a heart attack as those who didn't. Adding high blood pressure to the list more than tripled the likelihood of a heart attack.

Fortunately, the basic rules for keeping your heart healthy are simple, if not easy to follow: Eat low-fat foods, avoid being overweight, get enough exercise, and if you smoke, give it up. The goal is to keep those fatty deposits from building up on your arterial walls.

What clogs up the works faster than anything else are saturated fats. Meat, fried foods, and whole-milk dairy products are packed with them. Egg yolks and organ meats like liver will also send your cholesterol levels soaring. Cut down on these, and concentrate instead on the healthy stuff you've been hearing about for years: fruit, vegetables, and grains.

As for exercise, you don't have to be in training for the Olympics to achieve the desired results. You don't even have to take up a sport. Several studies have found that even

When You Need Treatment

You don't have to wait until you have a heart attack to find out that you're at risk for one. According to Louis J. Dell'Italia, M.D., professor of cardiovascular medicine at the University of Alabama in Birmingham, you should see a doctor about possible heart problems if you experience a diffused sense of discomfort through the chest area after any form of exertion. This discomfort can range from a feeling of pressure to a burning or squeezing sensation. It may also radiate into the arms—usually the left arm, although it could be both—or into the neck area. Shortness of breath after exercise may be another warning sign that the heart isn't pumping oxygen as efficiently as it should be.

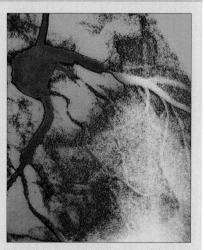

▲ This angiogram shows narrowing of the left coronary artery (where the red area becomes yellow).

Heart Attacks

One of the basic misconceptions about heart attacks is that they feel like somebody took a sledgehammer and smashed it into your chest. In truth, the majority of heart attacks are far more subtle affairs.

Most men describe them as being uncomfortable rather than painful—in fact, many heart attacks are mistaken for something else, such as a bout of indigestion or the flu. One study found that it takes most heart attack victims between five and six hours to get themselves to a hospital, usually because they don't realize (or don't want to realize) what's happening to them.

According to John Alpert, M.D., a cardiologist at the University of Arizona and author of *The Heart Attack Handbook*, typical symptoms of a heart attack are sensations of burning, heaviness, squeezing, tightening, or pressure in the middle of the chest, generally behind the breastbone. In some cases, these sensations spread to both arms, especially to the wrists, and up into the neck, jaw, or back—any one or all of these

the tamest forms of activity, from walking to gardening, can keep your cardiovascular system in good working order, as long as they're pursued five or more days a week. "The key is regularity," says John J. Duncan, Ph.D., a cardiology expert in Dallas, Texas, and former chief of clinical applications at the Cooper Institute for Aerobics Research. "It's just like

the pills the doctor prescribes: They work, but if you stop taking them, you don't get the benefit."

Nor need you worry about exercising for hours at a time, says Dr. Duncan. A regimen of 20 to 30 minutes of light to moderate exercise a day, five days a week, will do it. Men who exercise more strenuously can get away with less frequency.

The Facts about Cholesterol

Cholesterol is a soft, fatlike substance which the liver uses to help form cell membranes and hormones. Some of the cholesterol in our systems is produced by our livers, some of it we consume in the foods we eat. Eating foods that are rich in cholesterol and saturated fats, which many of us do, can lead to an excess of the stuff in our bloodstream.

Transported in the bloodstream, any excess cholesterol clings to artery walls as fatty deposits. The deposits may build up and obstruct the flow of blood to major organs, causing strokes and heart attacks. Given that some people have a genetic predisposition to developing abnormally high cholesterol levels, anyone over 20 ought to get a cholesterol test.

A reading of your total cholesterol level will usually do, although you can also get a full profile that will break out how much "good" cholesterol (HDL) you have versus "bad" (LDL).

A total cholesterol level of anything under 200 milligrams per deciliter (mg/dl) is considered "desirable." Readings that fall between 200 and 239 mg/dl are classified "borderline high," meaning your risk of heart attack in that category is twice as high as it is for men in the desirable range. Readings above 240 mg/dl will almost certainly call for substantial changes of lifestyle and, possibly, cholesterol-lowering drugs.

Many doctors advise that you have your cholesterol level tested every three years, and after 40 every two years.

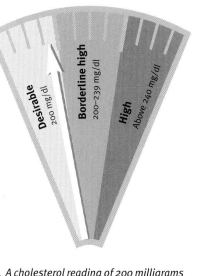

▲ A cholesterol reading of 200 milligrams per deciliter and below is desirable.

Heart Rate and Age

Did you know that we literally slow down as we get older? According to Gerald F. Fletcher, M.D., a cardiologist with the Mayo Clinic in Jacksonville, Florida, the rate of our heartbeat declines gradually through the course of our later life (although it may rise slightly in elderly people). That's because the heart's natural pacemaker—a cluster of cells called the sinoatrial node—begins firing at an increasingly mellower rhythm.

▶ *The graph shows how resting pulse rate declines with age. The cause? The heart's pacemaker gradually slows.*

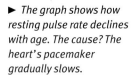

places may be involved. Sweating, nausea, or shortness of breath may also occur. The discomfort can last for several hours, which is why a heart attack can easily be mistaken for something less serious, such as a bad case of heartburn.

What should you do if you think you're having a heart attack? Get to a hospital without delay. "When the heart attack starts, every minute counts," says Paul Ridker, M.D., associate physician at the Brigham and Women's Hospital, Harvard Medical School. "Every single minute, cells are dying."

What actually happens during a heart attack? An overwhelming majority—like 85 percent—occur when an artery in the heart, already clogged by cholesterol deposits, gets blocked off entirely by a blood clot. The area of the heart supplied by that artery begins to die. The heartbeat is thrown into spasms, leading to cardiac arrest. At a hospital clot-busters can be given quickly.

Take the Heat Off Your Heart

When it comes to heart attacks, that old cliché can't be improved on as a piece of advice: Prevention is better than cure. By far the best way to lessen your risk of having a heart attack is to avoid narrowed arteries and other forms of heart disease in the first place. You can do that by controlling the risk factors that are within your control. Basically, that

Understanding Blood Pressure

Ever wonder how to decode those numbers when they take your blood pressure? The number on top (called the systolic pressure) represents the pressure of your blood when your heart is beating. The lower number (diastolic) represents the pressure when your heart's resting between beats.

When the systolic pressure is too high, it means your heart may be working too hard. If the diastolic pressure is too high, it's a sign the arteries aren't getting the break they need. In either case, high readings may be a sign of clogged arteries.

Blood pressure of less than 120 over 80 is considered a normal blood pressure reading for adults.

▶ *Your doctor uses an instrument called a sphygmomanometer to measure your blood pressure.*

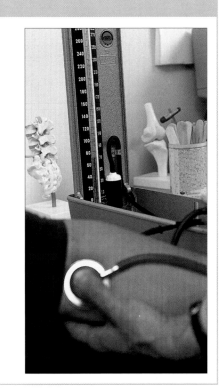

Threats to Your Heart's Health

Doctors don't always communicate with absolute clarity, so it's not surprising that they've come up with far more than the necessary number of names for the problems hearts can have. There's atherosclerosis (commonly called hardening of the arteries), angina (the official name is angina pectoris), hypertension (otherwise known as high blood pressure), and coronary heart disease (often called coronary artery disease or just plain heart disease), to name a few. One way to simplify this mass of terminology is to keep in mind that atherosclerosis occurs when cholesterol and other substances build up on the inner walls of arteries anywhere in the body. When the arteries in question are those that supply blood to the heart, you have heart disease. Heart disease manifests in various ways, which are described in the table below.

Condition	Symptoms	Causes	Treatment
Angina	Chest pain during exercise or stress.	Heart disease.	Drugs or surgery.
Arrhythmia	Fluttering sensations in chest or neck. In more severe cases, fatigue, lightheadedness, unconsciousness, death.	Misfiring of the heart's electrical system, often due to aging, high blood pressure, or atherosclerosis.	Medications. In more severe cases, implanting a pacemaker or various nonsurgical techniques.
Cardiac Arrest	Sudden, abrupt loss of heart function, leading rapidly to death.	All other heart conditions can lead to cardiac arrest. Differs from a heart attack in that the heart muscle typically doesn't die from a lack of blood supply—it abruptly stops beating, usually because of a disruption in the electrical signals that govern its beating (arrhythmia).	CPR; resuscitation within minutes by emergency medical workers.
Heart Attack	Feelings of heaviness, burning, or pressure in the middle of the chest, sometimes spreading to both arms and up into the neck or back. Sweating, nausea, or shortness of breath may also occur.	Blockage of coronary arteries due to atherosclerosis.	CPR; immediate emergency medical attention; clot-busters.
High Blood Pressure	None.	Unknown. Atherosclerosis a contributing factor.	Medication. In mild cases, reducing salt and alcohol consumption can help, as can exercise and losing weight.

means switching to a low-fat diet, getting regular exercise, and giving up smoking. And then there's stress.

THE DANGERS OF STRESS
Medical researchers are paying more and more attention to another potential risk factor: modern life. A number of major studies have shown that stress, anger, and anxiety can help set the stage for heart attacks. "Everyone has stress," says Stephen Hargarten, M.D., vice chairman of the department of emergency medicine at the Milwaukee County Medical Complex in Milwaukee, Wisconsin. "It's the management of stress that's the issue." Dr. Hargarten recommends the following regimen for de-stressing:

• Learn some relaxation techniques.
• Practice meditation.
• Get a hobby.
• Find some counseling.
• Ask your doctor about medication (in severe cases only).

Oh, and one more thing, says Dr. Hargarten, learn to look on the bright side: Don't forget to laugh every once in a while.

Stroke

Its name says it all: Short, sharp, powerful, and destructive, stroke is like a lightning strike. But like heart attacks—those other bolts from the blue—many strokes can be prevented by healthy living. And, like heart attacks, the quicker they're treated the better.

An Explosion in the Brain

They're called strokes, but perhaps a better way to think of them is "brain attacks." Just as a heart attack is an interruption of the supply of blood to the heart, so a stroke is usually caused by an interruption in the supply of blood to the brain.

Affected brain tissue starts to die, and the function of parts of the body controlled by the dead brain cells is impaired. The devastating consequences include weakness down one side, paralysis, loss of speech, and, of course, death. Surprisingly, though, stroke victims often have little idea of what's happening to them. "The brain is the organ that looks after you, and it's also the organ that's injured in a stroke," says John Marler, M.D., a neurologist at the U.S. National Institute of Neurological Disorders and Stroke, "so quite often the stroke victim is unaware that it's happened."

For that reason, it's often up to the people around stroke victims to recognize that there's a problem and to seek emergency treatment. Friends and families can also play a substantial role in helping stroke patients get the most out of rehabilitation.

Sad to say, in about 40 percent of all stroke cases, rehabilitation isn't an issue. Strokes are major killers, especially of men, ranking right after heart attacks on the list of mortality's Greatest Hits.

Who's at Risk?

- People who've had a heart attack, a previous stroke, or a transient ischemic attack.

- People with high blood pressure, high cholesterol levels, hardening of the arteries, or diabetes; smokers, the physically inactive, the obese, or heavy drinkers.

- Older people: Two-thirds of stroke victims are 65 or older.

- Men: They're 30 percent more likely to get strokes than women.

- People who've had episodes of atrial fibrillation (a type of irregular heartbeat), because they tend to have more blood clots in their system.

- People with high red blood cell counts: The thicker the blood, the more easily it clots.

- African-Americans: They have more than 60 percent greater risk of death and disability from stroke than white people.

- Those who have a family history of stroke.

Stroke's Angry Little Brothers

Sometimes strokes are preceded by little brothers, mini-strokes, which can serve as life-saving warnings of their bigger sibling to come.

They're called transient ischemic attacks, or TIAs. What happens is that an artery carrying blood to the brain gets blocked, but only briefly. Most TIAs last less than five minutes—one minute is the average—although they've been known to go on for 24 hours.

The symptoms of TIAs are pretty much the same as the symptoms of a full-fledged stroke. They include weakness or loss of feeling on one side of the body; vision problems, especially in one eye; problems talking or understanding; dizziness or loss of balance. The big difference is that with TIAs the symptoms go away without causing permanent brain damage.

Unfortunately, many people take the disappearance of symptoms after a TIA as a signal that nothing is wrong after all. Bad move. If you've had a TIA, you're 10 times more likely to have a stroke than someone who hasn't. It could come within a week, or within a few years, but don't gamble: Seek treatment immediately. Studies show that clot-busters can reduce the effects.

▶ *Transient ischemic attacks happen when an artery to the brain is blocked momentarily (top). The clot is quickly broken up, and normal blood flow resumes (bottom).*

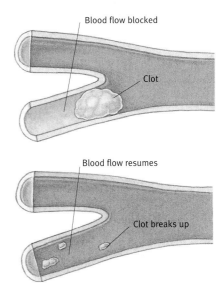

Blood flow blocked

Clot

Blood flow resumes

Clot breaks up

What Causes a Stroke?

There are two basic types of stroke: those caused by blockages—of which there are two kinds—and those caused by ruptures.

Blockages

By far the majority of strokes are caused when some obstruction—usually a blood clot—blocks an artery or vein that carries blood to the brain. There are two types. In one, the clot builds up on the blood vessel wall; in the other, the clot is swept into the blood vessel from elsewhere. The result is the same: The section of brain being served by that artery or vein then begins to die, which in turn disables whatever bodily function that portion of the brain was controlling.

Ruptures

The other major cause of stroke is when an artery or vein in the brain swells or breaks. These hemorrhagic strokes can be caused by high blood pressure, or because of a weak spot on the blood vessel wall. Such a weak spot is called an aneurysm. Some people are born with aneurysms, but they can also be caused by hardening of the arteries (atherosclerosis) or high blood pressure. Hemorrhagic strokes are dangerous not only because part of the brain's blood supply is lost, but also because blood from the ruptured vessel or artery spills into the tight confines of the brain cavity. That can create pressure—the brain is literally squeezed—which interferes with the brain's functions. The good news is that victims of hemorrhagic strokes often regain their capacities to function because the injured brain tissue can recover once the pressure is relieved.

Clot on blood vessel blocks blood

Clot from elsewhere blocks blood vessel

Blood vessel wall ruptures

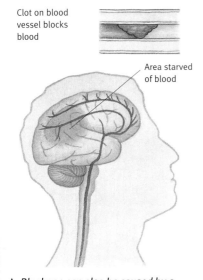

Area starved of blood

Area starved of blood

Area of bleeding

▲ *Blockage can also be caused by a buildup of clotting material on the side of a blood vessel wall. Again, the part of the brain served by the blood vessel is starved of blood and starts to die.*

▲ *A blood vessel to the brain can be blocked by a clot that's been swept in from elsewhere in the body. The blood supply to part of the brain is shut off, with potentially fatal consequences.*

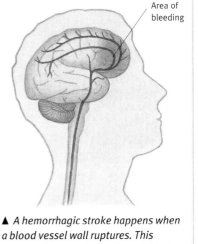

▲ *A hemorrhagic stroke happens when a blood vessel wall ruptures. This causes widespread bleeding within the brain or over its surface, resulting in pressure on the brain.*

An Old Man's Problem?

Doctors tell us that about two-thirds of the people who have strokes are over 65. Let's look at that figure another way. One-third of the people who have strokes are *under* 65. When you're talking about something that kills some 4.6 million people a year worldwide, that's not an insignificant number.

According to Thomas Brott, M.D., professor of neurology at the University of Cincinnati College of Medicine, young people usually have strokes for the same reasons older people do: blockages in arteries or veins that supply blood to the brain. Bad health habits are cumulative, but they can also kill you sooner rather than later.

Strokes caused by burst veins or arteries in the brain are more prevalent in young people than in old, Dr. Brott adds, because the weaknesses in blood vessel walls that cause such ruptures can be present from birth. Still, he says, that type of stroke is relatively rare.

Symptoms

- Weakness

- Numbness in the face, arms, or legs, especially on one side of the body

- Blurry vision or loss of vision, often in one eye

- Dizziness or loss of balance

- Difficulty speaking and understanding simple statements

- Severe headache

Prostate Problems

For such a little thing, the prostate seems to cause a lot of trouble—some guys end up wishing they could get rid of the thing. Perhaps it's best to be philosophical: As a man you don't have to mess around with having periods, do you? The prostate evens the score. It's part of the price you pay for being male.

The Worrisome Walnut

The prostate gland (technically, it's actually a cluster of glands) is about the size of a walnut. A lot of the trouble it causes stems from its location. It's lodged between the bladder and the penis, wrapped around the urethra, the tube through which urine is discharged.

That bear-hug proximity to the urinary tract means that when the prostate begins to grow (for unknown reasons), as it often does during middle age, the urethra gets squeezed, and men start stumbling around in the middle of the night, trying to find the bathroom.

Functionally, the prostate's position in the groin area makes sense, because its main purpose in life is to play a supporting role during sex. It's the prostate's job to manufacture the fluid that makes up about 90 percent of the milky semen you ejaculate when you have an orgasm.

Here's how it works. When you're aroused, sperm travels from the testicles upward through a tube called the vas deferens. The vas hooks into the urethra at the level of the prostate, where the sperm mingles with the prostate's reservoir of semen. At lift-off time—boom!—out they both shoot.

It's believed that the prostate's fluid assists sperm in transit and helps protect your sperm from some of the less hospitable female enzymes they're likely to encounter on their way to the uterus. Also, researchers believe the prostatic fluid contains chemicals that seduce the woman's cervix into relaxing.

The prostate gland also counts as a male erogenous zone: When it's busy churning out semen, it feels

Locating the Prostate

If your bladder were a blimp, the prostate gland would be the passenger cabin clinging to its underbelly. Like a doughnut, it surrounds the urethra—the tube through which urine runs from the bladder along the penis, which is why you can develop urination problems if your prostate starts growing larger in middle age. Most men's do. Note in the diagram how the vas deferens loops upward to carry sperm from the testicles so it can be mixed with the seminal fluid manufactured by the prostate.

▶ *The prostate gland sits under the bladder, in front of the rectum. Its job is to secrete fluid into the semen.*

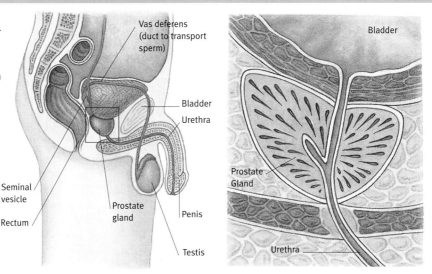

What Happens When the Prostate Starts to Grow

When the prostate gland enlarges in middle age, it can grow from the size of a walnut to the size of an orange. That can put a squeeze on your urethra that will narrow it from the diameter of a dime to that of a cocktail straw, a condition known as benign prostatic hyperplasia, or BPH for short. The condition varies greatly in severity. Treatment methods vary, but many doctors recommend treating BPH, at least initially, with a policy of "watchful waiting"—which basically means doing nothing, other than having regular checkups. That's because in some men the urination problems caused by BPH don't get significantly worse; in fact sometimes they even improve.

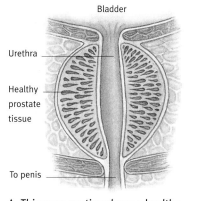

▲ *This cross-section shows a healthy prostate. Note how the urethra—the tube carrying urine and sperm from the penis—is wide and unblocked.*

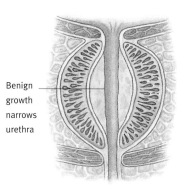

▲ *The prostate starts to grow, giving rise to benign prostatic hyperplasia, or BPH, in which the prostate puts the squeeze on the urethra. Shown above is a mild case.*

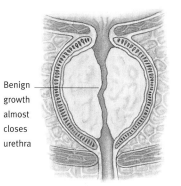

▲ *BPH may become so severe that only a very small part of the urethra remains unblocked. This leads to all sorts of problems with urination.*

good, and it's amenable to manual stimulation during sex by sliding a lubricated finger into the anus.

Heading Off Trouble

The prostate gland is basically a maintenance-free proposition until around middle age, but there are a few things you can do to help keep it in the best possible shape.

RELIEVE YOURSELF

Nature put the prostate in a crowded area of the body, so it's prone to getting squeezed for all sorts of reasons. For a sensitive gland, that can be very irritating. You can help keep the pressure off your prostate in three basic ways: Urinate regularly, don't sit in one place for too long, and—this is everybody's favorite—have regular sex.

STAY IN SHAPE

Research shows that men who are in good physical condition have fewer prostate problems. Our advice for heading off heart trouble holds for prostate health, too: Do 20 to 30 minutes a day of light to moderate exercise, five days a week.

EAT RIGHT

Your prostate will work best on a low-fat, low-cholesterol diet. It also craves vitamins A, C, and E. Get them by eating a wide variety of fresh fruit and vegetables, with special emphasis on green leafy vegetables like spinach, kale, and broccoli. Zinc also makes prostates happy: Oysters, soy, nuts, wheat germ, bran, eggs, pumpkin seeds, chicken, peas, and lentils are full of it.

Trouble with the Prostate

Recently, a middle-aged woman was overheard complaining to several of her female companions. "All my husband and his friends seem to talk about these days is their damn prostate glands," she said.

It is, admittedly, easy for guys in middle age to succumb to prostate preoccupation, if not prostate paranoia. According to James Hollander, M.D., associate director of the Beaumont Center for Male Sexual Function in Royal Oak, Michigan, men

Think about This

• Studies have shown that in some Western countries prostate cancer strikes about 12 percent of all men. About 50 percent have enlarged prostates. By age 85, those odds rise to about 85 percent.

• At last count there were some 193,000 deaths a year from prostate cancer worldwide. Of those yearly deaths, only 1,000 occurred in men who were less than 45 years old, and only 13,000 occurred in men less than 60 years old. After the age of 60, the number leaps to 179,000.

• More men in Eastern cultures such as Japan are adopting the high-fat diets of the West, so estimates are that by the year 2000 annual deaths from prostate cancer worldwide will have increased to 253,000.

Prostate Cancer: Prevention and Treatment

Since the causes of prostate cancer aren't known for certain, no one can say exactly how to prevent it, but several major studies suggest that eating a low-fat, low-cholesterol diet can help. Researchers specifically recommend eating more red tomatoes and soy products (tofu, soy flour, soy milk) and less red meat. Studies have also found that vitamins A, E, and D help inhibit the growth of prostate tumors in both animals and humans. Exercising regularly may also help.

Talk to your doctor about regular checkups. Many doctors recommend that men should have digital/rectal exams every year from age 40, and that you should start even earlier if you're African-American or have a family history of prostate cancer. As well, have a prostate-specific antigen (PSA) test every year from age 50.

With more and more men being tested for prostate cancer, doctors are finding that they can catch the disease at an

▶ *A cross-section of the prostate gland shows a cancerous growth, accompanied, as sometimes happens, by an area of benign growth.*

earlier stage, in younger men who have longer life expectancies. Because most prostate tumors grow slowly, older men with shorter life expectancies often choose to forgo surgery, partly because it can cause impotence. A new "nerve-sparing" technique has been developed for prostate surgery which can preserve potency, but it is more consistently effective at doing so for men in their forties and fifties, rather than those 60 and older. New techniques are also reducing the impotency rates in radiation treatment for prostate cancer.

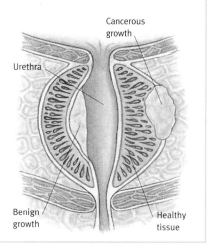

Cancerous growth

Urethra

Benign growth

Healthy tissue

condition. Other men elect to take medications which can shrink the prostate chemically. If the inconvenience becomes great enough, surgery—conventional, laser, microwave or ultrasound—is a common option.

As its name suggests, BPH is a benign condition. It isn't cancer, nor does it lead to cancer. You can reduce the nuisance factor by reducing your need to urinate, especially at night, by cutting out all fluids after 7:00 P.M. or so, especially coffee and alcohol, which tend to irritate the urinary tract. The same thing goes for spicy foods and cough medicines.

PROSTATE CANCER

Let's relieve some tension right now. Most men who have prostate cancer survive it. If you catch it early, before it has a chance to spread to other parts of the body, your chances of survival are almost 100 percent.

An even better reason for optimism is that most prostate tumors grow extremely slowly, so slowly that many men have prostate cancer for decades without knowing it. Gerald Hoke, M.D., chief of urology at Harlem Hospital Center in New York City, says the cliché among urologists is that more men die with prostate cancer than of it.

In fact, the odds that some other health problem will kill you before prostate cancer does leads many doctors to believe that there's no reason for men to be regularly checked for the disease, unless they have symptoms suggesting they have it.

Other doctors disagree, saying it's a good idea to start having prostate checkups every year after you turn 40. "Probably the best recommendation is that each man discuss the risks and benefits of testing and treatment with his physician so he can make his own, informed decision," says Otis W. Brawley, M.D., a medical oncologist who specializes

tend to have the same level of apprehension about their prostates as women do about their breasts. In truth, the odds are high that your prostate's bark will be much worse than its bite.

Two things may happen to prostates as men get older: They get bigger, or they develop cancer. Let's take them in order of likelihood.

ENLARGED PROSTATE

Nobody knows why prostate glands decide to start growing as men hit middle age, but they do. It may be caused by a change in hormones in the prostate. It's a condition doctors call benign prostatic hyperplasia, or BPH for short.

After a certain age most men have signs of it. Studies show that less

than 5 percent of men under 40 have BPH. That number rises to about 50 percent of men over age 60; by the age of 85 the odds hit 90 percent.

You may have BPH and not even know it. Often, however, a swelling prostate will begin to squeeze the urethra, causing problems with urination. These can include a feeling that you need to pee all the time (trips to the bathroom three or four times a night are not uncommon); feeling as if you haven't completely emptied your bladder; feeling that you need to forcibly push the urine out; feeling as though you want to pee but can't get started; and dribbling at the end of urination.

Most men simply put up with BPH, making annual or semi-annual trips to the doctor to keep an eye on the

Threats to Your Prostate's Health

The prostate is an oddball organ in many respects. It's the only one that continues to grow in adulthood, for example, and it shows an alarming propensity for developing cancer. In both cases, nobody knows why.

The good news is that the squeaky wheel gets the grease. The prostate makes a nuisance of itself with enough regularity that

medical researchers and doctors worldwide pay a lot of attention to it. That's shown by the fact that in many industrialized countries, prostate surgery is one of the most common operations there is.

That's the comforting thing about the prostate. If yours starts giving you trouble, you'll have plenty of company.

Condition	Symptoms	Causes	Treatment
Enlarged Prostate	Problems with urination (see below, "Prostate Cancer" symptoms).	Natural growth of prostate gland in middle age puts pressure on urethra.	Drugs; surgery. Many men elect to have no treatment.
Prostate Cancer	None in its early stages. Eventually problems with urination may develop, including a constant feeling that you need to urinate; a feeling that you have urine yet to pass even though there's none left; wanting to pee but not being able to; feeling that you need to forcibly push the urine out; and dribbling after peeing. Advanced cases may lead to impotence; blood in urine; swollen lymph nodes in groin area; pain in the pelvis, spine, hips, or ribs.	Unknown. Genetics and diet may be factors. The growth of the cancer tumor restricts the urethra.	Depends on age of patient and stage of disease. Surgery or radiation, if cancer is deemed life-threatening; drug therapies if cancer has spread beyond the prostate.
Prostate Infections	Fever; severe pain in lower abdomen and groin; chills; discharge from penis; painful or frequent urination.	Often unknown. Bacterial and viral infections; inflammation of urinary tract; sexually transmitted disease; stress.	For bacterial infections, antibiotics; for nonbacterial inflammation, warm baths, ibuprofen.

in research into the prostate, at the National Cancer Institute in Bethesda, Maryland.

Having a prostate examination isn't the way most of us would choose to spend an afternoon. The route to the prostate is via the rectum, which is exactly where your doctor will place a gloved index finger. He or she will be feeling for any lumps that might indicate a tumor. In addition to that annual indignity, many doctors recommend that men over 50 have an annual blood test called a PSA (for prostate-specific antigen), which screens for any signs of cancer that might be circulating in the system.

Prostate Infections

An organ as intimately connected to both sex and urination as the prostate is can be prone to infections, and in many cases doctors can't tell exactly what the source of the trouble is. "Prostate infections can hit at any age for lots of different reasons: a bacterial infection, a virus, inflammation of the urinary tract, even stress," says Gerald Hoke, M.D., chief of urology at Harlem Hospital Center in New York City. "Some men get prostate infections when the stock market goes down."

Whatever the cause, the symptoms are a high fever, severe pain in the prostate area, chills, and a frequent need to urinate. The penis may emit a puslike

discharge and you may have a burning sensation when you pee.

These symptoms may make you suspect that your supposedly monogamous lover has been playing around, but see a doctor—promptly—before making any accusations. A sexually transmitted disease could be responsible, but so could that cough medicine you've been taking, or those extra cups of coffee, even a stray bug from the swimming pool. If your doctor suspects it's a bacterial infection, he or she will treat it with antibiotics; otherwise you may just have to wait it out taking warm baths and ibuprofen to comfort yourself.

Cancer

Cancer is scary, but it's far from the hopeless killer it once was. Not only can it be cured, it can be detected early, before it gets too dangerous. Better yet, many cancers can be prevented. Of all the options available, not getting the disease in the first place has an excellent chance of being voted most popular.

It's Preventable, It's Curable

There are more than 100 different forms of cancer. All are characterized by one thing: Renegade cells override the body's natural control mechanisms and begin to proliferate unchecked. The cancer cells then spread through the body and work their way into healthy tissues, blocking off pasageways such as veins, eroding bone, and destroying nerves.

Enough of the grisly details. Cancer prevention is all about avoiding exposure to known cancer-causing substances, living a healthy lifestyle, and getting regular medical checkups to catch any malignancies that do develop while they're still in the easily curable stage. For specific tips on how to do all of the above, see the boxes throughout this section.

What Causes Cancer?

Often doctors don't know why cancer develops, but there are many causative factors. The two basic ones are genetic and environmental; both can work at the same time.

Some people inherit a predisposition to certain types of cancer that tend to run in families. Colon and stomach cancers are in this category.

Environmental causes are significant factors in a number of cancers. We can be consistently exposed to something that causes cancer (a carcinogen): Tobacco is one obvious example; direct exposure to high doses of nuclear fall-out is another.

Whatever the cause, how well you take care of yourself makes it more or less likely that a cancerous growth will develop. "We feel that

Who's at Risk?

• Smokers: About 85 percent of lung cancers in men worldwide are related to smoking; smoking is also a major cause of mouth, larynx, esophagus, pancreas, and bladder cancer.

• Those who eat poorly: Studies show that men who eat a lot of fats and few fresh vegetables are at greater risk of developing colon cancer and prostate cancers.

• Heavy drinkers: They have an increased risk of liver, mouth, throat, esophagus, and larynx cancer.

• People who've been exposed to radiation: Excessive exposure to medical x-rays can increase your risk of cancer, as can exposure to radon (a natural radioactive gas that seeps from the ground) in the home.

• Sun worshippers, especially those who are light skinned: They have a significantly greater chance of developing skin cancer if they don't protect themselves.

• People who've been exposed to certain industrial and chemical substances: These carcinogens include asbestos, arsenic, benzene, vinyl chloride, and PCPs.

Think about This

• The World Health Organization predicts that the number of recorded cancer cases will double in most countries during the next 25 years. A 40 percent increase in the worldwide incidence of prostate cancer is expected to be a significant part of that growth.

• Nearly a million men a year contract lung cancer. In most of the countries of the world, that rate is increasing, although in nations where smoking is no longer as prevalent as it used to be—the United States, Britain, and Finland, for example—the rate is falling.

• Cancers of the lung, colon, and prostate are the most common among men worldwide.

• The incidence of stomach cancer among men in most industrialized countries has fallen steadily during the last 30 years. Epidemiologists attribute the decline to better nutrition from fresh fruit and vegetables and less consumption of cured, preserved, and salted foods.

▶ The microscope reveals one of cancer's many forms—leukemia. At the top is a cancerous blood cell; below it is a normal one.

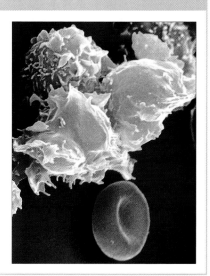

changes in people's lifestyles could reduce the incidence of cancer by about 70 percent," says LaMar McGinnis, M.D., a medical consultant and past president of the American Cancer Society. That means not just quitting smoking, but living a healthier life in general.

Researchers are paying a lot of attention to the roles diet and fitness play in the development of cancer. Diet seems to be particularly important. It's known, for example, that consistently eating high-fat, low-fiber foods increases your risk of developing cancer of the colon. Other studies have found that people whose diets include little fruit and vegetables have twice the rate of lung cancer as people who eat a lot of fruit and vegetables. That may be because of the presence in leafy vegetables of a nutrient called beta-carotene, or because of the vitamin E found in many vegetable oils. A third possibility is the fact that healthy diets are lower in fat, and fat is a suspected risk factor for lung cancer.

THE KNOWN CARCINOGENS
More than half of all cancer cases can be attributed to exposure to cancer-causing substances.

Probably the best-known carcinogen is tobacco smoke, which is the main reason that lung cancer is the most common cause of cancer deaths in the world today. Some

other carcinogens are radiation, radon (a naturally occurring radioactive gas seeping from the ground), ultraviolet radiation in sunlight, alcohol, and such chemical and industrial substances as asbestos, arsenic, vinyl chloride, PCPs, and benzene.

The likelihood of developing cancer increases proportionately with the duration and intensity of exposure to the carcinogen. For example, someone who smokes two packs of unfiltered cigarettes a day for 40 years is more likely to develop lung cancer than someone who smokes half a pack of filtered cigarettes a day for 10 years.

THE SUSPECTS
There's a long list of things that experts believe contribute to cancer, but they haven't yet been able to prove the connection. Air pollution is in that category. "There's a difference between what we know and what we think," says Otis W. Brawley, M.D., an oncologist and epidemiologist at the National Cancer Institute in Bethesda, Maryland.

Cancer Warning Signs
Cancer sends out a vast range of warning signs and symptoms. If you have any one of the symptoms, listed here, don't panic. All can be signs of

---

Is It Benign or Malignant?

A tumor is an abnormal growth of tissue that serves no physiological purpose. There are two types: malignant (cancerous) and benign.

Once individual cancer cells start growing, they form into tumors, which crowd out and eventually kill off healthy surrounding tissue. Many times cancer cells metastasize, meaning they migrate through the bloodstream or the lymphatic system to other parts of the body, forming tumors there. Benign tumors, those that don't have the potential to migrate, aren't cancer. All cancer tumors are by definition malignant.

The major goal of cancer detection is to catch tumors before they metastasize; once that happens, chances of a cure are more remote. The rate at which cancers grow and metastasize varies, although most cancers take years to spread.

Although it's important to watch for warning signs of cancer, the truth is that cancer symptoms are usually a sign that the disease is already at an advanced stage. That's one reason why trying to prevent cancer by living a healthy lifestyle and avoiding the known carcinogens is the smartest bet by far.

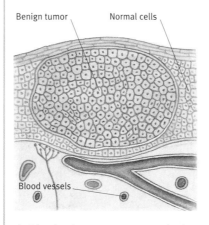

▲ A benign tumor grows among body tissue (here, the skin), but does not spread to the rest of the body.

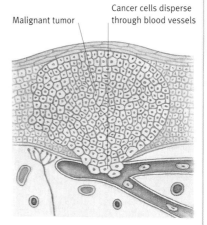

▲ A malignant tumor not only grows but migrates to other parts of the body, in this case, through the bloodstream.

How Doctors Fight Cancer

The first step doctors take in treating cancer is to assess how far the disease has progressed, a process called staging. Treatment strategies vary depending on the type of cancer, what stage it is in, how aggressive the cells look, and the personal characteristics of each patient. For example, an old man with heart disease may elect not to treat a slow-growing prostate tumor, whereas a younger man with a longer life expectancy would.

The basic cancer treatment methods are surgery, where the goal is to cut the tumor out of the body; radiation therapy, which attempts to kill the tumor by zapping it with highly concentrated beams of radiation; and chemotherapy, in which the patient takes strong anticancer drugs that stop the cells from dividing. Surgery and radiation therapy are used to treat localized tumors, meaning those that haven't spread to other parts of the body. Chemotherapy goes after cancer cells which have spread through the

blood or lymphatic systems. Often doctors attack the cancer on more than one front by using these methods in combination with one another.

Some experts believe that a newer form of treatment called immunotherapy will become an increasingly important weapon in the anticancer arsenal. The idea is to help the body's own immune system fight the malignancy by injecting anticancer vaccines.

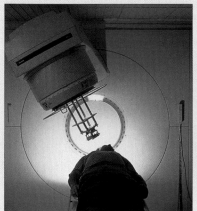

▲ This radiation machine may look ominous, but it's on your side.

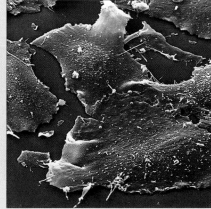

▲ What a human cell looks like after treatment—back to normal.

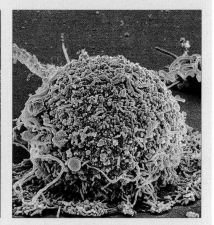

▲ Cancer cells like this one are the targets of all cancer-fighting strategies.

---

other problems, but they call for a visit to your doctor.

• Any change in bowel or bladder habits. Such a change can be a sign of cancer of any one of the colon, bladder, or prostate.

• A sore that doesn't heal can suggest mouth or skin cancer.

• Any obvious change in a mole or wart can signal skin cancer.

• Unusual bleeding or discharge. Blood in the urine, for example, could be a sign of bladder or kidney

> **"Cancer will always be with us. Prevention remains the best strategy for managing it, and that depends on the integrity of the healing system."**
>
> Andrew Weil, M.D., author of
> *Spontaneous Healing*

cancer. Blood in the stool may be a sign of colon cancer. Spitting up blood can indicate lung cancer.

• A thickening or lump anywhere on the body, including the testicles.

• Persistent indigestion or difficulty in swallowing food or drink can point to cancers of the stomach, esophagus, or throat.

• Chronic hoarseness or a cough that won't go away is a warning sign of lung cancer.

• Persistent, low-grade fever.

• A consistently pallid complexion.

• Unusual tiredness.

• A tendency to excessive bruising.

• Persistent headaches.

• Loss of appetite or loss of weight for no apparent reason.

• Any nagging pain that's felt in the bones or elsewhere, without apparent reason.

Every Man's Nightmare

Among the things we should all be grateful for is the fact that cancer of the penis is, as one expert put it, "incredibly rare."

Otis W. Brawley, M.D., a medical oncologist and epidemiologist at the National Cancer Institute in Bethesda, Maryland, says it's a condition that usually appears in uncircumcised men. That's why it's more common (though still incredibly rare) in Asia and South America than it is in the United States and Europe.

Penile cancer is also associated with chronic infections due to poor hygiene or sexually transmitted disease. Symptoms, Dr. Brawley says, include anything that looks abnormal on the surface of the penis, including a rash, a bump, a boil, or a sore.

Lung Cancer

Symptoms

As with many cancers, the appearance of lung cancer symptoms often indicate the disease is relatively advanced. Watch for a persistent cough and for blood in the phlegm. Chronic bronchitis, chest pains, and breathlessness can also be warning signs of lung cancer.

Treatments

Surgery; radiation therapy; chemotherapy.

► *The red splotches are cancerous areas in this x-ray of a man's lungs.*

Causes

Cigarette smoking is far and away the leading cause of lung cancer. Light smokers are 10 times more likely to develop lung cancer as nonsmokers; heavy smokers are 25 times more prone to the disease. Second-hand tobacco smoke is also considered a risk factor. Other, rarer causes of lung cancer include prolonged exposure to such chemical or industrial substances as arsenic, radon, and asbestos.

Prevention

• Don't smoke. Lung cancer kills more men worldwide than any other cancer, and 85 percent of all cases in men are tobacco related.

• Eat well. There's no proof yet, but some research suggests that beta-carotene, which your body converts into vitamin A, can help prevent lung cancer. There's also some evidence that selenium and vitamins C and E help protect the lungs against cancer. The best way to get the protection vitamins may offer is to eat five to nine servings of fruit and vegetables each day; the effectiveness of vitamin supplements has not been confirmed.

• Drink moderately. Studies have shown that heavy drinkers are more prone to lung cancer.

• Dodge pollutants. Avoid exposure to such environmental pollutants and chemicals as radon, arsenic, asbestos, air pollution, and second-hand tobacco smoke.

Colon Cancer

Symptoms

Any change in bowel habits which lasts for more than a week can be a warning sign of colon cancer. Blood in the stool is an even stronger indication of a problem and should be reported to your doctor. Watch also for any lumps or pain in the lower abdomen and for unexplained weight loss.

Treatments

Surgery; radiation therapy; chemotherapy.

► *The small, greenish area in this x-ray of the colon is cancer.*

Causes

Colon cancer usually develops from polyps in the colon. There is a strong genetic link as well: If anyone in your immediate family has a history of colon cancer, you are at greater risk. A history of inflammatory bowel disease is another risk factor.

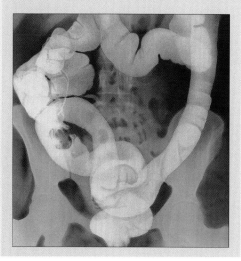

Prevention

• Know your history. If you or anyone in your family has a history of colon cancer or inflammatory bowel disease, greater vigilance against colon cancer is advisable.

• Get tested. All doctors recommend that all men over age 50 should be tested annually for microscopic signs of blood in the stool. Ask for a fecal occult blood test. Other, more invasive tests (rectal exam, proctoscopy, colonoscopy) are also recommended by some doctors, especially if you have a family history of the disease, or if polyps are suspected.

• Eat fiber. Numerous studies show that eating a diet that's high in fiber decreases your risk of developing colon cancer. Fiber-filled foods include grains, legumes (such as pinto beans), fruit, and vegetables.

Prostate Cancer

Prostate cancer generally has no symptoms in its early stages, but after a while problems with urination develop, including a constant feeling that you need to urinate, feeling that you have to really push out the urine, not being able to urinate, and dribbling after peeing. See pages 240 to 241 for full details on prostate cancer's symptoms, causes, and treatment.

Stomach Cancer

Symptoms

Stomach cancer usually has no symptoms until its later stages. Warning signs include vague discomfort in the abdomen, usually above the navel; a sense of fullness in the upper abdomen, just below the chest bone after eating a small meal; heartburn, indigestion, or ulcerlike symptoms; nausea; vomiting; swelling of the abdomen. All these can be signs of less serious problems as well.

Treatments

Surgery; radiation therapy; chemotherapy.

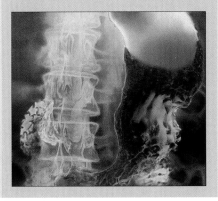

▶ The cancer-affected part of the stomach is obvious in this colored barium meal x-ray.

Causes

The exact causes of stomach cancer are uncertain. Risk factors include diets high in smoked foods, salted fish and meat, pickled vegetables, and starch. Smoking and alcohol abuse also increase your risk of stomach cancer. People who have a family history of stomach cancer are more likely to contract the disease, and roughly twice as many men as women develop it, probably because of poor lifestyle habits.

Prevention

• Eat right. Eating fresh fruit and vegetables that contain vitamins A and C appears to lower the risk of stomach cancer. It's also recommended that your diet contain plenty of bread, cereals, pasta, rice, and beans.

• Cut down on deli food. People whose diets contain large amounts of smoked foods, salted fish and meat, pickled vegetables, and foods high in starch have a higher risk of stomach cancer.

• Avoid bad habits. Smoking tobacco and abusing alcohol increase your risk.

• Forewarned is forearmed. Men are about twice as likely as women to develop stomach cancer. Extra caution is therefore advisable. Other predisposing factors to watch out for include having a family history of stomach cancer and (for reasons no one yet understands) having blood type A.

Liver Cancer

Symptoms

Loss of weight and appetite in addition to pain and swelling in the upper abdomen. Jaundice and anemia may also appear. A blood test can reveal elevated enzymes indicating the presence of a liver tumor.

Treatments

Surgery; chemotherapy; liver transplant.

Causes

Liver cancer is rare and often secondary to a malignancy elsewhere in the body. The two main causes of primary liver cancer are cirrhosis caused by alcoholism (more common in industrialized countries) and infection with a chronic hepatitis virus (more common in Africa and Asia). In some countries there are molds and fungi in certain foods (the aflatoxin mold on peanuts, for example) which can cause liver cancer.

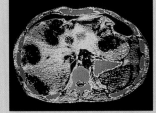

▶ This CT scan shows the liver (colored yellow) riddled with dark, cancerous growths.

Prevention

• Avoid hepatitis. The vast majority of liver cancer cases worldwide—some 83 per cent—are attributable to hepatitis B infections. Its close cousin, hepatitis C, has also been shown to be a risk factor for liver cancer. Avoid catching these viruses by practicing safer sex and staying away from dirty hypodermic needles. There's a vaccine available for hepatitis B, which people at risk of exposure (intravenous drug users and those practicing unsafe sex) should discuss with their doctors. There is as yet no vaccine for hepatitis C.

• Drink in moderation. Most liver tumors in the West are related to cirrhosis, which is usually caused by heavy drinking. Limit yourself to two drinks a day.

Testicular Cancer

Symptoms

The most common sign is a small, hard lump on one of the testicles, about the size of a pea. Other possible symptoms include feelings of soreness or heaviness in the scrotum or scrotal swelling. All these symptoms can be signs of problems less serious than cancer, such as bacterial infection or cysts.

Treatment

Surgical removal of testicle. Since the other testicle is unaffected, fertility is not usually compromised.

Causes

The exact cause isn't known. Testicular cancer, though rare, tends to strike men between the ages of 15 and 39. It may be spurred by the hormonal changes that occur at puberty. Men with an undescended testicle or testicles are at greater risk of developing testicular cancer, especially if the condition wasn't surgically corrected in childhood. Also liable are men with a family history of the disease.

▶ *Check yourself monthly for testicular cancer. You're looking for hardness, lumps, or swelling—things that could indicate the presence of a tumor.*

Prevention

• Examine yourself. If detected early enough, testicular cancer has a cure rate of about 90 percent. Watching for early warning signs involves no invasive tests; you simply give yourself an examination every month or so. A good time for it is right after a warm bath or shower, because the heat relaxes your scrotum, making it easier to get a grip on the situation. Stand in front of a mirror if one's available. Examine each testicle with both hands, rolling it gently between your thumbs and finger. Look for any lumps, swelling, or hardening—anything that seems unusual. Don't panic if you find something—not all such changes are cancerous—but do have it checked out by a doctor.

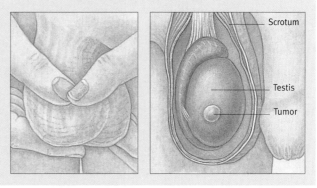
Scrotum
Testis
Tumor

Skin Cancer

The three main types of skin cancer

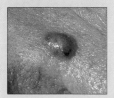

▲ *Basal cell carcinoma*

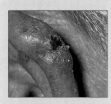

▲ *Squamous cell carcinoma*

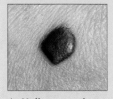

▲ *Malignant melanoma*

Symptoms

Any change on the skin, especially a change in the size, color, or shape of a mole or other dark spots and growths. These changes can include scaliness, oozing, bleeding, itchiness, tenderness, or pain.

Treatments

Surgery; radiation therapy; cryosurgery (tissue destruction by freezing); electrodessication (tissue destruction by heat); laser therapy. In rare, advanced cases, chemotherapy or anticancer vaccines (immunotherapy) may be used.

Causes

Excessive exposure to ultraviolet radiation, including sunlight, can cause skin cancer, especially in men who have fair complexions. Other risk factors include a family history of skin cancer and prolonged exposure to such substances as coal tar, pitch, creosote, and arsenic.

▶ *If you want to go out in the sun, remember to take some protection along.*

Prevention

• Protect yourself from the sun. The best way to avoid contracting skin cancer is to avoid sunburn, which means using sunblock and wearing protective clothing. To find out more, see "Don't Let the Sun Catch You Frying" on page 7.

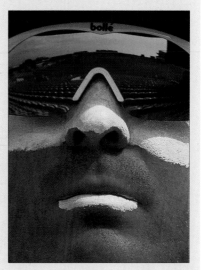

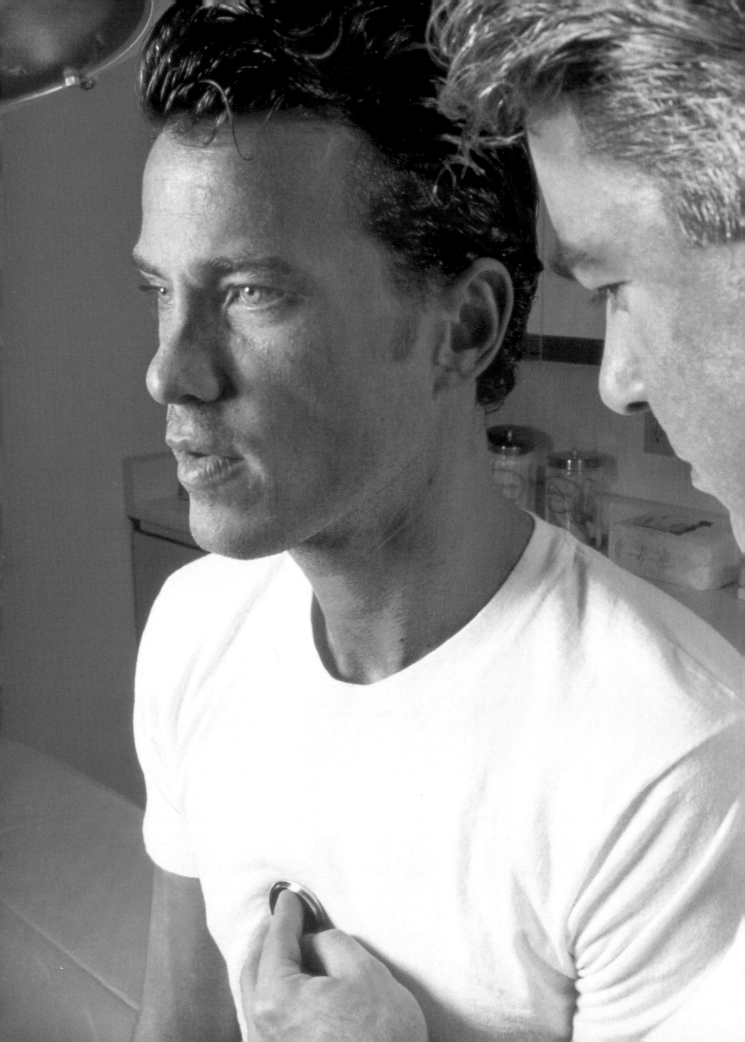

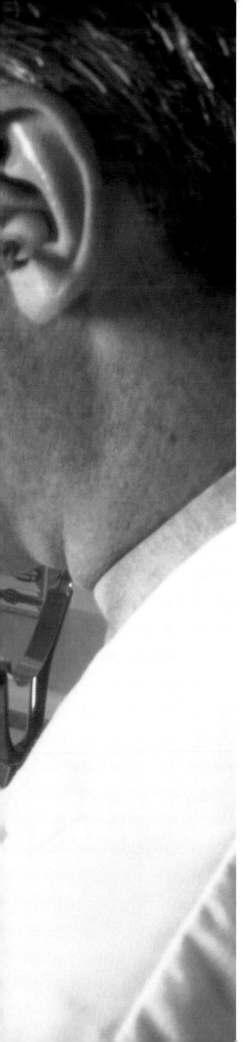

Getting
Medical Help

When Medical Help Is Needed

It's part of being male to try to tough it out on your own—to ignore pain, fatigue, anxiety, headache, sore muscles. There's one tiny flaw, though: We're simply not superhuman. Admitting our limitations is crucial to continued good health, as is the advice and support of a good doctor.

Look After Yourself

Many men go from age 20 to 40 without ever seeing a doctor. In our twenties, we don't go because we think we're invincible—nothing can hurt us. In our thirties, we imagine ourselves too busy with work and family. And when we hit our forties we're no better. "Middle-age men in particular are reluctant to call up for even an annual checkup," according to Margaret Lytton, M.D., a family practitioner at the Thomas Jefferson University Hospital in Narbeth, Pennsylvania. "We have to wriggle them in here."

The statistics bear her out. Men make 135 million fewer doctor visits a year than women, according to the National Center for Health Statistics. Surveys show that 30 percent of men have not been to a doctor in more than a year. For many men, seeing a doctor is often the last resort. And when they go, they hamper their own health care by tending to ask too few questions and convey too little information.

Unfortunately, these particular masculine foibles can be hazardous to health. On average, men die seven years before most women. The death rate from heart disease is twice as high for men as it is for women. Men also have higher death rates for a host of other causes, including accidents, suicide, murder, and alcohol-related conditions.

Why Men Hate Doctors

There's no shortage of theories about why men have an aversion to doctor's offices. Here are some you may hear in medical circles.

• We don't think it's manly. A man tends to see it as a sign of weakness if he even pays attention to a health problem, let alone get it taken care

Symptoms You Should Never Ignore

Don't try to decide whether you should or shouldn't seek medical help if you have any of these symptoms. Get to a doctor as soon as you can.

Chest Pain
Symptoms of heart problems can range from a crushing, squeezing pain that lasts for several minutes to vague chest discomfort, according to the American Heart Association. Let the doctor decide if it's only a case of heartburn.

Severe Shortness of Breath
It's normal to get winded from running up a flight of stairs, but if you're struggling for breath for no apparent reason, the American Heart Association says seek urgent medical help.

Unexplained Bleeding
When blood shows up in places where it doesn't belong, like the urine or stool, that's a red flag. "Rectal bleeding is always a reason to consult a physician," says Arvey Rogers, M.D., a professor of medicine at the University of Miami.

Dizzy Spells
Don't worry about that unsteadiness you may feel when you jump off the couch too fast to answer the phone. But, says Brian Blakley, M.D., an otolaryngologist in Winnipeg, Manitoba, "Dizziness can be a symptom of many underlying things." That includes stroke, so if your dizziness is severe or regular, Dr. Blakley suggests prompt medical attention.

Impotence
If you persistently have trouble getting and maintaining erections, that's reason enough to seek medical advice. But there's more. "Erectile dysfunction is a good indicator of diabetes or cardio-vascular disease," says Aaron Vinik, M.D., Ph.D., director of research at the Diabetes Institute in Norfolk, Virginia. "So it can be fatal."

Excessive Thirst, Frequent Urination
These symptoms, especially coupled with fatigue or weight loss, are warning signs for diabetes, according to the American Diabetes Association.

Failure to Heal
A cut that takes longer than usual to heal could be a sign that your immune system isn't working properly.

Lingering illness
Even normally manageable conditions like cold symptoms or a slight fever call for a doctor's visit if they don't go away after three days. "It doesn't matter if the symptoms are severe or mild," says Joseph Marzouk, M.D., of the Infectious Disease Medical Group in Oakland, California. "If they persist, you should call the doctor."

Top 10 Reasons Why Men See Their Doctor

- Persistent cough
- General medical exam
- Follow-up visit
- Throat problems
- Back pain, earache, fever, or skin rash*
- Vision problems

- Head cold or knee symptoms*
- Nasal congestion
- Stomach pain, headache, or high blood pressure*
- Depression

*Equal numbers of visits for these complaints.

of. After all, he's been told since childhood to "take it like a man." "It's just the way they're socialized," says Lorraine Fitzpatrick, M.D., associate professor of medicine at the Mayo Clinic in Rochester, Minnesota. "A woman is much more likely than a man to come in just because she's just not feeling right."

• We just haven't got the message. A man isn't told to think much about his body, so he tends to ignore the signals it puts out until symptoms are advanced. "Women have been taught by the media that they're supposed to come in for, say, mammograms," Dr. Lytton says. "Men aren't made aware of similar compelling reasons for them to come in, although there are plenty."

• We don't know the territory. With pap tests, birth control, breast exams, pregnancy, and childbirth, women are used to dealing with doctors. Men aren't. And the medical and economic systems seem to reflect that, according to Dr. Lytton. "It's accepted that women need to go for gynecological or obstetrical care," she says. "But the system may not bend as much to allow a male factory worker time off for equivalent medical care."

• We want to keep control. Our first instinct may be to try it our way. If we're having trouble urinating, we might think, "This will start clearing up if I just cut back on the coffee." So we try whatever we can before phoning for an appointment because

once we're in that office, the doctor's calling the shots.

• We're embarrassed. A lot of men don't feel comfortable talking about their health concerns, especially if they involve impotence, prostate problems, colon trouble, or urination. We're squeamish about doctors poking around the lower parts of our anatomy.

• We're afraid. "The effects of aging are something nobody likes to face," Dr. Fitzpatrick says. "Your first experience with chronic medication is a disturbing passage."

Change Your Mindset

Break down your resistance to medical care. A doctor isn't just someone to fix you when you're not well. Through preventive medicine, he or

Routine Tests for Men

There's no consensus among doctors and insurers on exactly what tests are necessary or how often they should be carried out. Futhermore, symptoms and family history are key to determining when testing should be done.

If those factors are absent, however, Kenneth A. Goldberg, M.D., medical director of the Male Health Institute at Baylor Health Center, Irving-Coppell, Texas, offers the following table as a rough schedule of routine medical tests for the health-savvy male, according to age group. Remember, though, that family history, medical history, or current symptoms change everything.

Begin in Your Twenties

History and physical: Twice in the decade; at 30, three times; at 40 every 2 years; at 50 every year

Complete blood count: Twice in the decade; at 30, three times; at 40 every 2 years; at 50 every year

Blood glucose: Twice in the decade; at 30, three times; at 40 every 2 years; at 50 every year

Blood pressure: Twice in the decade; at 30, three times; at 40 every 2 years; at 50 every year

Cholesterol: Twice in the decade; at 30, three times; at 40 every 2 years; at 50 every year

Urinalysis: Twice in the decade; at 30, three times; at 40 every 2 years; at 50 every year

Vision: Twice in the decade; at 30, three times; at 40 every 2 years; at 50 every year

Testicular self-exam: Every month

EKG: Baseline once per decade

HIV: Depending on sexual activity

Tuberculin skin test: Twice in the decade; at 30, three times; at 40 every 2 years; at 50 every year

Begin in Your Thirties

Hearing: Only if difficulties emerge

Chest x-ray: Only if you are a smoker

Begin in Your Forties

Glaucoma: Every 2 years

Digital/rectal prostate exam: Every year

After Age 50

Sigmoidoscopy: Every 5 years (with family history, substitute colonoscopy every 5 years at 40)

Blood in the stool: Every year

PSA screening: Every year (African-Americans or those with a family history of prostate cancer start at 40)

she can keep you healthy in the first place. Try thinking of your doctor as your coach taking you through the game of life—a trained professional who knows how to keep you healthy. The two of you should form a kind of partnership whose objective is to keep you active and productive to a ripe old age.

Pick a regular doctor and make an appointment for a physical examination. This usually means once a year or once every other year. Depending on your age, a routine physical will include recording your height and weight, checking your vital signs such as blood pressure, heartbeat and respiration; examination of your ears, nose, throat, and lymph glands; and routine screening tests appropriate for your age, such as cholesterol, hearing, or vision tests, and the dreaded digital/rectal exam of your prostate gland. The physical exam should include an interview with the doctor to discuss any concerns you may have.

Alternative Therapies

Remember when the only health-care choice you had to make was between this doctor and the other one? These days we're faced by an array of practitioners, experts in everything from acupuncture to Zen therapy.

While conventional medicine is most effective at treating acute conditions, especially emergency situations or grave illnesses, it's often less successful at managing chronic conditions, such as arthritis or migraine. That's where alternative therapies come in, and many are rapidly gaining credibility. The question is no longer a clear-cut choice between conventional medicine or alternative medicine, but how to integrate the treatments of both to maintain good health. The best care should take all options into consideration.

Use caution and good sense when selecting an alternative therapy.

In particular, always check a practitioner's credentials with his or her registering body, and never give up a conventional form of treatment in favor of an alternative one.

Here are three of the most popular and accepted alternative therapies.

Acupuncture
Used for at least 5,000 years in traditional Chinese medicine, acupuncture involves a therapist inserting very fine needles just under the skin at specific points. These points are believed to coincide with the body's "energy pathways" or *ch' i*, which flow along 14 invisible and interconnected channels.

Acupuncture can be used for a variety of health problems, but in Western cultures it's used primarily for pain control and to ease withdrawal from substance abuse.

Chiropractic
The largest category of alternative medicine, with some 50,000 practitioners nationwide, chiropractic therapy involves manipulation of the spine and joints to influence the body's nervous system and natural defense mechanisms. It's most commonly used to treat back problems and headaches.

Homeopathy
Greek physician Hippocrates first observed in the fourth century B.C. that large amounts of certain natural substances can produce symptoms in healthy people resembling those caused by disease, while smaller doses of these same substances can relieve those symptoms.

Samuel Hahnemann, a German doctor, developed a therapeutic approach based on this theory in the eighteenth century in which extremely small amounts of substances derived from plants, minerals, and animals are taken to enhance the body's resistance to disease and to alleviate symptoms.

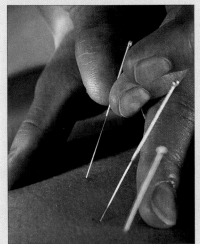

▲ *Acupuncture needles are said to stimulate energy pathways called* ch'i *when inserted into the skin.*

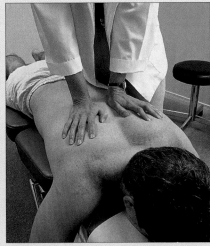

▲ *Chiropractors relieve pain—especially insistent back pain—by skillfully manipulating the spine and joints.*

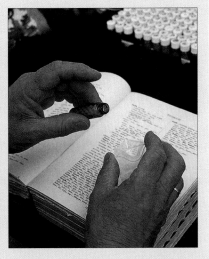

▲ *Based on a formula, a homeopath measures out pills which contain tiny amounts of herbal and other remedies.*

Top 10 Reasons Why Men Are Hospitalized

1 Cardiovascular surgery

2 Digestive system operation

3 Musculoskeletal operation

4 Arteriography and angiography

5 Urinary system operation

6 Cardiac catheterization

7 CT scan

8 Ultrasound

9 Respiratory system surgery

10 Skin and tissue surgery

It may sound elementary, but speaking up when you see the doctor is crucially important. Researchers have found that men are much more passive during doctor visits than women and may suffer poorer health as a result. Patients who are more effective at communicating with their physicians have better health outcomes. In studies of visits to the doctor, men asked fewer questions, gave less information, and displayed less emotion than women. In an office visit lasting 15 minutes, men typically didn't ask a single question, while women asked six.

Surveys also show that men are tongue-tied when it comes to discussing their sex lives with their doctors. But sexual functioning is a barometer of your general health, so it's important that you speak up about any changes or problems, says Aaron Vinik, M.D., Ph.D., director of research at the Diabetes Institute in Norfolk, Virginia. And don't wait for the doctor to bring up the subject. "It would be wonderful if physicians themselves asked the questions," Dr. Vinik says. "But very few do."

When There's a Problem

When you have a health problem, there are basically four ways to respond, according to Kenneth A. Goldberg, M.D., medical director of the Male Health Institute at Baylor Health Center, Irving-Coppell, Texas: You can ignore the symptom and wait for it to go away on its own; if it's a little more serious, you can treat it yourself, like bandaging a cut or taking a painkiller; you can also call the doctor; or you can rush to the emergency room.

TURN A BLIND EYE

Some symptoms are so mild that, with exceptions, if you're otherwise healthy you can safely put them to the back of your mind. A wait-and-see approach allows the body to heal itself without any interference.

There are, however, some seemingly minor symptoms that should be seen to immediately (for details, see "Symptoms You Should Never Ignore" on page 250). Apart from these, if your mild symptom fails to disappear after a week or so, see a doctor to be on the safe side.

TAKE TWO ASPIRIN . . .

Some symptoms, although still mild, require you to take action to relieve discomfort, like downing a painkiller or even just getting a little extra rest.

While treating the symptom usually results in temporary relief, you can also guess at the underlying cause and in some instances address that. For example, if you find yourself popping antacids every time you drink more than three cups of coffee, maybe it's time to cut back.

The vast majority of minor health symptoms can be handled this way. More serious health problems, however, defy self-diagnosis and treatment, and require the expertise of a professional. And while the list of symptoms you can treat yourself is very long, all can require a physician's attention if they persist or intensify. Learn to listen to the signals that your body sends out.

TIME TO CALL THE DOCTOR

When mild symptoms don't get better on their own, or with a little help from us, it's time to call the doctor. How do you know if a symptom has crossed the line and needs a doctor's attention? Joseph Marzouk, M.D., of the Infectious Disease Medical Group in Oakland, California, offers this rule of thumb: "If you have new and severe symptoms, or a persistent symptom, you should call a doctor," he says.

In other words, Dr. Marzouk says, take aspirin for a garden-variety headache. "But if it's a headache that's so severe you've never experienced anything like it before, you should seek a doctor's advice," he says. And if that headache doesn't go away for days, get thee to a doctor.

Keep a record and monitor your symptoms. Be objective, and resist the urge to minimize or exaggerate. The record can be a useful tool to assist your doctor with a diagnosis.

Don't ignore serious symptoms, such as shortness of breath, dizziness, severe pain, or unexplained bleeding, If symptoms are interfering with your ability to perform ordinary day-to-day tasks, you need to see a doctor.

IT'S AN EMERGENCY

When a symptom strikes that is suddenly debilitating or indicates a life-threatening situation, such as a heart attack, race to the emergency room. If you experience intense chest pain or shortness of breath, don't waste precious minutes waiting to see if it will go away. Time is vital to saving your life when an emergency strikes.

Checking Out the Doctor

Choosing a doctor is one of the most important health-care decisions you can make. It's important to find not just a doctor, but the right doctor—a medical expert who you can talk to easily. Establishing a long-term relationship with a doctor can help you live a longer, more satisfying life.

> **"Patients are less likely to volunteer symptoms if the doctor is trying to act like their parent. Male patients respond better if they feel like the doctor is a business partner."**
>
> Dr. Richard Honaker,
> Family Medicine Associates of Texas

Goodbye Marcus Welby

It's common to talk about choosing a doctor (singular), these days, but it's likely you'll select not a sole practitioner of the Marcus Welby type but a practice managed by a health-care system, which employs anywhere from three to a dozen doctors. If you belong to a health maintenance organization (HMO), you may find that your choices are limited to its selection of primary-care physicians. Even when your choices are restricted, however, you should still keep a watchful, informed eye on the medical care you're getting.

Training and Qualifications

Here's what Timothy B. McCall, M.D., a practicing internist and author of *Examining Your Doctor*, says about his fellow medical practitioners: "The quality of doctors varies enormously, and the quality of the doctor is the primary determinant of the quality of the medical care. Blind faith in physicians is like Russian roulette. If you want to get consistently good medical care, you should begin by examining your doctor." And the first part of that exam is to look at a prospective doctor's training and qualifications.

All doctors endure a rigorous education that includes college, four years of medical school, and usually at least three or four years of training. But not all are equally qualified. Board certification and hospital affiliation are especially important.

BOARD CERTIFICATION

Two-thirds of practicing physicians in the United States are board-certified. This means that the doctor has received extra training in a specialty and passed an exam. Research shows that you are most likely to receive care that meets at least minimal treatment standards from board-certified doctors. And, as Margaret Lytton, M.D., a family practitioner at Thomas Jefferson University Hospital in Narbeth, Pennsylvania, says, "You may want to know if a physician has a particular expertise in an illness you might have."

Check the credentials of doctors who claim to be certified in a specialty. And just how do you do that? "Patients are intimidated about asking," says Lorraine Fitzpatrick, M.D., associate professor of medicine at the Mayo Clinic in Rochester, Minnesota. "But there are ways to do it." She suggests: Call the American Medical Association office near you, or contact the American Board of Medical Specialties (ABMS) either by mail (47 Perimeter Center East, Suite

---

The Good-Doctor Checklist

Here are some questions that Kenneth A. Goldberg, M.D., medical director of the Male Health Institute at Baylor Health Center, Irving-Coppell, Texas, recommends you think about when choosing a doctor.

• Is the doctor board-certified in a specialty? Is his or her knowledge up-to-date through continuing education?

• Is the doctor affiliated with a hospital? If so, which one?

• If you need a procedure, ask about the doctor's training and how many of the procedures he or she has done.

• Does the doctor examine you thoroughly before deciding to order tests?

• Tests should be used prudently and sparingly. Does your doctor start with the least invasive tests?

• Is your doctor a good communicator?

• Does he or she explain things in ordinary language? Are you made to feel able to say what you want?

• Are cleanliness levels high?

• Does your doctor prescribe drugs sparingly and advise you about the possible side effects? Are the drugs prescribed the safest, most cost-effective choice?

• Does your doctor counsel you about a healthy lifestyle? Does he or she do routine screening tests to detect treatable diseases?

• Is there a hidden agenda? Do money matters appear to be the incentive in offering more or fewer services? Does the doctor seem preoccupied with being sued? Is the doctor mainly interested in research instead of treatment?

How a Doctor Reaches a Diagnosis

Doctors learn the pattern at medical school: interview, examination, diagnosis. Understanding this process may help you to get more out of your next interview.

The doctor starts by listening as you describe your symptoms. This becomes a dialog as the doctor asks questions aimed at finding out the details of the symptoms—their onset and intensity, for example. Depending on the illness, he or she may want to know about your medical history.

As this is going on, the doctor is mentally forming a rough diagnosis. A physical exam follows, based on what you've said. That will rule out at least some of the possibilities your doctor's been considering. If more information is needed, the doctor may order lab tests, such as x-rays or blood tests.

The interview and the exam are where a doctor collects the bulk of the data crucial to an accurate diagnosis. But because both are time-consuming, some doctors may rush through an interview, or fail to complete a thorough physical exam. Or worse yet, work backwards by simply ordering a battery of tests and "seeing what comes up." Timothy B. McCall, M.D., practicing internist and author of *Examining Your Doctor*, says that you can tell if the interview is inadequate if the doctor asks mostly yes or no questions, uses medical terms you can't understand, or seems rushed or distracted.

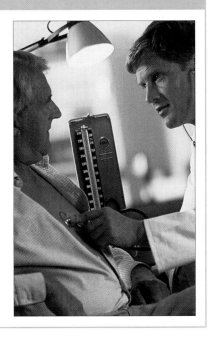

▶ *After listening to his patient, a doctor starts the physical examination.*

500, Atlanta, GA 30346) or through their Public Education Program Web site (www.certifieddoctor.org).

HOSPITAL AFFILIATION

If a doctor is not on staff at any hospital, or the hospital of your choosing, then he or she won't be available to treat you in a crisis. If the doctor is hospital-affiliated, then which hospital? Not all hospitals are created equal; some are better equipped than others, especially when it comes to dealing with emergencies and acute surgery. Also, check if the hospital is convenient for you.

Find the Right Fit

"Board certification shows you a certain level of competence," says Dr. Fitzpatrick. "But it doesn't tell you all you want to know about a doctor." It doesn't tell you if you and the doctor make a good fit. "You should find a doctor you like," Dr. Fitzpatrick says. " If a partnership is going to work the partners should feel comfortable with each other."

Set up a face-to-face interview with a prospective physician. Ask for a few free minutes of the doctor's time. If the doctor won't talk to you for free, either treat the first consultation as an interview or look for another doctor. A few well-planned interview questions can offer insight into the physician's style and personality.

According to Dr. Fitzpatrick, your "gut feeling" can help you judge how well the two of you will click. But you're also looking for two specific traits during the interview: an ability to communicate clearly and a willingness to treat you like a partner, not a child. You might want to ask questions like these:

• To what degree do you think patients should be informed about the nature of their medical conditions and treatment?

• What preventive programs do you recommend for a person my age?

• How do you feel about involving patients in decision-making?

Dr. Fitzpatrick also recommends getting other opinions. "Ask your friends what they like about their doctor, and what they don't like," she says. "You get a lot of insights that way."

You Deserve an Explanation

At one time, physicians often made all the decisions for their patients, but a new culture has developed in which patients are on equal terms. "In the past, patients took everything that a doctor said as the word from on-high," says David Vining, M.D., assistant professor of radiology at Wake Forest University's Medical Center in Winston-Salem, North Carolina. "But now they're much more skeptical and demanding."

Doctors are now required by law to inform you of your options before performing tests or beginning treatment. You have the right to expect your doctor to explain everything about your medical condition. If tests are ordered, your physician should review the risks and purpose of the procedure. When a diagnosis is made, the condition should be explained in understandable terms, as well as how you got it and what needs to be done to either cure it or treat it. The doctor should also point out alternative approaches and their risks and benefits, even the option of doing nothing.

Screening Tests for Good Health

A host of serious diseases and conditions—from high blood pressure to various forms of cancer—can damage your body before showing any symptoms at all. That's where screening comes in. Screening tests are designed to detect medical conditions before trouble starts.

Get Checked Out

The screening tests you need depend on your age and on various risk factors, and also on the philosophy of your physician. There's no consensus among doctors about which tests are needed, when men should start having them, and how often they should be done. Talk with your doctor to see what's best for you. For a suggested schedule of tests, see "Routine Tests for Men" on page 251. Tests will also be ordered if you report a specific symptom.

Family history is an important factor in determining when and what tests will be administered, according to Kenneth A. Goldberg, M.D., medical director of the Male Health Institute at Baylor Health Center, Irving-Coppell, Texas. Your doctor should order as few tests as possible to confirm or rule out a diagnosis, says Dr. Goldberg.

It's Just Routine. . .

Beginning in your twenties, a routine physical exam will include a complete blood count and tests to monitor the levels of cholesterol and glucose (to check for diabetes) in your blood. Your blood pressure is taken. Untreated high blood pressure can lead to heart attack, stroke, blindness, or kidney failure. A normal reading is less than 140 over 90.

"Fill this," you'll be told, as the doctor hands you a tiny jar. Analysis of your urine yields information about the overall state of your body, screening for diabetes, kidney function and kidney stones, urinary tract infections, the health of your liver and gallbladder, and more.

These routine screening tests are generally done with your scheduled physical exams. Depending on your age, a man's health regimen should normally include an electrocardiogram, a digital/rectal exam, prostate-specific antigen (PSA) screening, and checking the stool for blood.

Your regular self-testing should include a testicular self-exam (see page 247), a skin exam, an oral exam, and breast exam, Dr. Goldberg says. Inspect your skin regularly, checking for what the American Cancer Society calls the ABCDs: A spot that's Assymetrical, Border-irregular, Color-varied, or with a Diameter bigger than a pencil's eraser. "For the oral exam you run your tongue along the inside of your mouth, inside and outside the teeth," Dr. Goldberg recommends. "Feel for bumps." Your self-examination for your breasts is much like the test women do, Dr. Goldberg explains. Feel for lumps. "Actually, breast cancer is more lethal with men than women because it's picked up later," Dr. Goldberg says.

Blood Tests: What They're Looking For

With each heartbeat, blood interacts with every organ of the body, shipping nutrients and carrying away wastes. This intimacy means that most diseases and disorders affect the blood in some way, and also explains why doctors are so keen on getting your blood for a test. Here are some common blood tests and what they measure.

Complete Blood Count
The most basic test, it establishes the number and appearance of the various cells and components of the blood, how much oxygen they can carry, and how well they fight disease.

Blood Glucose
Elevated levels of this simple sugar, the body's main energy source, may indicate diabetes.

Bilirubin
A high level of this pigment, which is released when old blood cells are destroyed, may be an indication of liver disease or anemia.

Potassium
High levels may indicate kidney failure.

Sodium
An excessive amount in the blood can be due to dehydration or congestive heart failure.

Chloride
Low levels can be a sign of infection, intestinal obstruction, or severe diabetes.

Carbon Dioxide
Elevated levels suggest a lung problem, such as emphysema or pneumonia.

How Medical Imaging Shows the Inner Man

Sometimes diagnosing a disease or condition needs more than just a blood test. Doctors have at their disposal a range of sophisticated techniques that allow them to look inside your body without reaching for the scalpel. Here are some of the most common.

X-rays
Because x-rays have a shorter wavelength than light, they can pass through the body to produce a photographic image. They're mainly used to diagnose problems of hard tissue, such as bones and teeth. Sometimes doctors use a dye or other substance that is impervious to x-rays so that blood vessels and internal organs will show up.

Ultrasound Scanning
Like a depth-sounder on ships, an ultrasound scanner uses high-frequency sound waves to build up a picture of the hidden depths. The sound waves bounce off tissues of differing densities to build up a view of your internal organs. You're probably most familiar with it from its use in fetal monitoring. With men, it's used especially to view the heart, kidneys, liver, and eyeballs.

Computerized Tomographic (CT) Scanning
In CT scanning, a series of x-rays is taken from a source that rotates around the patient. Analyzed by computer, the x-rays are used to produce a clear cross-sectional image of body tissue, including bones and organs. A CT scan can detect tumors as small as a millimeter.

Magnetic Resonance Imaging (MRI)
In MRI, the patient lies on a couch surrounded by a huge electromagnet and is exposed to bursts of strong magnetic fields and radio waves. This causes atoms in the patient's body to give off radio signals, which are analyzed by computer and made into an extremely clear image that is basically a "slice" though the body. MRI is particularly useful for showing the brain and spinal cord in detail, and changes in the heart muscle following a heart attack.

▲ A chest x-ray is one of the most common of all tests.

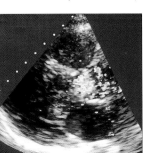
▲ Ultrasound relies on high-frequency sound waves.

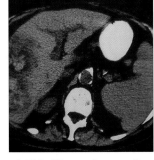
▲ This CT scan shows a slice through the abdomen.

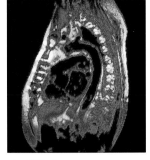
▲ MRI gives a cross-sectional view of the thorax.

ELECTROCARDIOGRAM
Electrodes attached to your wrists, ankles, and chest pick up the heart's electrical activity. Abnormal readings can indicate heart disease.

Have a baseline EKG every decade starting in your twenties. Family history and symptoms such as cholesterol or blood pressure will determine how early you should take a stress EKG, Dr. Goldberg says.

A baseline EKG, done while you are lying down, will show the electrical activity of your heart at rest. It shows what's normal for you at that age, and becomes a very useful standard against which subsequent EKGs can be compared.

A stress EKG is taken while you're placing stress on your heart, usually by walking on a treadmill. It shows whether the heart is working normally during physical activity.

DIGITAL/RECTAL PROSTATE EXAM
It has to be done: A doctor inserts a finger into the rectum to check for (among other things) prostate swelling, an early sign of prostate cancer, and for rectal cancer. Experts disagree about when you should start having this test. The American Cancer Society recommends a yearly exam for men over age 40, while others say it should be done every two years. Discuss it with your doctor.

PSA SCREENING
The PSA blood test is usually recommended annually after 50. Higher risk groups—African-Americans and those with a family history—should start at age 40. The PSA test measures the level of prostate-specific antigen in your blood. This is a type of protein often found in high levels in men with prostate cancer. Unfortunately, PSA test results can be less than accurate, so as a back-up you should have a digital/rectal exam at the same time.

If elevated PSA levels are found, that doesn't necessarily mean prostate cancer is present, Dr. Goldberg points out. They could be signalling an infection, or simply prostate enlargement. They could even possibly be elevated due to an ejaculation in the last 48 hours. But your doctor will want to do more tests.

Drug Treatments

The range and number of medical drugs today is staggering: Over 8,000 are available, and another new drug is approved every two or three weeks. Millions of people experience their benefits, but drugs are not "magic bullets"; they're powerful chemicals that need to be handled with care.

Take Your Medicine—Wisely

Drug treatments are used either to cure an ailment, as is the case when you eliminate infection with antibiotics, or to treat a symptom, which is often the situation with chronic conditions, such as arthritis and asthma. Whatever they're used for, drugs should be prescribed sparingly and with a rundown of the side effects. Next time you're prescribed a drug, ask yourself these questions: Do you come away from your doctor understanding exactly why you've been given this particular drug? Or why you had to have medication at all? Or what the risks of side effects are? Many people don't.

When you're next offered a prescription, make sure to get all the facts; that way, can you make an informed decision about whether to take your medicine. If you decide you do need it, always follow directions. And ask your doctor about foods or drugs (including alcohol) that you should avoid during the course of the treatment.

How Drugs Do Their Stuff

When you pop a pill, you're setting up a kind of partnership between your body and the drug. All drugs, in other words, interact with your body in some way to achieve their intended effect. They do this in three main ways: by changing the way the body's cells react, by destroying invading organisms, or by causing a chemical reaction.

Many of the most commonly prescribed medicines, including some used for heart disease, ulcers, allergies, and glaucoma, act either on or in the cells of the body. Like a finger fits in a glove, such drug compounds have physical and chemical properties that fit a receptor site on certain cells in the body. Depending on how

How Drugs Work

When you swallow a tablet, you set off a complex chemical event in your body. Normally, a drug taken by mouth takes about an hour to be absorbed and distributed to its target in the body.

With the help of a little water and some muscle contractions, the pill travels down your esophagus to your stomach.

The acids in the stomach begin to break down the pill into molecules. Some pills are coated, and stay intact through the assault of stomach acids. Drugs of this type travel further down the digestive tract to the intestine before being converted into a molecular form.

The molecules pass into blood vessels surrounding the stomach and intestine, and go to the liver to be broken down further.

From the liver, the drug is distributed around the body by the bloodstream.

A tiny percentage of the drug reaches its target.

Esophagus

Liver

Stomach

Bloodstream

Intestine

Blood vessels

The 10 Most Commonly Prescribed Drugs

Well-informed patients know exactly what they're putting into their bodies. The table below lists 10 of the nation's most commonly prescribed drugs, their generic name, what condition a drug is prescribed for, and a list of adverse reactions and side effects experienced by more than 1 percent of people who take a drug.

Brand Name	Generic Name	Reason for Use	Adverse Reactions/Side Effects
Amoxil	Amoxicillin	Antibiotic for treatment of infections of the ear, nose, throat, genitourinary tract, and lower respiratory tract.	Diarrhea, nausea, vomiting. Possible allergic reaction to penicillin.
Coumadin	Warfarin	Anticoagulant prescribed to treat blood clots and reduce the risk of death in recurrent heart attacks and strokes.	Hemorrhage.
Lanoxin	Digoxin	To treat heart failure and regulate heart rate.	Change in heartbeat, headache, dizziness, vision disturbances, lower stomach pain, weakness, loss of appetite.
Prilosec	Omeprazole	Ulcer medication to suppress gastric acid secretion.	Abdominal pain, constipation, diarrhea, flatulence, nausea, vomiting, acid regurgitation, headache.
Procardia	Nifedipine	Calcium channel-blocker used to treat angina.	Cough, dizziness, headache, heartburn, low blood pressure, light-headedness, flushing, weakness, muscle cramps, palpitations, swelling of the hands and feet, nausea, nervousness, nasal congestion, sore throat.
Prozac	Fluoxetine hydrochloride	Antidepressant used for the treatment of depression and obsessive–compulsive disorder.	Skin rash, hives, fatigue, sweating, gastrointestinal complaints; may interfere with cognitive and motor performance.
Vasotec	Enalapril maleate	For treatment of high blood pressure.	Fatigue, headache, dizziness; less frequently, diarrhea, nausea, impotence, ringing in the ears, cough, skin rash.
Zantac	Ranitidine hydrochloride	For treatment of duodenal and gastric ulcers.	Headache, constipation, diarrhea, nausea, vomiting; in rare instances, impotence.
Zocor	Simvastatin	Cholesterol-lowering agent.	Abdominal pain, constipation, diarrhea, flatulence, nausea, headache.
Zoloft	Sertraline hydrochloride	Antidepressant.	Dry mouth, increased sweating, palpitations, chest pain, headache, dizziness, tremor, twitching, skin rash, nausea, diarrhea, constipation, dyspepsia, vomiting, flatulence, increased appetite, abdominal pain.

the drug fits the receptor, it will either stimulate the cell to react in a certain way or block chemicals that are producing an undesirable effect in the cell, such as pain.

A second category of drugs works by destroying disease organisms in the body. Penicillin cures infection this way by preventing bacteria forming a new cell wall, causing them to burst and die. Other antibiotics produce equally lethal results by preventing the bacteria's cell wall from dividing during reproduction.

The third way that drugs work is on chemicals—those that are either invaders or products of the body. Ordinary sodium bicarbonate works this way by neutralizing excess acid produced by the stomach. Symptoms are relieved as the chemical reaction yields water, salt, and carbon dioxide, which are all easily eliminated from the body.

How Side Effects Happen

Drugs are potent chemicals and can cause side effects—known unwanted reactions—in addition to their intended effects. This is because the drug is distributed throughout the whole body (not just the target area) and because no two people react in exactly the same way to the same dosage of the same drug.

The potential for side effects is not confined to a few heavy-duty chemotherapy drugs either. "There's no such thing as a drug without side effects," says Bernard Mehl, R.Ph., D.P.S., director of the department of pharmacy at Mount Sinai Medical Center in New York City. "It's just a matter of how serious they are and how often they happen."

Side effects range from the merely annoying—like the diarrhea caused by antibiotic treatment—to the life-threatening. Some of the most common side effects include nausea, dry mouth, appetite loss, constipation, drowsiness, loss of sex drive, insomnia, headache, dizziness, depression, and bleeding. People who have liver or kidney disease have a higher than normal risk of experiencing side effects because medications can build up to toxic levels when these organs fail to break down and eliminate drugs properly.

Most side effects are related to the amount of medicine given in a dose and the amount of drug circulating in your body. Getting the dosage right for each patient can be difficult for a doctor since no two people respond to medicine in exactly the same way.

FINDING THE RIGHT WINDOW

A doctor bases a drug dosage on very specific "windows" in which the medication is concentrated enough to be effective, yet causes as few side effects as possible. Some drugs have small windows—this means they're very difficult to prescribe without causing side effects of some kind—while other drugs have large windows. Factors such as age, weight, your general health, and even your emotional state can affect drug dosage and with it your tendency to develop side effects.

IS IT WORTH THE RISK?

The Food and Drug Administration says that 7 out of 10 doctors never tell their patients about the risks of drugs they prescribe. If your doctor doesn't tell you, ask. Only then can you weigh up the benefits against the risks. Allergy medicine, for instance, often causes drowsiness, but people who are plagued by frequent sneezing may feel it's a small price to pay for relief.

Some side effects can be managed or offset by when or how you take your medication. For instance, if a drug makes you drowsy, take it when you won't have to drive. If you tend to become constipated by a drug, add fiber to your diet.

Expecting the Unexpected

Adverse reactions, unlike known side effects, are unexpected. They are infrequent, but virtually anyone can have one. Even under the best conditions the right drug, prescribed for the right condition, in the right dose, can cause an unexpected reaction in a patient.

For the most part, an adverse reaction depends on a person's distinctive body chemistry. You are at a higher risk for an adverse reaction if you have a history of allergies or have had a previous drug reaction.

Reactions can range from mild skin rashes, indigestion, and constipation to psychotic episodes, blood disorders, coma, or death. Sometimes adverse reactions occur when medications build to toxic levels in

---

Did You Know?

Studies show that 75 percent of visits to the doctor result in a prescription for at least one drug.

What to Ask Your Doctor about Drug Treatments

Studies show that many doctors aren't giving their patients the full story when it comes to the drugs they're prescribing. One thing you can do, says Kenneth A. Goldberg, M.D., medical director of the Male Health Institute at Baylor Health Center, Irving-Coppell, Texas, is to use the same pharmacy consistently. "They usually keep everything on a computer," he says, "and that makes it easier for you to keep track." Also, Dr. Goldberg says, ask the following questions the next time your doctor pulls out the prescription pad:

• What is the dosage and how often should I take the medication?

• What time of the day should I take it?

• Should I avoid certain foods?

• Should I take it with food or on an empty stomach?

• What side effects are associated with this medicine, and what should I do if I experience any of them?

• Is the drug likely to interact with any over-the-counter or prescription drugs that I am currently taking?

• Will it interact with alcohol?

• What should I do if I miss a dose?

• Is there a drug that costs less that can do the same job?

• What are the trade and generic names of the drugs prescribed?

• Are there any alternative treatments that don't involve drugs?

the bloodstream and can be reversed by a dosage adjustment. But more often they happen as a result of drug interactions with food or alcohol.

ALLERGIC REACTIONS

While most adverse reactions take time to build up in your system, allergic reactions happen almost immediately. Some people are hypersensitive to particular drugs—penicillin is a common one.

Allergic reactions need fast medical help. Anyone who thinks they might be having one should see their doctor, or if symptoms are especially serious, go immediately to the nearest emergency room. Symptoms of an allergic reaction include:
• Coughing, wheezing, or a sensation of something closing up in your chest
• Difficulty breathing or a feeling of swelling in the throat
• Uneasiness
• Agitation or loss of consciousness
• Rapid pulse, low blood pressure, fainting, or shock
• Flushing, itching, swelling, or rash
• Abdominal pain, nausea, vomiting, or diarrhea

The Drug That's Best for You

The best drug may be no drug, according to Kenneth A. Goldberg, M.D., medical director of the Male

I Missed a Dose!

What do you do if you miss a dose of medication? For most drugs, according to Kenneth A. Goldberg, M.D., medical director of the Male Health Institute at Baylor Health Center, Irving-Coppell, Texas, you should take a missed dose as soon as you remember, unless it's almost time for the next dose. In that case, just skip the missed dose. Don't try to "catch up" by doubling the next dose. It's best to ask the doctor who prescribed the medicine.

Drugs and Food

Certain foods and drugs can sometimes interact in ways that will throw your treatment off-course; some interactions are downright dangerous.

Speak to your doctor about whether you need to lay off your favorites for a while. Here are some common problem foods and the damage they may do.

• Dairy products interfere with the effectiveness of certain antibiotics and laxatives coated to dissolve in the lower intestine.

• Soft drinks and citrus juices should not be taken with antibiotics because they interfere with absorption and effectiveness.

• Licorice can cause people taking diuretics to develop dangerously low potassium levels and can also cause the heart to beat abnormally (arrhythmia) when eaten by those taking digoxin (Lanoxin).

• Orange juice can cause the body to absorb aluminum when taken with aluminum-containing antacids.

• Oatmeal, bran, and other high-fiber foods can interfere with the absorption of some drugs, making them less effective. The drugs include digoxin (Lanoxin), a heart medication; levothyroxine, a thyroid hormone; and certain antidepressants.

Health Institute at Baylor Health Center, Irving-Coppell, Texas, and author of *How Men Can Live as Long as Women*. Many conditions can be managed quite successfully by changing your lifestyle.

High blood pressure and elevated cholesterol levels are two examples of conditions that can be treated by changing your diet and taking up some form of regular exercise. Even if you have to take drugs for a while, you may reach a point where you can make lifestyle changes and ease off the medication. All of this, of course, should be discussed with your doctor first.

If you've got no choice and you have to take medication, keep in mind that the drug that's best for you balances effectiveness against the risk of serious side effects, says Dr. Goldberg.

Sometimes that means that the drug you're prescribed by your doctor may not be the most effective at treating your condition; the risk of side effects outweighs the benefits of that particular drug. The less severe your condition, the less risk of serious side effects you should be willing to take.

ARE GENERICS OKAY?

You'll likely pay a whopping price for a new, brand-name drug. Sometimes a generic can be just as effective. But are they safe?

In one respect, at least, they're actually safer, because by the time the original manufacturer's patent expires and a generic equivalent can be produced, the drug's side effects have been well documented. And the quality of most generics is good, too.

Problems arise with drugs whose effectiveness depends upon precise amounts being in your bloodstream. These include digoxin (a heart drug), warfarin (a blood thinner), and phenytoin (a drug to treat epilepsy). Although generics must by law be exactly the same drug as the brand-name type and must be absorbed in a similar way by the body, generics can be formulated differently so that they are absorbed at a somewhat different rate. That means that the blood levels of one drug may not be exactly the same as for its brand-name equivalent.

The best advice is to ask your doctor if there's an effective, cheaper, generic alternative. Then stick to doctor's orders.

Preparing Yourself for Surgery

No one likes the idea of going under the knife. Not only is surgery scary but it creates a feeling that you've lost control of your own body. Don't take it lying down! The success of any operation—whether it's a heart bypass or a cyst removal—hinges to a large extent on physical and mental preparation.

Know the Risks

We don't want to frighten you, but all operations—no matter how seemingly minor—carry some risk. That's why you need to weigh the benefits of the surgery against the risks of complications and side effects. Don't be afraid to ask your surgeon how often complications occur, and how the complication rates in his or her operations compare with those of other surgeons. A competent surgeon should be happy to give you this information.

Find out exactly what might happen if you don't have the operation. Is your surgery considered to be optional, elective, necessary, essential, or emergency? The categories give a general indication of the level of urgency.

Optional and elective procedures, including many types of cosmetic surgery, are not necessary for your health. With necessary surgery, a clear medical problem, like a torn knee cartilage, exists and should be fixed, but there is not usually a level of great urgency.

By contrast, operations such as hernia repair, gallbladder removal, and coronary artery bypass are considered essential surgery, and in most cases must be performed quickly before a patient's condition deteriorates. Treatment for any immediately life-threatening condition, such as severe bleeding, is emergency surgery.

ARE YOU LISTENING?

When you talk with your surgeon about what's in store, it's up to you to be an active listener. Your surgeon can share a wealth of information and advice with you, but if you don't listen and understand, then you're less likely to make a speedy recovery.

Don't be reluctant to ask a question. If you don't understand a term, get some clarification. It's a good idea to bring a pad and pen to your appointment—you'll probably be surprised at what you may not remember once you leave the surgeon's office. And sometimes even the smallest detail is important.

If you have an appointment that may have a critical outcome, bring along someone to give feedback and support. A second set of ears may also pick up something you missed.

Avoid These Before Surgery

You'll get lots of pieces of advice from your surgeon, and one of them undoubtedly will be to stop taking any aspirin or other nonsteroidal anti-inflammatory medicines before surgery. These drugs interfere with the blood's ability to clot. You should also avoid the following common nutritional supplements, which have the same effect:

- Vitamin E
- EPA (fish oil)
- Garlic
- Hawthorn berry
- Selenium

Psyching Yourself Up

You can aid healing, reduce your risk of complications, and lessen the pain and anxiety of surgery by being psychologically prepared, says Kenneth A. Goldberg, M.D., medical director of the Male Health Institute at Baylor Health Center, Irving-Coppell, Texas.

- Gather information and develop an understanding of the operation to give you a feeling of control.

- Use imagery to quell fears and tap into the power of the mind. The night before the operation imagine yourself in the operating room peacefully asleep while a skilled surgeon successfully completes the procedure. Picture yourself in the recovery room afterwards, becoming alert. Picture your pain. Give it a size, shape, color, and texture. Then transform it into a liquid and allow it to flow out of you.

- Practice relaxation techniques. See "10 Ways to Relax" on page 23.

▶ *One way to combat presurgery jitters is to picture the operation in progress.*

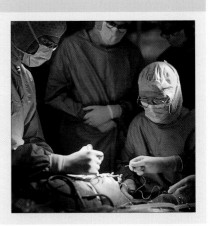

Be Prepared

A regimen of physical and mental self-preparation is crucial to reducing the risks of surgery and promoting a rapid recovery.

We'll get to the mental part later, but for now let's look at the physical considerations your doctors will take into account—what you can eat and drink, your level of fitness, whether you smoke, and so on.

Doctors will also give you a list of instructions to follow in the lead-up to the big day. Here's what you might expect.

FOOD AND DRINK RESTRICTIONS

Topping your doctor's list will probably be restrictions on what you may eat or drink after midnight prior to surgery. This is important because of the possibility of life-threatening complications under anesthesia.

The long-established precaution "NPO after midnight"—the abbreviation for the Latin phrase, *nil per os* (nothing by mouth)—was thought to prevent the back-up of stomach contents during surgery. Evidence now suggests that you can safely consume clear liquids, such as water, apple juice, or black coffee, up until two hours prior to surgery. Depending on the type of surgery, your physician may ease up on the NPO restriction, but be sure to ask first.

FITNESS CONSIDERATIONS

You don't need to be a world-class athlete—able to run marathons—to face surgery, but you usually should be fit enough to walk a mile or climb a couple of flights of stairs briskly without becoming excessively short of breath. Your doctors will probably want to know what level of exertion you can manage.

NUTRITION

The complex healing process of fighting off infection, tissue repair, and replacement of lost fluids requires an ample supply of protein, fats, and carbohydrates. If these are not supplied by proper nutrition, then the body will use its own tissues, resulting in poor healing.

SMOKING

Doctors need to know if you're a smoker. People who smoke are six times more likely to suffer from post-operative chest complications than

The View through the Keyhole

In the old days, most operations, no matter how minor, were traumatic to some degree. In the most invasive procedures, such as major abdominal surgery, a long incision through skin and muscle led to a long recovery period while the wound healed, and increased the risk of complications and infections. Fortunately, advances in surgery have led to less invasive techniques that are easier on the body.

Keyhole, or laparoscopic, surgery is only about 10 years old. It's performed in an increasing number of mainly abdominal procedures, including appendectomies, gallbladder removal, and the repair of peptic ulcers. You'll first be given a general anesthetic, then the abdomen is inflated with carbon dioxide to create space for surgical instruments. The surgeon makes a small incision and through it inserts a fiberoptic endoscope, an instrument that is about half an inch across. It has its own light source and miniature video camera, which allows the surgeon to view the abdominal cavity on a television monitor. The endoscope also has a channel through which instruments can be passed, enabling the surgeon to carry out the entire operation without having to make a long incision.

Keyhole surgery minimizes pain, blood loss, and incapacitation. Operations that once meant a week's stay in hospital can now be performed on an outpatient basis. And because there's no large wound, the recovery period and risk of infection are substantially less than for conventional surgery.

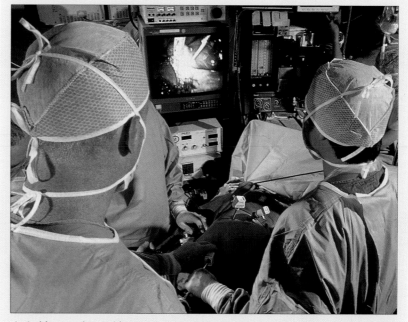

▲ *A video monitor guides surgeons as they carry out an abdominal operation using an endoscope. Only a small, "keyhole" incision is necessary, making recovery faster.*

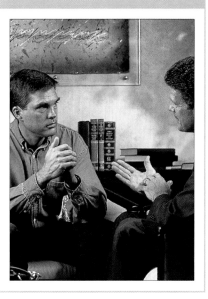
those who don't. Wound healing is also slower because there is less oxygen present in the blood.

ALCOHOL CONSUMPTION

If you have more than one or two drinks a day, you may require more anesthesia, so you will probably be asked how much you drink. Be honest. That way, the anesthesiologist can be prepared for how your body will respond when you're under.

Your Mental Attitude

Don't underestimate the role your mind plays in the success of surgery and the healing process. Studies have shown that patients who take an active role in their surgery by developing an understanding of what they will experience are able to reduce anxiety and stress and are less likely to suffer complications. Patients who lay back helplessly and lament their condition tend to have longer hospital stays and suffer more setbacks.

Ask your surgeon to describe exactly what will be done during the procedure. Although this may alarm you initially, eventually it will help you establish a reassuring sense of control. Try using a technique called imagery, which helps promote relaxation and a positive mental outlook by visualizing the event. For details, see "Psyching Yourself Up" on page 262.

What to Expect after Surgery

Recovery times vary depending on the type of procedure and your general health; your surgeon will give you some indication. Before the operation, find out what kind of supplies, equipment, and any other help you'll need when you go home. Ask when you'll be able to return to work and when you can resume regular exercise. Knowing what to expect can help you cope better.

To avoid complications, you will be encouraged to get up and move around as soon as possible, usually within 24 hours of surgery. This discourages the formation of life-threatening blood clots caused by being in bed too long. It also helps to prevent common respiratory complications, such as pneumonia. Once home, most people are on the way to recovery, but setbacks do occur. Call your doctor if you experience nausea, constipation, or diarrhea, or if you have increased bleeding or pain.

The Road to Recovery

No one likes being an invalid. Whether you've just weathered major open-heart surgery or are trying to shake off a bad cold, your goal is a speedy recovery. What you do for your body, as well as your mind, can have a big effect on how fast you regain full health and fitness.

Get Well Soon

If it's flu, you'll probably feel like you've been through your washing machine's spin cycle: dizzy, groggy, and achy. If you've had an operation, you may find a drip in your arm or even a catheter "down there" to drain urine. In both cases, you want a rapid recovery with no setbacks.

The old advice retains its power, according to Kenneth A. Goldberg, M.D., medical director of the Male Health Institute at Baylor Health Center, Irving-Coppell, Texas: Rest up, eat well, drink lots of fluids, and take prescribed medication. Follow those maxims and your body's healing powers will come into play.

REST AND EXERCISE

There's no question that your body needs more rest during recovery to restore good health. But there's a fine line between recharging your batteries and staying in bed so long that the blood congeals in your veins. How much rest is enough? If you resume normal activities too soon, you risk a relapse. If you stay in bed too long, you risk complications from inactivity such as blood clots or pneumonia, especially after undergoing surgery.

The best approach is to take cues from your body, Dr. Goldberg says. As soon as you're able, get up and walk around for a short period a few times a day. Research shows that people who resume activity faster recover faster and are discharged from the hospital sooner. Even heart patients are encouraged to get up the day after surgery.

Dr. Goldberg suggests that you slowly build up your level of endurance over a period of time.

Light exercise, such as walking, will raise your heart rate, improve circulation, and promote healing.

Don't overdo it by forcing the pace. Listen to your body. If you experience pain or extreme fatigue, it's a signal that you're probably exerting yourself too much.

THE ROLE OF GOOD NUTRITION

Good nutrition gives your body the building blocks it needs to get well. When you're sick, though, it may be difficult to stomach three square meals a day, so Dr. Goldberg suggests these tips for getting the most from your diet.

• Eat light and eat often. Regular-size meals can make you uncomfortable, especially following surgery. Eat five or six mini-meals a day. Some easy-to-digest favorites are fortified fruit/protein shakes, whole-wheat toast, pudding and custard, yogurt, fruit, and chicken soup, which actually helps break up the congestion of the common cold,

Top 10 Tips for Making a Good Recovery

Here are some things that Kenneth A. Goldberg, M.D., medical director of the Male Health Institute at Baylor Health Center, Irving-Coppell, Texas, suggests you might do in the recovery stage. Keep in mind that the the first suggestion takes precedence over all the others.

1 Follow your doctor's instructions.

2 Eat a healthy, fiber-filled diet.

3 Double the normal requirement of six to eight glasses of water a day.

4 Rest.

5 Take all medications as prescribed.

6 Get up and walk around as soon as possible to help prevent pneumonia and blood clots in the legs.

7 Use analgesics and relaxation techniques to minimize pain.

8 Listen to music that encourages a sense of wellness.

9 Avoid stress.

10 Believe in yourself.

Coping with Relapses

Doctors say that even if you're making steady progress overall, you can still suffer a relapse along the way. Relapsing isn't just a physical setback, it's a psychological blow that can sometimes trigger tension, anxiety, depression, and despair. There's much you can do to deal with the situation positively, according to Kenneth A. Goldberg, M.D., medical director of the Male Health Institute at Baylor Health Center, Irving-Coppell, Texas.

Ask yourself why. What might you have done to cause the relapse? Did you do too much too soon? Not take your medicine as instructed? Don't chastise yourself, but it's better to light a candle than curse the darkness. Here are some other things to keep in mind.

• Acknowledge that relapses are normal, and that you're still going to recover.

• Take difficulties one step at a time, instead of becoming overwhelmed.

• Lean on a loved one for emotional support or find a support group.

• Listen to restful tapes, such as ocean sounds, or watch a relaxing video.

• Occupy yourself. Do a crossword puzzle, write a letter, or read a good book.

• Remember to look beyond. Don't allow your health condition to be the center of your universe.

▶ *When a relapse happens, don't hold back from asking for help.*

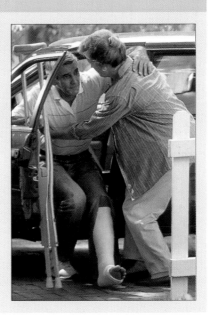

according to medical researchers at the Mount Sinai Medical Center in Miami Beach.

• Fill up with fiber. The bowels are often sluggish after surgery or when you're ill. In the hospital, moving your bowels following surgery is a much-anticipated event—a sign that your digestive system is in working order. In the outside world, keep things moving by eating an adequate amount of fiber from sources such as prunes, prune juice, fruit, vegetables, legumes, bran, and whole grains.

DRINK UP
Make sure to drink plenty of fluids, says Dr. Goldberg. Normally, you need six to eight, eight-ounce glasses of fluid a day. When you're sick, you can easily lose a quart or more of fluid as your body does battle with an infection. So double your fluid intake, especially if you're congested. This will help trap viruses in the moist mucus of your throat so that they can travel to the stomach where the powerful digestive juices will destroy them.

FOLLOW DOCTOR'S ORDERS
If your doctor has prescribed medication, it's important to take it as directed, especially when it comes to antibiotics, which are prescribed for bacterial infections.

Normally, antibiotics are taken for 7 to 10 days. After a day or two, though, chances are that you'll begin to feel better, and by the third or fourth day you may actually feel cured. This is where the urge to stop

The Recovery Workout

Light exercise will promote general healing by increasing your heart rate and circulation. Going for a walk or riding a stationary bicycle are the best low-impact workouts when you're recuperating from an illness or an operation.

If you're facing a long convalescence, you don't have to wait until you're up and around to stretch and tone your muscles. The following exercises are recommended to improve blood flow and promote healing while you're still confined to bed. You'll need a bungee cord, or elastic exercise cord.

Caution: If you're recuperating from surgery, follow your doctor's advice before beginning any exercise program. Stop exercises if they cause pain, especially around the surgical site.

Exercise 1
Attach the bungee cord behind you at the head of the bed. Holding each end of the cord, extend your arms to your sides so that your hands are even with the shoulders. To the count of four, slowly pull forward until arms are extended in front of your body. Return your arms to the side position to the count of four. Do eight times to work the arms and back.

Exercise 2
Attach the bungee cord to the foot of the bed. Holding the ends of the cord with your hands facing the ceiling, rest your arms on your lap. Keeping the upper arms stationary, slowly pull both hands to your chest to the count of four. Then return to the resting position to a slow count of four. Do eight times to exercise the biceps, triceps, and abdominals.

> "'Exercise is good for the physical self and the psychological self by letting you re-establish control of your body."
>
> D. W. Edington, director of the University of Michigan Fitness Research Center

taking your medicine kicks in. But to kill all of the bacteria lurking in your body effectively, you have to take all the antibiotics as prescribed. If you stop taking your medication too soon and the infection re-establishes itself, it may be more difficult to kill the bacterial invaders the second time around.

If you're experiencing pain, don't try to tough it out; talk to your doctor about painkillers. Pain control is necessary, not only because it keeps you more comfortable, but because the body is better able to heal itself when it's relatively pain-free. And pain is more easily controlled if extinguished early before it escalates to an intolerable level.

Most pain can be treated with the usual over-the-counter analgesics, including ibuprofen, acetaminophen, and aspirin.

Pain can also be controlled by a number of methods that don't employ medications. These include visualization, relaxation techniques, biofeedback, and self-hypnosis.

The Healing Powers Within

The mind, if stressed and anxious, can have a negative effect on your body and your recovery. Just imagine how a good case of stage fright makes you feel—heart palpitations, a dry mouth, and sweaty palms. On the flip side, the body can derive many benefits from a mind that's calm and relaxed, benefits that

"Each of us has within ourselves more mending and healing powers than most of all the medicines put together."

Dr. Robin A. J. Youngson, author of *Operation: A Handbook for Surgical Patients*

include relief from pain and anxiety, and faster healing.

An increasing number of doctors acknowledge that the mind has enormous power over the body. In various medical studies, music therapy, relaxation techniques, visualization, and even prayer have been found to speed recovery. So, in addition to your doctor's prescription for a little R&R, put your mind to work to stimulate your body's ability to heal itself. For information about relaxation exercises, see page 23.

Supplements to Speed Healing

Vitamin supplements are not a substitute for good nutrition, but the body's need for nutrients goes way up when it's fighting disease. And research has shown that additional amounts of certain vitamins and minerals can speed the healing process and boost the immune system. Listed below are some of the most versatile supplements, together with the normal daily requirement and safe supplemental dosages. These supplemental dosages are meant for short periods only, so as soon as you feel like you're back to your normal self, stop taking them and rely on your diet (we're assuming it's a healthy one) to provide you with all the nutrients you need. Check with your doctor before taking any supplements.

Nutrient	Normal Daily Requirement	Supplemental Daily Dosage	Healing Effects	Caution
Vitamin A	5,000 IU	15,000 IU	Supplemental dosage improves wound healing, especially in patients who have to take steroids. It also improves tendon, fractured bone, and intestinal healing, and slows the progression of HIV infection.	Vitamin A can be toxic at high levels (including 15,000 IU) if taken for extended periods.
Vitamin C	600 mg.	500—2,000 mg.	Supplemental dosage can speed healing. Since the body quickly excretes vitamin C, you should take large dosages in 250–500 mg. increments throughout the day.	Dosages in excess of 1,200 mg. a day can cause diarrhea in some people; high dosages can also interfere with medical test results.
Zinc	15 mg.	15 mg.	A nutrient necessary for the production of collagen, the connective tissue that allows scars to form, zinc speeds tissue repair. Take zinc citrate, an easily absorbed form, following surgery.	Dosages in excess of 15 mg. a day can be toxic.

Index

Boldface page references indicate main discussion. *Italic* references indicate illustrations. <u>Underscored</u> references indicate boxed text, tables, and charts.

PC (pubococcygeal) muscles, 145, 148, _148_
Pheromones, _31_
Phobias, _177_
Phosphorus, _52_
Physicals. _See_ Checkups and screening tests
Physicians. _See_ Doctors
Pimples and acne, 25, _25_
Pinch test, _61_
Places/venues for sex, _131_, _151_
Plaque, dental, 32, 33, 35
Plateau phase, 144–45, _145_
Pleurisy, _189_, _191_, 228, _229_
Pneumonia, 190, _191_, 229, _229_
PNF (proprioceptive neuromuscular facilitation) stretching, _99_
Pollution, air, 227
Polyps, in colon, 202–3
Polysporin, 25
Polyunsaturated fats, _63_
Positive thinking, when meeting new partners, _134_
Posture, 214, 216
    during sleep, _217_
    postural problems, with office equipment, _122_
    test, _98_, _98_
Potassium, 53, _256_
Potency, **138**
Pressing (massage technique), _141_, _141_, _142_
Prickly heat, 183
Prilosec, 259
Problem sleep, _16_, _17_, _169_, 170, _170_
Procardia, 259
Propecia, 15, 27
Proprioceptive neuromuscular facilitation (PNF) stretching, _99_
Prostate cancer, _239_, 240–41, _241_, _242_, _246_
Prostate gland, 238, _238_, _238_
    digital/rectal examination, 241, 257
    problems and disorders, 225, **238–41**
Prostate infections, _241_
Protein, 49, 50
Prozac, _179_, 259

PSA screening, 241, 257
Psoriasis, 182, _182_
Pubococcygeal (PC) muscles, 145, 148, _148_
Pulp, dental, _34_, _34_, 37
Pulse rate. _See also_ Heart rate
    daily variations, _18_
Pyramid, Food Guide, 54, _55_, 55

Q
Quickie sex, _148_

R
Racket sports, 77
Radiation therapy, _244_
Radicals, free, _14_
Raised leg crunches, 116
Ranitidine hydrochloride, _259_
Rapid eye movement (REM) sleep, 16, _17_
Rashes, **182–83**
Razor bumps, 40, 41
Razors, 40, _41_
Rear entry positions (sexual position)
    classic, kneeling, _153_
    rear window, _155_
    seated, _154_
    seated wheelbarrow, _157_
    spoon, _154_
    standing, _154_
    standing wheelbarrow, _156_
Recovery
    from illness, **265–67**
    from surgery, 264
    rest and recovery, from exercise, 117
Rectal bleeding, _155_, _167_
Rectus abdominis muscles, _110_, _110_, _111_
Refractory period, _149_
Relapses, _266_
Relationships. _See also_ Sex
    being accepting in, 5
    conflict resolution in, _133_
    effective communication in, **126–27**
    love, passion, and romance in, **130–33**
    marriage, benefits of, 5, _132_
    re-entering the singles scene, **134–35**

understanding a partner's needs, **128–29**, _139_
Relaxation. _See also_ Stress reduction
    exercises, 23, _23_
    headache treatment, 173
REM (rapid eye movement) sleep, 16, _17_
Resistance training. _See_ Weight training and lifting
Resolution phase, 145
Respiratory system, _184_, _184_, 188–89, _226_. _See also_ Breathing disorders, 225, **226–29**. _See also specific diseases_
Rest and recovery
    from exercise, **117**
    from illness, **265–67**
    from surgery, 264
Retin-A, 15
Reverse curls, _112_
Reverse missionary position (sexual position), _152_
Rheumatoid arthritis, _210_, _211_, 212, _213_, _213_
Riboflavin, _51_
Ribs, bruised, _207_, _209_
RICE (rest, ice, compression, elevation), _118_, _221_, _221_
Risk factors, for disease. _See specific diseases_
Rogaine. _See_ Minoxidil
Romance, passion, and love, **130–33**
Root canal, _34_
    surgery, 37
Rosacea, 25
Rowing
    as aerobic exercise, 90, _90_
    benefits and drawbacks, _77_
    calories burned up, _89_
    injury prevention, _120_
    machines, _84_
Running
    as aerobic exercise, 90–91, _91_
    benefits and drawbacks, _77_
    calories burned up, _89_
    endurance events, 107, _107_
    injury prevention, _120_

skin disorders, 25, 25
  cancer, 7, 24, 247
  effect of stress, 20
  rashes, **182–83**
  structure, 24–25, 25, 25
  wrinkles, 13, 14–15
Sleep, **16–17**
  posture during, 217
  problems, 16, 17, 169, 169
  snoring, 170, 170
  requirements, 9, 16–17
Slow squats, 73, 73
Slow-wave (deep) sleep, 16, 17
Small intestines, role in digestion, 48, 193
Smell. *See also* Odor
  sense of, 30, 31
Smoking
  as carcinogen, 242, 243
  effect on
    back pain, 216
    breath and teeth, 33, 33, 35
    lungs, 189–90, 189, 227, 227
    skin, 24, 25
    surgery, 263–64
  quitting, 6, 228
Snacks, 56, 65
Sneezes, 184, 185, **186**, 186, 187
Snoring, 170, 170
Snowboarding, 77
Socks, 83
Sodium, 53, 232, 256
Sore throats, sneezes, and coughs, **184–87**
Sperm, 147
SPFs (sun protection factors), 7, 13, 14, 24
Spinal stenosis, 215
Spinal tumors, 215
Spine, 214–15, 215. *See also* Back
Spleen, 193, 193
Spoon (sexual position), 154
  facing, 155
Sports. *See also specific sports*
  sport and exercise injuries
    prevention, **118–21**, 206–7, 208–9, **218–21**
    safety tips, 81
Sprains, 207, 210, 211, 212, 219
  and back pain, 215
  ice treatment for, 213

Squats, 96
  slow, 73, 73
Squatted kneeling (sexual position), 155
SSRIs (selective serotonin reuptake inhibitors), 179
Stained teeth, 35
Stairclimbing
  benefits and drawbacks, 77
  equipment, 85
  injury prevention, 121
  stair-stepping, as warm-up, 86
Standing (sexual position), 157
  rear entry, standing, 154
  standing wheelbarrow, 156
Starches, 48
Static stretching, 98–99
Stationary bikes, 84, 87
STDs (sexually transmitted diseases), 158, 160, 161
Stenosis, spinal, 215
Step test, 73, 73
Stitch, 207
Stomach
  how to flatten it, 14
  problems. *See specific diseases*
  role in digestion, 48, 193
Stomach cancer, 242, 246
Strains, 207, 215, 219
Strength, 72, 218–19
  in emergencies, 80
  exercises. *See also* Weight
    training and lifting
      age-related choices, **78–80**, 92
      chair dips, 73, 73, 123
      fitness test, 73, 73
      slow squats, 73, 73
Stress, **18–20**. *See also* Stress
    reduction
  and aging process, 13, 14
  effects of
    fatigue, 169
    illness, 20
    weight fluctuation, 20, 204
  as heart attack risk factor, 235
Stress reduction, **20–23**
  at work, 122, 123
  importance of, 5, 9, 11
    heart attack prevention, 235
  role of sex, 9

through exercise, 21, 73
  to slow down aging process, 14
Stretching exercises, 77, 77, **98–99**, 209, 219–20
  age-related choices, **78–80**
  for the buttocks, 102
  for the calves, 103
  ceiling reach, 98, 98
  chair twist, 98, 98
  for the chest, 104
  for the groin, 101
  for the hamstrings, 101
  for the hips, 100, 104
  for the lower back, 100, 102, 103
  for the neck, 105
  posture test, 98, 98
  for the shoulders, 99
  for the sides, 103
  for the thighs, 102, 104
  toenail touch, 98, 98
  toe touches, 73, 73
  for the triceps, 105
  warming up, 86
Stroke, **236–37**
Strokes, massage, 141
Stroking (massage technique), 141, 141, 142
Styles and styling
  beards, 41–42, 42
  clothes, **43–45**
  hair, 27–28, 28, 29
    when balding, 26, 26, 27
Subcutaneous fat, 61
Sugars, 48, 54
Suits, 43, 44
Sun
  exposure to, 7, 7
    effect on skin, 13, 14, 24
  protection from, sunscreens and sun protection factors (SPFs), 7, 13, 14, 24
  sunburn, 25
Supplements, vitamins and minerals, 8, 57, 147, 265, 267
Support belts, 209
Suppressants (cough medicine), 186, 187
Surgeons
  communicating with, 262, 264
  second opinions, 264

Acknowledgments

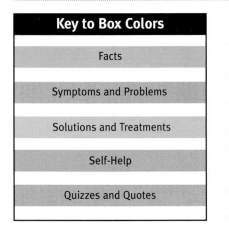

Key to Box Colors
Facts
Symptoms and Problems
Solutions and Treatments
Self-Help
Quizzes and Quotes

The Mitchell Beazley Team

Senior Editor	**Penelope Cream**
Executive Art Editor	**Emma Boys**
Executive Editor	**Samantha Ward-Dutton**
Editor	**John Mapps, Arlene Sobel**
Design	**Lovelock & Co**
Design Assistance	**Russell Miller**
Picture Research	**Jenny Faithfull**
Production	**Paul Hammond**
Index	**Susan Bosanko**
Illustrations	**Jim Robbins, Halli Verrinder**
Special Photography	**Steve Gorton**
Medical Consultants	**Dr Abi Berger, MRCGP, Kenneth A Goldberg, MD**
Sports and Fitness Consultant	**Mark Williams**

The publishers would like to thank the following for their assistance in the production of this book: Ged Allen, Hughton Campbell, Guy Croton, Debbi Finlow, Kelly Garrett, Ian Hinde, Ruth Hope, James Hoskins, Marc Raymond, John Round, Simon Spalding, and Alexa Stace; Angela Hampton, Bob Gerheart, and Rose Benedick at Rodale Images; Julie Dinsdale, Brandon Boll and all at the Science Photo Library; Bodyactive at Charing Cross Concourse, London WC2; The Metropolitan Health & Fitness Club; Sports Division at Selfridges, London W1, and Bauer in-line skates.

Picture Credits

AKG, London/Berlin, SMPK, Gemäldegalerie 12; Allsport/Stu Forster 108, /Doug Pensinger 209, /Ben Radford 247 right, /Pascal Rondeau 77 left, 109; Biophoto Associates 242, 244 center, 244 right; Anthony Blake Photo Library/Gerrit Buntrock 55 bottom left, /Maximilian Stock Ltd 55 top center left, 55 bottom center left, 55 center top right 1, 55 center top right 2, 55 center top right 3, 55 bottom center right, 55 bottom right, /Rosenfeld Images 55 top left, /J Topps 55 top right; Corbis UK Ltd 4 bottom, /Owen Franken 26 bottom left, /Matt Mendelsohn 27 top, /Pacha 28 bottom right; Gold's Gym home fitness equipment supplied by CSA Fitness 800 995 3875 for stockist 82 top right; Mary Evans Picture Library 140 top; Frank Lane Picture Agency/Chris Mattison 177 bottom; Angela Hampton 38 left, 38 right; Robert Harding Picture Library/Photoworld 1993 16, /Sharpshooters 76 right; Hulton Getty Picture Collection 171 top; Image Bank/Barros & Barros 264, /Romilly Lockyer 255, /Butch Martin 169, /Yellow Dog Productions 208; Kobal Collection 11, 13 bottom, 28 top left, 140 bottom, /Columbia, 1965 68, /Columbia/TriStar Motion Picture Companies/ Melinda Sue Gordon 28 top right, /MGM 22, 126, /1995 New Line 28 bottom left, /Paramount 9 top; Medical Illustration Group 194, 201, /Imperial College School of Medicine 182 center; Octopus Publishing Group Ltd Picture Library/Steve Gorton vii, 9, 14, 20, 21, 24, 33, 36 top, 40, 41, 48, 56, 73 top left, 73 top right, 73 bottom left, 73 bottom right, 82 top left, 82 bottom, 83, 85, 86 left, 86 center, 86 right, 87 left, 87 right, 93 top left, 93 top right, 93 bottom left, 93 bottom right, 94 top left, 94 top right, 94 bottom left, 94 bottom right, 95 top left, 95 top right, 95 bottom left, 95 bottom right, 96 top left, 96 top right, 96 center, 96 bottom left, 96 bottom right, 97 top left, 97 top right, 97 bottom left, 97 bottom center, 97 bottom right, 98 left, 98 center left, 98 center right, 98 right, 99 top, 99 bottom, 100 top, 100 center left,

100 center right, 100 bottom left, 100 bottom right, 101 top, 101 center left, 101 center right, 101 bottom left, 101 bottom right, 102 top left, 102 top right, 102 center, 102 bottom, 103 top left, 103 top center, 103 top right, 103 bottom left, 103 bottom right, 104 top left, 104 top right, 104 bottom left, 104 bottom right, 105 top, 105 center left, 105 center, 105 center right, 105 bottom left, 105 bottom right, 111 top left, 111 top right, 111 bottom left, 111 bottom right, 112 top left, 112 top right, 112 bottom left, 112 bottom right, 113 top, 113 center, 113 bottom left, 113 bottom right, 114 top, 114 center left, 114 center right, 114 bottom, 115 top left, 115 top right, 115 bottom left, 115 bottom right, 116 top, 116 bottom left, 116 bottom right, 118, 119 left, 119 center, 119 right, 120 top, 120 center, 120 bottom, 121 top, 121 center top, 121 center bottom, 121 bottom, 122 left, 122 right, 123 top left, 123 top right, 123 bottom left, 123 bottom center, 123 bottom right, 167, 172, 175, 177, 190, 192, 193, 198 center, 200, 207, 215, 217 top left, 217 top right, 217 center left, 217 center right, 217 bottom, 219, 221 top left, 221 top right, 221 bottom left, 221 bottom right, 228 bottom, 258; Nicholas Ogden 34; Rex Features/Nils Jorgensen 42, /Sipa Press/Roussier 15 bottom; Rodale Images 1 top, 4 top, 32, 46–47, 79 center left, 90 left, 129, 133, 163 center bottom, 222–223, /Tim De Frisco i, 77 right, 84 left, 91 left, /T L Gettings 183, /John P Hamel ii, iv–v, vi bottom, 1 center bottom, 23, 30, 43, 57, 70–71, 72, 76 left, 77 center, 85 bottom, 90 center, 90 right, 91 center, 91 right, 107, 130, 163 top, 199, 248–249, /Ed Landrock 79 center right, 80, 205, /Mitch Mandel vi top, 2–3, 15 top, 62, 84 right, 149, 162, 164–165, /Ron Modra 124–125, 135, /Margaret Skrovanek viii, 1 center top, 7, 127, 131, 136–137, 159, 163 center top, 163 bottom, /Kurt Wilson 1 bottom, 18, 26 top, 31, 45 top, 60, 67, 173; Science Photo Library 182 left, 196, 245 bottom, /Biology Media 8, /Chris Bjornberg 198 right, /BSIP, LECA 244 left, /BSIP, Chassenet 55 center bottom

right, /Scott Camazine 228 top, /CDC 188, /Department of Nuclear Medicine, Charing Cross Hospital 171 bottom right, 171 bottom left, /CNRI 245 top, 257 right, /John Smith/ Custom Medical Stock Photo 257 left, /Schleichkorn/Custom Medical Stock Photo 257 center left, /Martin Dohrn/Royal College of Surgeons 189, /John Durham 211, /Eye of Science 185 left, 185 right, /GCa/CNRI 246 bottom, /John Greim 179, /Dr P Marazzi 247 top left, 247 center left, /Maximilian Stock Ltd 262, /Matt Meadows/ Peter Arnold Inc 257 center right, /Ouellette & Theroux, Publiphoto Diffusion 252 center, /David Parker 55 center bottom left, /Salisbury District Hospital 246 top, /Science Pictures Ltd 147, /Simon Fraser 233, /James Stevenson 182 right, 247 bottom left, /St Bartholomew's Hospital 202, /Andrew Syred 27 bottom, /Geoff Tompkinson 263, /Jonathan Watts 186, /Hattie Young 252 right; Tony Stone Images/ Al Bello 79 right, /Stewart Cohen 177 top, /Ben Edwards 234, /Jerry Gay 13 top, /Zigy Kaluzny 252 left, /David Madison 79 left, /Bill Roberts 37; The Stock Market Photo Agency Inc 266, /R Duchaine 26 bottom right; Dr Tim Watson, Guy's Dental Hospital, London 36 bottom. The diagram on page 62 is reproduced by permission from JH Wilmore, 1986, *Sensible Fitness* (Champaign, IL: Human Kinetics), 30; the diagram on page 88 is from *Towards Better Coaching: the art and science of sports coaching*, ed Frank S Pyke, published by the Australian Government Publishing Service, 1984; Commonwealth of Australia copyright reproduced by permission.